CULPEPER'S COLOUR HERBAL

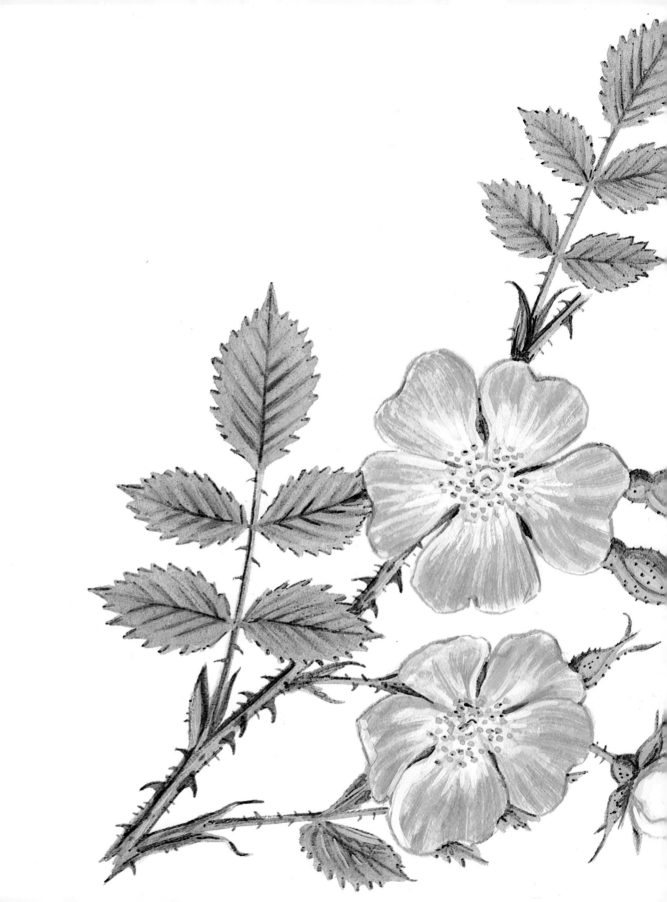

CULPEPER'S COLOUR HERBAL

Edited by David Potterton

Foreword by E. J. Shellard
Emeritus Professor of Pharmacognosy, University of London

Illustrated by Michael Stringer

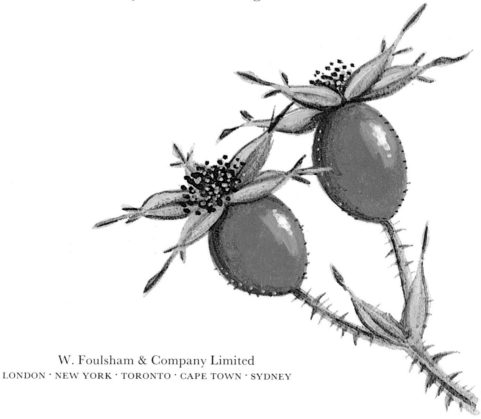

W. Foulsham & Company Limited
LONDON · NEW YORK · TORONTO · CAPE TOWN · SYDNEY

W. Foulsham & Company Limited
Yeovil Road, Slough, Berkshire, SL1 4JH

Editor:	David Potterton ND, MBNOA, MNINH
Pharmacognostical Consultant:	Professor E. J. Shellard BPharm. PhD (Lond), Hon DSC (Warsaw Med Acad), FPS, CChem, FRSC, FLS
	Honorary Member Egyptian, Hungarian and Polish Pharmaceutical Societies
	Emeritus Professor of Pharmacognosy, University of London
	President, Section for the Study of Medicinal Plants, International Pharmaceutical Federation
Botanical Consultant:	J. R. Press MPhil

ISBN 0-572-01152-0

Photoset in Great Britain by Rowland Phototypesetting Limited, Bury St Edmunds,
Suffolk and printed in Hong Kong.

CONTENTS

Foreword   6

Preface   8

Alphabetical List of Herbs   9

Glossary   206

Illnesses and Their Herbal Cures
According to Culpeper   207

Illnesses and Their Modern Herbal Cures   214

Index   219

FOREWORD

The use of plants in the treatment of disease has its origins in the antiquities of man's evolution from his more primitive forms. At first all the experiences of these early societies were passed from one generation to another by word of mouth, and it was not until many thousands of years had gone by that communication from one person to another was made possible by means of the written or printed word. Many of these earlier forms of communication are available for consultation today and it is clear that with the development of different societies based on different ideologies, so the use of plants for medicinal purposes became related to superstitions and religious beliefs currently held in those societies. Not only that, but new developments often arose out of the conflicts between different groups within the societies.

There were few exceptions to this, and when the struggle in England between the old landowning class and the new class of industrialists became intensified in the early seventeenth century it was inevitable that the practice of medicine and the use of plants should reflect this struggle to a considerable extent. It was a period which saw the growth of a proletarian population in the developing industrial areas at the expense of a depopulated countryside. It was a period which saw a conflict between the physicians, who preferred to attend to the needs of the wealthy, and the herbalists – and some apothecaries – who exploited the needs of the poor working classes. Many of these people, when living in the country, would have treated themselves when ill by collecting plants from near their homes, but now that they lived in urban areas they had to rely on herbalists – many of whom were charlatans – for their medicines.

This is the background to Nicholas Culpeper's *The Complete Herbal* published in 1649. Nicholas Culpeper was the son of a Surrey clergyman who was himself the son of a landowner, Sir Thomas Culpeper. He studied at Cambridge and was considered a bright scholar but, because of a personal tragedy – his bride-to-be was killed in a thunderstorm – he gave up his studies in medicine and started a long apprenticeship with a London apothecary. He was greatly influenced by the contrast between the life of his family and that of the working people in London, and at the end of his apprenticeship he set himself up as an apothecary in Spitalfields. He supplied plant medicines at very low cost to his impoverished clients and in contrast to the practice of physicians he never prescribed more than one plant medicine if only one was needed. Furthermore, he preferred the English plants over the more exotic imported plant materials and frequently indicated to his clients where in the nearby countryside the appropriate plants could be collected. He insisted on using the common English names rather than the Latin names used by the physicians and to emphasise this need to communicate with his clients he translated the London Pharmacopoea from Latin into English.

His decision to publish a herbal was taken because the herbals of John Gerard, published in 1597 and of John Parkinson in 1640 were based on Latin and included too many imported drugs. It was, in a sense, a poor man's dispensatory – not that the poor of his day could afford to buy it even if they could have read it. Nevertheless it proved a most popular book and over the years since 1649 there have been 41 different editions, while in 1979 a facsimile of the original text was published.

Culpeper lived at a time when astrology was a kind of religion – not an alternative to the religions based on God – but certainly complementary to them. It was a belief firmly held by the majority of people, so it was inevitable that, like Parkinson, his concept of disease and his ideas about plants useful in the treatment of disease should be based on astrology. It is impossible today to comprehend how diseases and plants could be classified on an astrological basis, even though in this age of science and technology there are still many people who look to the stars for an explanation and understanding of their lives. Such people must be warned that the use of plants for the treatment of

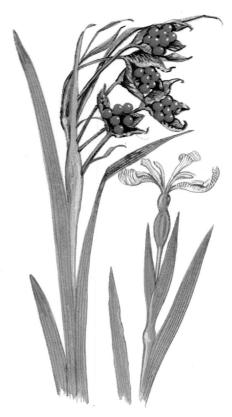

Gladwin IRIS FOETIDISSIMA

symptoms as given by Culpeper is quite valueless although any similarities which might occur between his use and the modern indications are not entirely coincidental.

Parkinson and Culpeper were not the first 'herbal practitioners' to base their use of plants on astrology. Astrology is an ancient belief with its true origins unknown but there can be no doubt that the ancients, looking for an explanation as to why certain plants were efficacious in the treatment of certain diseases and others were not, turned to astrology to provide a theoretical basis. And why not! To the agrarian communities there was an obvious relationship between the growth of their crops and the behaviour of animals with the changing seasons and the position of the heavenly bodies. Thus an explanation could be given, based on the long experience of the people, as to why those plants were efficacious. But an irrational development – though undoubtedly considered to be rational at the time – extended this ideological approach to relate each disease to a planet and then search for a plant, never before used for medicinal purposes but having an association with a different planet, with which to treat the disease. The fact that it would be quite useless was of no consequence because with the new concept, practice was based on theory and not vice versa.

Thus the irrational use of plants became mixed up with the rational use and as the years went by it became impossible to distinguish between them. The same sequence of events took place many years later in connection with Paracelsus' Doctrine of Signatures. A firm believer that God had placed plants on earth for the benefit of man, he was able to discern a broad relationship between the disease and the plant which cured it, for example, shape, number, colour, habitat. This theory was subsequently stood on its head so that people deliberately looked for plants with which they could discern some connection with the disease. It was a development which has led to much confusion ever since.

Culpeper does not seem to have been influenced by this idea – it had probably not spread to England by the beginning of the seventeenth century. His herbal is firmly based on astrology, as was his entire understanding of medicine, and he put forward a guide as to the correct choice of plants as follows.

First of all, decide which planet is responsible for the disease. In this connection he had already published a guide entitled *Judgement of Disease*.

Then ascertain which part or parts of the body were affected by the disease, referring particularly to the flesh, the blood, the bones or the heart. Reference to the *Judgement of Disease* would then indicate which planet or planets governed the affected part or parts of the body and treatment would then be based on the use of plants governed by the planets in opposition to those associated with the particular parts of the body.

Culpeper pointed out, however, that in addition to the use of 'opposites', some diseases could be cured by 'sympathy'. This supported the fact that some diseases could be treated rationally but by plants which did not have a different governing planet. According to Culpeper the planet associated with the disease could also nominate one of its own plants to cure one of its own diseases. Thus he was able to take advantage of the two conflicting theories of medicine which had developed over the centuries.

Culpeper was undoubtedly a popular apothecary and although he died at the early age of 38 his ideas and methods persisted for a long time. Even today there are some people who accept Culpeper's philosophy.

Foulsham has therefore made a useful contribution to present-day herbal medicine by producing this modern Colour Herbal based on the original text of Nicholas Culpeper but pointing out quite clearly the real value of each plant. Readers will be able to compare with great interest the ideas of the sixteenth and seventeenth centuries with those currently held. It makes

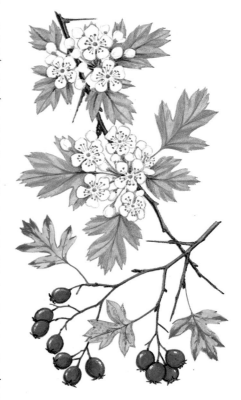

Hawthorn CRATAEGUS MONOGYNA

fascinating reading, but more than that, in these days when there is such a resurgence of interest in herbal medicine, it enables the reader to differentiate between the rational and the irrational use of plants.

There is a widespread belief that because plants are part of nature, they are harmless. Nothing is further from the truth. Plants can be both useful and harmful – even poisonous – and everything depends on the preparation and the dose. David Potterton has clearly indicated those plants from which the reader can make simple, safe preparations – provided the plant is correctly identified – and those which should only be taken following the advice of a qualified herbal practitioner. As a conclusion to this foreword may I strongly urge everyone not to disregard this.

E. J. Shellard
Emeritus Professor of Pharmacognosy
University of London

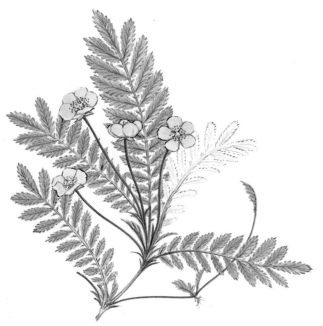

Silverweed POTENTILLA ANSERINA

PREFACE

This is the essence of Culpeper's work on herbal medicine. We have retained the famous herbalist's caustic comments and many of his colourful descriptions of herbs, but have included the present-day uses of herbs in the light of modern practice. It is interesting to note how many herbs used in Culpeper's time still occupy a prominent position in herbal dispensaries today.

Because the uses of some herbs may have changed considerably, readers are recommended to obtain professional advice rather than treat themselves. It should be remembered that herbalists undergo a long training in the selection and use of herbal medicines.

David Potterton
Editor

ACONITE

A decoction of the root is a good lotion to wash the parts bitten by venomous creatures.

We have many poisonous Aconites growing in the fields, of which we ought to be cautious; but there is a medicinal one kept in the shop. This is called Anthora, the Wholesome Aconite, or Wholesome Wolf'sbane.

It is a small plant, about a foot (30 cm) high with pale, divided green leaves and yellow flowers. The stem is firm, angular and hairy. The flowers, large and hooded, grow on top of the branches in spikes. The root is tuberous.

Where to find it: It is a native of the Alps, but it is planted in gardens.

Flowering time: The seeds ripen towards the end of the summer.

Astrology: The plant is under the government of Saturn.

Medicinal virtues: The shoot only is used, and that not often. However, it is said to be very serviceable against vegetable poisons. A decoction of the root is a good lotion to wash the parts bitten by venomous creatures, but it is not much regarded at this time, and should be cautiously kept out of children's way, for there is a farina in the flower, which is very dangerous if blown in the eyes; the leaves also, if rubbed on the skin, will irritate and cause soreness.

Modern uses: All species of Aconite should be regarded as being poisonous and, on no account, used medicinally by the unqualified. Modern herbalists make use only of the root of *Aconitum napellum* in the form of a lotion, but this also has restricted applications. Homoeopathic physicians use a specially made tincture of the whole plant of *Aconitum napellum*. The dose given, however, is so minute that no danger arises.

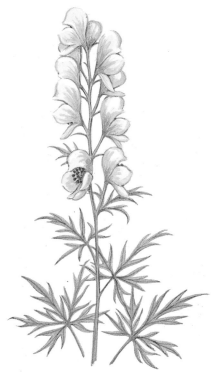

Aconite ACONITUM ANTHORA

ADDER'S TONGUE

It is given with good success unto those that are troubled with casting, vomiting, or bleeding at the mouth and nose, or otherwise downwards.

This herb has but one leaf which grows with the stalk a finger's length above the ground. Its appearance resembles the tongue of an adder serpent.

Where to find it: It grows in moist meadows.

Flowering time: It flowers not, being a fern, but it appears in mid to late spring. It quickly perishes in warm weather.

Astrology: It is under the dominion of the Moon and Cancer, and therefore, if the weakness of the retentive faculty be caused by an evil influence in any part of the body governed by the Moon, or under the dominion of Cancer, this herb cures it by sympathy. It cures these diseases after specified, in any part of the body under the influence of Saturn, by antipathy.

Medicinal virtues: The juice of the leaves drank with the distilled water of Horsetail, is a singular remedy of all manner of wounds in the breasts, bowels or other parts of the body. The said juice given in the distilled water of oaken buds, is very good for women who have their usual courses, or whites flowing down too abundantly. It helps sore eyes. Of the leaves infused or boiled in oil, omphacine, or unripe olives, set in the sun for certain days, or the green leaves sufficiently boiled in the said oil, is made an excellent green balsam, not only for green and fresh wounds, but also for old and inveterate ulcers. It also stayeth and refresheth all inflammations that arise upon pains by hurts and wounds.

Modern uses: Its main use is as a remedy for wounds, but it is not in general use these days. More popular today is the homoeopathic medicine Arnica which is taken for shock in drop doses or in tablet form, or St John's Wort which has an affinity for nerve endings and will alleviate pain. The tincture is available from herbalists. Adder's Tongue can be infused in oil to make an application for burns, ulcers and cuts. The infusion – 1 oz (28 g) dried herbs to 1 pt (568 ml) of boiling water – is taken in doses of 2 fl oz (56 ml).

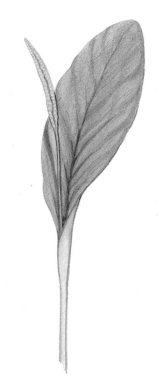

Adder's Tongue OPHIOGLOSSUM VULGATUM

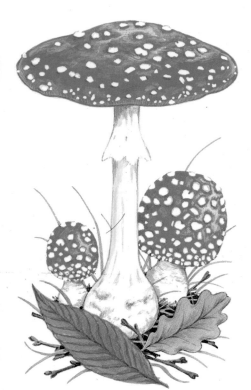

Agaric AGARICUS

AGARIC

It evacuates phlegm, and is given in defluxions and disorders of the chest, but that only to strong people.

This is a fungus which may grow from the size of a man's fist to the size of his head. There are a great variety of these excrescences and they differ both in virtue and the substance on which they grow.

Where to find it: One kind grows at the foot of Oak trees and is pleasant to eat, tasting like the meat of a lobster's claw. Touchwood, or Spunk, is made from another kind of fungus growing on Willows. A third kind grows on the trunks of Larch trees.

Flowering time: No flower is produced, it being a fungus.

Astrology: It is under the government of Mercury in the sign of Leo.

Medicinal virtues: It evacuates phlegm, and is given in defluxions and disorders of the breast, but that only to strong people. It is reckoned a useless medicine, or rather noxious, for it loads the stomach, distends the viscera, creates a nausea, and causes vomiting. Its powder has been prescribed from half a dram (890 mg) to two drams (3.5 g).

Modern uses: There are several species of *Agaricus*, some being poisonous, some being edible mushrooms. Homoeopaths make use of *Amanita muscaria*, *Agaricus emeticus*, and *Amanita phalloides*. It is employed as a remedy for acute sensitiveness to cold and damp when there is itching and redness and a burning sensation in the hands and feet. In days gone by it was in constant use during the winter months, but less now since the advent of central heating.

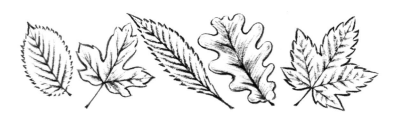

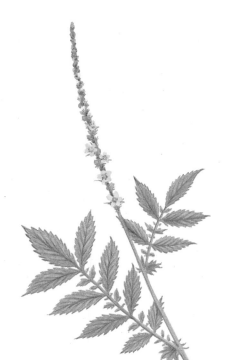

Agrimony AGRIMONIA EUPATORIA

AGRIMONY

It draweth forth thorns and splinters of wood, nails, or any other such thing gotten into the flesh.

This has long leaves, dented about the edges, green above and greyish underneath, and a little hairy; a strong, round, hairy brown stalk, two or three feet (61 or 91 cm) high, and small yellow flowers one above another in long spikes.

Where to find it: It grows upon banks near the sides of hedges.

Flowering time: Midsummer, the seed being ripe shortly after.

Astrology: It is under Jupiter and the sign of Cancer. It strengthens those parts under the planet and sign, and removes diseases in them by sympathy; diseases under Saturn, Mars and Mercury are removed by antipathy if they happen in any part of the body governed by Jupiter, or under the signs Cancer, Sagittarius or Pisces, and therefore must be good for the gout, either used outwardly in oil or ointment, or inwardly in an electuary, or syrup, or concerted juice.

Medicinal virtues: It openeth and cleanseth the liver, helpeth the jaundice, and is very beneficial to the bowels, healing all inward wounds, bruises, hurts and other distempers.

The decoction of the herb made with wine, and drank, is good against the biting and stinging of serpents, and helps them that make foul, troubled or bloody water, and makes them part with clear urine speedily. It also helpeth the colic, cleanseth the breast, and rids away the cough.

A draught of the decoction taken warm before the fit, first removes, and in time rids away the tertian or quartan agues.

The leaves and seeds taken in wine stays the bloody flux. Outwardly applied, being stamped with old swine's grease, it helpeth old sores, cancers and inveterate ulcers. The juice dropped in helpeth foul and imposthumed ears.

Modern uses: A valuable herb in modern practice used mainly as a gastro-intestinal tonic. It is also a useful remedy for coughs, skin eruptions and cystitis. As all the medicinal properties are fully soluble in water, the best way to administer it is as an infusion – 1 oz (28 g) of the dried herb to 1 pt (568 ml) of boiling water. Small doses are given frequently. A fluid extract is available from herbalists, the dose being from 10 to 40 drops.

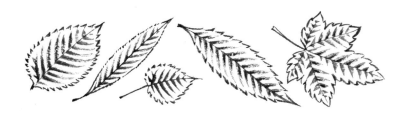

BIDENS TRIPARTITA

AGRIMONY (Water)

It kills worms and cleanseth the body of sharp humours which are the cause of itch and scab.

A common plant also known as Bur Marigold, Water Hemp, Bastard Hemp and Bastard Agrimony; Eupatorium and Hipatorium because it strengthens the liver. This is a short to medium height annual, with dull, yellowish-brown flowers borne on erect stems.

Where to find it: Look for it by the sides of ponds and ditches and by running water.

Flowering time: Midsummer. The seed ripens shortly after.

Astrology: It is a plant of Jupiter and belongs to the sign of Cancer.

Medicinal virtues: It healeth and drieth, cutteth and cleanseth thick and tough humours of the breast, and for this I hold it inferior to few herbs that grow.

It helps the cachexia or evil disposition of the body, the dropsy and yellow jaundice. It opens the obstructions of the liver and mollifies the hardness of the spleen, being applied outwardly. It breaks imposthumes taken inwardly. It provokes urine and the terms. It strengthens the lungs exceedingly.

Modern uses: A valuable herb with a wide range of properties and used for the treatment of fevers, urinary tract disorders and renal and respiratory diseases. The plant contains natural antiseptics. Some herbalists recommend it for menstrual problems, particularly where there is an excessive loss of blood. The way to take it is as an infusion – 1 oz (28 g) to 1 pt (568 ml) of boiling water. The dose is 2–3 fl oz (56–85 ml) three to four times a day.

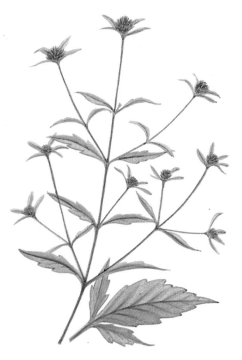

Agrimony (Water) BIDENS TRIPARTITA

11

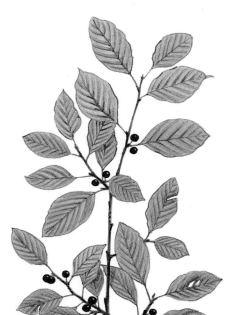

Alder (Black) FRANGULA ALNUS
(= ALNUS NIGRA)

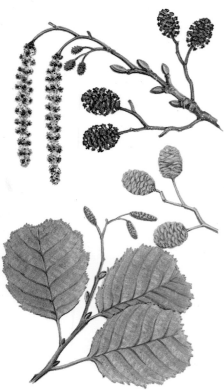

Alder (Common) ALNUS GLUTINOSA

FRANGULA ALNUS (= ALNUS NIGRA)

ALDER (Black)

It purgeth and strengtheneth the liver and spleen, cleansing them from such evil humours and hardness as they are afflicted with.

The Black Alder or Alder Buckthorn does not grow to any great height, but spreads its branches like a hedge-bush. The outer bark is of a blackish colour. The leaves are like the Common Alder and the flowers are white. Berries are produced which at first are green, then red and blackish when thoroughly ripe. They contain two small round, flat seeds.

Where to find it: In woodland.

Flowering time: It flowers in late spring and the berries are ripe in early autumn.

Astrology: It is a tree of Venus and perhaps under the celestial sign of Cancer.

Medicinal virtues: The dried inner yellow bark purgeth downwards both choler and phlegm and the watery humours of such as have the dropsy. It strengthens the inward parts again by binding. If the bark be boiled with Agrimony, Wormwood, Dodder, Hops, and some Fennel with Smallage, Endive and Succory roots, and a reasonable draught taken every morning for some time, it is very effectual against the jaundice, dropsy and evil disposition of the body, especially if some suitable purging medicines have been taken before to void the grosser excrements.

The fresh green bark taken inwardly provokes strong vomitings, pains in the stomach and gripings in the belly. If the decoction stands and settles for two or three days until the yellow colour be changed black, it will not work so strongly as before, but will strengthen the stomach and procure an appetite to meat.

The outer bark doth bind the body and is helpful for all laxes and fluxes thereof. It must be dried first whereby it will work better. The inner bark boiled in vinegar is an approved remedy to kill lice, cure the itch and take away scabs by drying them up in a short time. It is singularly good to wash the teeth, and to take away the pains, to fasten those that are loose, to cleanse them and keep them sound.

In springtime take a handful of each of the herbs before mentioned, add a handful of Elder buds, bruise them all and boil them in a gallon (4.5 l) of ordinary beer when it is new. Boil for half an hour and then add three gallons (13.5 l) more. Drink a draught of it every morning, about half a pint (284 ml). It is an excellent purge for the spring to consume the phlegmatic quality the winter has left behind, and to keep your body in health. Esteem it as a jewel.

Modern uses: Not popularly used in modern practice. The Common Alder is used, however. See below.

ALNUS GLUTINOSA

ALDER (Common)

The leaves gathered while the morning dew is on them and brought into a chamber troubled with fleas will gather them thereunto, which being suddenly cast out, will rid the chamber of these troublesome bedfellows.

The Common Alder grows to about 65 feet (20 m) in height. It produces purplish-red catkins which change to greenish-yellow.

Where to find it: It grows in moist woods and watery places.

Flowering time: From mid to late spring. It yields a ripe seed in early autumn.

Astrology: It is under the dominion of Venus, and of some water sign, one supposes Pisces.

Medicinal virtues: The decoction, or distilled water of the leaves, is excellent to bathe inflamed or burnt skin and wounds with. It is especially recommended for that inflammation of the chest, which the vulgar call an ague.

In winter make use of the bark in the same manner. The leaves and bark are cooling, drying and binding. The fresh leaves laid upon swellings dissolve them and stay the inflammations. The leaves put under the bare feet galled with travelling are refreshing to them.

Modern uses: The bark and leaves are used as a tonic. A decoction is made from 1 oz (28 g) of the dried bark to 1 pt (568 ml) of boiling water. This has astringent properties and is used as a gargle for sore throats and pharyngitis in doses of 2–3 fl oz (56–85 ml). The bark can be taken as a tonic powder in doses of a half to one teaspoonful or mixed with a little Goldenseal and infused in a pint (568 ml) of water and taken in doses of 2 fl oz (56 ml) for dyspepsia.

GLECHOMA HEDERACEA

ALEHOOF

The juice dropped into the ear doth wonderfully help the noise and singing of them, and helpeth the hearing which is decayed.

It is also called Cat's-foot, Ground-ivy, Gill-go-by-ground, Gill-creep-by-ground, Turn-hoof and Hay-maids.

This well-known herb spreads and creeps along the ground. Roots shoot forth at the corners of tender-jointed stalks, set with two round leaves at every joint. The hollow, long flowers are of a blueish-purple colour with small white spots on the lips that hang down.

Where to find it: It is found under hedges, on the sides of ditches, in shadowy lanes and on waste land.

Flowering time: Early to late spring. The leaves stay green until the winter.

Astrology: It is a herb of Venus and therefore cures, by sympathy, the diseases she causes; and those of Mars by antipathy.

Medicinal virtues: A herb for all inward wounds, exulcerated lungs, or other parts, either by itself, or boiled with other similar herbs. It easeth griping pains, windy and choleric humours in the stomach, spleen or belly; it helps the yellow jaundice by opening the stoppings of the gall and liver, and melancholy by opening the stoppings of the spleen. It expels venom or poison and also the plague.

It provokes urine and women's courses. The decoction of it in wine drank for some time eases those that are troubled by sciatica, or hip gout, and also the gout in the hands, knees or feet. If you add to the decoction some honey and a little burnt alum, it is excellent as a gargle for any sore mouth or throat, and to wash the sores and ulcers in the privy parts of man or woman.

It speedily helps green wounds, if bruised and bound thereto. The juice of it boiled with a little honey and verdigris doth wonderfully cleanse fistulas, ulcers and stayeth the spreading or eating of cancers and ulcers. It helpeth the itch, scabs, wheals and other breakings out in any part of the body.

The juice of Celandine, Field Daisies, and Ground-ivy clarified and a little fine sugar dissolved therein, and dropped into the eyes, is a sovereign remedy for all pains, redness and watering of them; also for the pin and web, skins and films growing over the sight. It helps beasts as well as men. The juice dropped into the ear helpeth the hearing.

Modern uses: Generally known as Ground-ivy among modern herbalists, the herb is collected in late spring when the flowers are still fresh. It is used in the treatment of dyspepsia, kidney disease, abscesses, gatherings and tumours, eye problems and freckles. For abscesses, it is combined in equal parts with Chamomile flowers and used as a poultice. For treating coughs, it is combined in equal parts with Horehound and Colt's Foot and made into a syrup. An infusion can be made by adding 1 oz (28 g) of the herb to 1 pt (568 ml) of boiling water. Strain and administer in doses of 2 fl oz (56 ml) three times a day.

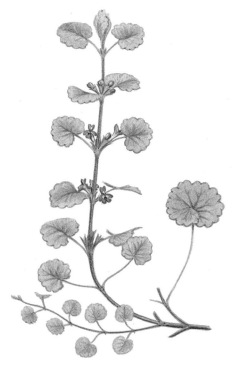

Alehoof GLECHOMA HEDERACEA

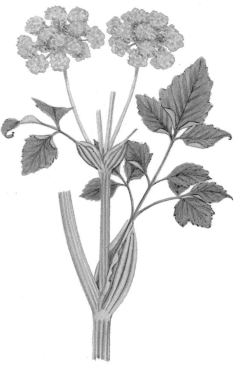

SMYRNIUM OLUSATRUM

ALEXANDERS

It warmeth a cold stomach and openeth a stoppage to the liver and spleen.

It is also called Horse Parsley, Wild Parsley and the Black Pot-herb. Similar to Wild Angelica, it is sometimes mistaken for it by collectors. It is a biennial growing to about four feet (1.2 m) high and producing yellowish-green flowers.

Where to find it: It is usually cultivated in gardens, but prefers coastal regions.

Flowering time: Early to midsummer. The seed is ripe in late summer, and is almost black, hence the name Black Pot-herb.

Astrology: It is a herb of Jupiter and therefore friendly to nature.

Medicinal virtues: It is good to move women's courses, to expel the afterbirth, to break wind, to provoke urine, and helpeth the strangury. These things the seeds will do likewise. Boiled in wine or bruised and taken in wine the herb or seeds are effectual in the biting of serpents.

Modern uses: This herb is not used by professional herbalists at the present time; other remedies for flatulence, such as Fennel and Aniseed, are more popular.

Alexanders SMYRNIUM OLUSATRUM

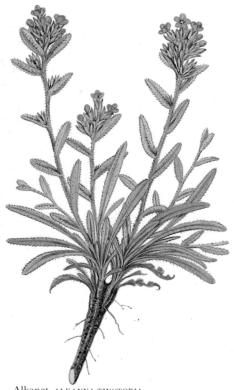

ALKANNA TINCTORIA

ALKANET

If you apply the herb to the privities, it draws forth the dead child.

Besides the common name, it is called Orchanet and Spanish Bugloss, and by the apothecaries, Enchusa. It has a great and thick root of a reddish colour, long, narrow hairy leaves, and small blue or reddish-purple flowers.

Where to find it: It grows in weedy places along the verges of roads and on waste land. It likes a dry sandy soil. It is cultivated commercially for the red dye extracted from the roots.

Flowering time: It flowers from mid to late summer, but the root is in its prime, as are Carrots and Parsnips, before the herb runs up to stalk.

Astrology: It is under the dominion of Venus, and is indeed one of her darlings.

Medicinal virtues: It helps old ulcers, hot inflammations, burnings by common fire and St Anthony's fire, by antipathy to Mars. For these uses your best way is to make it into an ointment. If you make a vinegar of it, as you make Vinegar of Roses, it helps the morphy and leprosy. It helps the yellow jaundice, spleen and gravel in the kidneys. Dioscorides saith, it helps such as are bitten by venomous beasts, whether it be taken inwardly or applied to the wound; nay, he saith further, if any that hath newly eaten it do but spit into the mouth of a serpent, the serpent instantly dies.

It stays the flux of the belly, kills worms and helps the fits of the mother. Its decoction made in wine, and drank, strengthens the back, and easeth the pains thereof. It helps bruises and falls, and is as gallant a remedy to drive out the smallpox and measles as any is. An ointment made of it is excellent for green wounds, pricks or thrusts.

Modern uses: The red dye is used to colour ointments. The flowers, roots and seeds have expectorant properties. It is also used by some as a blood purifier. But it is not in general use and not recommended for internal use domestically.

Alkanet ALKANNA TINCTORIA

AMARANTHUS

I wonder in my heart how the virtue of herbs came at first to be known, if not by their signatures. The moderns have them from the writings of the ancients; the ancients had no writings to have them from.

Amaranth is also called Flower-gentle, Flower-velure, Floramor, Velvet-flower and Prince's Feather. It runneth up with a stalk which is streaked and somewhat reddish towards the root. It has long, broad reddish-green leaves and flowers which are more like tufts, very beautiful to behold.

Where to find it: A garden plant, commonly known as Love Lies Bleeding.

Flowering time: Continues in flower from late summer till the frost nips it.

Astrology: It is under the dominion of Saturn and is an excellent qualifier of the unruly actions and passions of Venus, though Mars should also join with her.

Medicinal virtues: The flowers, dried and beaten into powder, stop the terms in women. The flowers stop all fluxes of blood, whether in man or woman, bleeding either at the nose or wound.

There is also a sort of Amaranthus that bears a white flower, which stops the whites in women, and the running of the reins in men, and is a most gallant anti-venereal, and a singular remedy for the French pox.

Modern uses: Classified today as an astringent and used to check diarrhoea, dysentery and rectal bleeding. Also used for treating heavy menstrual periods. The flowering herb is used for these purposes in the form of a decoction – 1 oz (28 g) of herb to 1 pt (568 ml) of boiling water – in doses of 2 fl oz (56 ml). The same can be used as a mouthwash for ulcerated conditions, and as a vaginal injection for leucorrhoea.

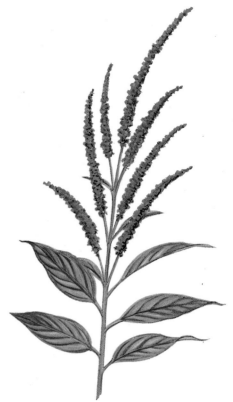

Amaranthus AMARANTHUS HYBRIDUS
(= A. HYPOCHONDRIACUS)

ANEMONE

And when all is done, let physicians prate what they please, all the pills in the dispensary purge not the head like to hot things held in the mouth.

It is called the Wind-flower because they say the flowers never open unless the wind bloweth. But it is also known as the Wood Anemone of Great Britain.

Where to find it: A beautiful low-growing plant which naturalises itself in open woodland beneath leaf-losing trees and in shady places in rock gardens.

Flowering time: Spring.

Astrology: It is under the dominion of Mars.

Medicinal virtues: The leaves provoke the terms, being boiled, and the decoction drank. The body bathed with the decoction cures the leprosy. The leaves stamped, and the juice snuffed up the nose, purgeth the head mightily; so doth the root, chewed in the mouth, for it procureth much spitting and bringeth away watery and phlegmatic humors and is therefore excellent for the lethargy.

Made into an ointment and the eyelids anointed with it, it helps inflammations of the eyes. The same ointment is excellent to cleanse malignant and corroding ulcers.

Modern uses: Medical herbalists use the Pasque Flower, *Pulsatilla vulgaris*, as a nervine and anti-spasmodic for nervous headaches and asthma. The tincture available from them is given a few drops at a time, in water every two or three hours.

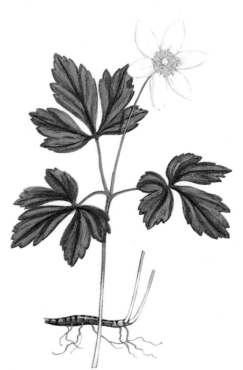

Anemone ANEMONE NEMOROSA

ANGELICA

Our physicians . . . blasphemously call Tansies or Heart's Ease, an herb for the Trinity, because it is of three colours, and they call a certain ointment, an ointment of the Apostles, because it consists of 12 ingredients. Alas! I am sorry for their folly and grieved at their blasphemy. God send them wisdom the rest of their age, for they have their share of ignorance already. Some call this an herb of the Holy Ghost; others more moderate called it Angelica, because of its angelical virtues.

A perennial plant growing five or six feet (1.5 or 1.8 m) high with large leaves and flat heads of greenish-white flowers.

Where to find it: A common garden plant, but it also grows wild, preferring humid habitats.

Flowering time: It flowers from early to late summer.

Astrology: It is a herb of the Sun in Leo. Gather it when he is there, the Moon applying to his good aspect. Let it be gathered either in his hour, or in the hour of Jupiter.

Medicinal virtues: For all epidemical diseases caused by Saturn. It resists poison by defending and comforting the heart, blood and spirits. It doth the like against the plague. The root is taken in powder to the weight of half a dram (890 mg) at a time with some good treacle in Carduus water, and the party laid to sweat in his bed. The stalks and roots candied and eaten fasting are good preservatives in time of infection, and will warm and comfort a cold stomach. The root steeped in vinegar and a little of the vinegar taken fasting and the root smelled is good for the same purpose. A water distilled from the root, as steeped in wine and distilled, and drank two or three spoonfuls at a time easeth all pains and torments coming of cold and wind, and taken with some of the root in powder, helpeth the pleurisy, as also all other diseases of the lungs and breast, as coughs, phthisic and shortness of breath. A syrup of the stalks doth the like.

It helps pains of the colic, the strangury and stoppage of the urine, procureth women's courses, and expelleth the afterbirth, openeth the stoppage of the liver and spleen, and briefly easeth and discusseth all windiness and inward swellings.

The decoction drank before the fit of an ague, that they may sweat, if possible, before the fit comes will, in two or three times taking, rid it quite away. It helps digestion and is a remedy for a surfeit. The juice or the water dropped into the eyes or ears helps dimness of sight and deafness. The juice put into the hollow of the teeth easeth their pain. The root in powder, made up into a plaster and laid on the biting of mad dogs or any other venomous creature doth wonderfully help. The juice or water dropped into dead ulcers, or the powder of the root in want of either, doth cause them to heal quickly by covering the naked bones with flesh.

The distilled water applied to places pained with gout or sciatica doth give a great deal of ease.

Modern uses: Angelica is still widely used as an anti-dyspeptic, and for flatulence. For this an infusion is made from the bruised root or whole herb. Use 1 oz (28 g) to 1 pt (568 ml) of boiling water and administer in doses of 2 fl oz (56 ml).

An ointment can be made from the root by boiling it in paraffin wax and straining it before it cools. Use for minor skin problems and for rheumatic pain. The stems preserved with sugar are used as a confection.

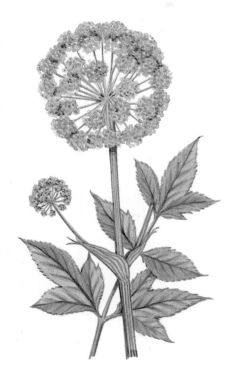

Angelica ANGELICA ARCHANGELICA

ARCHANGEL

To put a gloss on their practice, the physicians call an herb (which country people vulgarly know by the name of the Dead-nettle) Archangel.

The White, with the Red and Yellow Dead-nettles, are nettles that do not sting. Yet except their flowers they resemble the Stinging Nettle.

Where to find them: They grow almost everywhere unless it be in the middle of the street. The Yellow is most usually found in the wet grounds of woods.

Flowering time: From the beginning of spring and through the summer.

Astrology: The chief use of them is for women, it being a herb of Venus.

Medicinal virtues: The Archangels are somewhat hot and drier than the Stinging Nettles and better used for the stopping and hardness of the spleen. Flowers of the White Archangel are preserved or conserved to be used to stay the whites, and the flowers of the Red to stay the reds, in women. It makes the heart merry, drives away melancholy, quickens the spirits, is good against the quartan agues, stauncheth bleeding at the mouth and nose if it be stamped and applied to the nape of the neck. The herb bruised and with salt and vinegar and hog's-grease laid upon a hard tumour or swelling, or that vulgarly called the king's-evil, do help to dissolve or discuss them. In like manner applied, it doth much allay the pains and give ease to the gout, sciatica and other pains of the joints and sinews. It is also very effectual to heal green wounds and old ulcers. It draweth forth splinters and is very good against bruises and burnings. The Yellow Archangel is most commended for old, filthy, corrupt sores and ulcers, although they be hollow, and to dissolve tumours.

Modern uses: The flowering tips of the White Dead-nettles are prescribed for menstrual problems and leucorrhoea in women, and for prostatitis in men. It is also used for catarrhal conditions and where liver stimulation is required. It is given in the form of an infusion which is made by steeping 1 oz (28 g) of the dried flowers in 1 pt (568 ml) of boiling water for 20 minutes, straining and administering in doses of 2 fl oz (56 ml) three times a day.

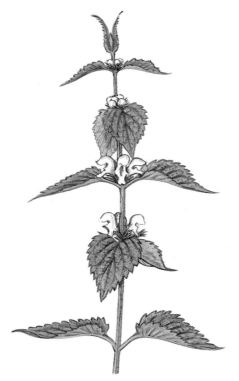

Archangel LAMIUM

ARRACH (Garden)

It is so commonly known to every housewife it were labour lost to describe it.

It is also called Orach and Arage and Mountain Spinach. Occasionally it is grown as a vegetable. A tall erect plant, it has large leaves.

Where to find it: It grows naturally in Western Asia, but otherwise is cultivated.

Flowering time: From early to late summer.

Astrology: It is under the government of the Moon, cold and moist like her.

Medicinal virtues: Being eaten, it softeneth and looseneth the body of man, and fortifieth the expulsive faculty in him. Whether bruised and applied to the throat, or boiled and similarly applied, it matters not much. It is excellent for swellings in the throat. The best way is to drink the decoction and apply the herb outwardly. The decoction is an excellent remedy for the yellow jaundice.

Modern uses: It is not now used in medicine.

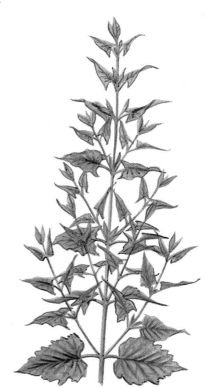

Arrach (Garden) ATRIPLEX HORTENSIS

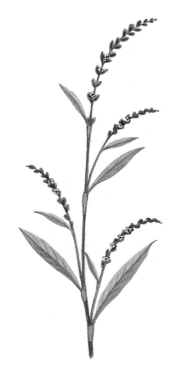

Arssmart POLYGONUM

ARSSMART

The Hot Arssmart is called also the Water-pepper. The Mild Arssmart is called Dead Arssmart, or Peachwort. Our college Physicians mistake the one for the other in their New Master-piece, whereby they discover their ignorance, their carelessness; and he that hath but half an eye may see their pride without a pair of spectacles.

A very common creeping weed, the Mild Arssmart (also called Redshank) has broad leaves at the great red joints of the stalks, with semicircular blackish marks on them. The root is long with many strings and perishes yearly. The taste is rather sour like Sorrel.

Where to find it: It grows in watery places, ditches and the like, which for the most part are dry in summer.

Flowering time: It flowers in early summer and the seed is ripe at the end of the summer.

Astrology: As the virtue of both of these is various so also is their government; for that which is hot and biting is under the dominion of Mars, but Saturn challengeth the other as appears by that leaden-coloured spot he hath placed on the leaf.

Medicinal virtues: The Mild is very effectual for putrid ulcers in man or beast, to kill worms and cleanse putrefied places. The juice, dropped in, or applied, consumeth all cold swellings and dissolveth the congealed blood of bruises by strokes, falls etc.

A piece of the root, or some of the seeds bruised, held to an aching tooth, taketh away the pain. The leaves bruised and laid to the joint that hath a felon thereon, taketh it away. The juice destroyeth worms in the ears, being dropped into them. The Mild Arssmart is good against all imposthumes and inflammations at the beginning, and to heal all green wounds.

The Hot Arssmart groweth not so high or so tall as the Mild, but hath many leaves of the colour of Peach leaves, seldom or never spotted. If you will be pleased to break a leaf of it across your tongue, it will make your tongue smart.

If the Hot Arssmart be strewed in a chamber, it will soon kill all the fleas. A good handful put under a horse's saddle will make him travel the better, although he were half tired before.

Modern uses: A homoeopathic tincture is made from the hot *Polygonum hydropiper* and used for diarrhoea and dysentery. The milder *Polygonum persicaria* is not widely used, but an infusion of the plant has been recommended for lung disorders, rheumatism, eczema and liver disease. The plants contain an irritant oil.

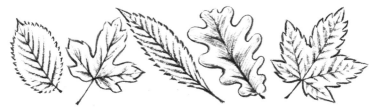

ASARABACCA

I fancy purging and vomiting medicine as little as any man breathing doth, for they weaken nature, nor shall ever advise them to be used unless upon urgent necessity. If a physician be nature's servant, it is his duty to strengthen his mistress as much as he can, and weaken her as little as may be.

A creeping perennial plant, Asarabacca is now rare in most places, but still grows abundantly in South America. It has many small leaves each upon its own foot-stalk and the roots are small and whitish, spreading divers ways but not running or creeping under the ground. It hath dull purple, solitary flowers.

Where to find it: It grows in gardens, but its natural habitat is woodland.

Flowering time: Spring. The seed ripens about midsummer on.

Astrology: 'Tis under the dominion of Mars and therefore inimical to nature.

Medicinal virtues: This herb being drunk not only provoketh vomiting, but purgeth downward, and by urine also, purgeth both choler and phlegm. The common use is to take the juice of five or seven leaves in a little drink to cause vomiting. The roots have the same virtue, though they do not operate so forcibly. I shall desire ignorant people to forbear the use of the leaves. The roots purge more gently and may prove beneficial to such as have cancers, putrefied ulcers, or fistulas upon their bodies.

Modern uses: Many over-the-counter medicines contain an emetic to prevent overdosage. Asarabacca was an official emetic, but has now been replaced by Ipecacuanha. It is not recommended for domestic use as it is an abortefacient. It also causes internal bleeding and gastro-enteritis. A homoeopathic tincture of Asarum is used to treat gastro-enteritis.

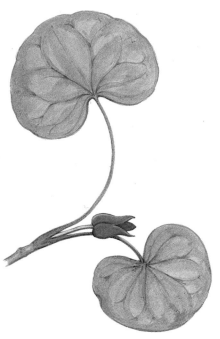

Asarabacca ASARUM EUROPAEUM

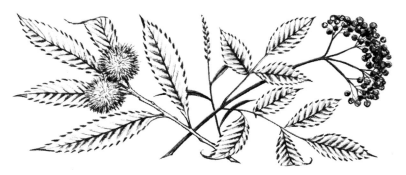

FRAXINUS EXCELSIOR

ASH TREE

This is so well known that time will be misspent in writing a description of it; and therefore I shall only insist upon the virtues of it.

Where to find it: It is a large, deciduous woodland tree common throughout Europe.

Flowering time: Mid to late spring.

Astrology: It is governed by the Sun.

Medicinal virtues: The young tender tops, with the leaves taken inwardly, and some outwardly applied, are singularly good against the biting of an adder, viper or any other venomous beast. The water distilled therefrom and taken in small quantity each morning fasting is a singular medicine to those that are subject to the dropsy, or to abate the greatness of those that are too gross or fat.

The decoction of the leaves in white wine helpeth to break the stone and expel it, and cure the jaundice. The ashes of the bark made into lye and those heads bathed therewith which are leprous, scabby or scald, they are thereby cured. The kernels within the husks, commonly called ashen key, prevail against stitches and pains in the side, proceeding of wind and voiding away the stone by provoking the urine.

I can justly except against none of this, save only the first – that Ash Tree tops and leaves are good against the biting of serpents and vipers. The rest are virtues something likely, only if it be in winter when you cannot get the leaves, you may safely use the bark instead. The keys you may easily keep all the year, gathering them when they are ripe.

Modern uses: It has laxative and diuretic properties. Also useful for intermittent fever. An infusion of the dried leaves is used in rheumatic disease and gout.

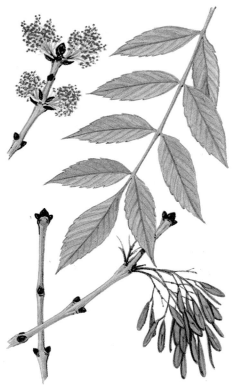

Ash Tree FRAXINUS EXCELSIOR

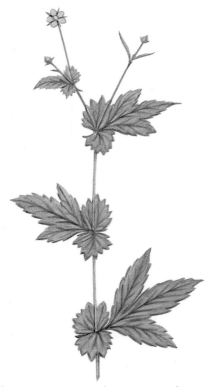

ASPARAGUS OFFICINALIS and SATIVUS

ASPARAGUS

The decoction taken fasting several mornings together, it stirreth up bodily lust in man or woman, whatever some have written to the contrary.

Asparagus officinalis is the well-known vegetable; *sativus* is the Prickly Asparagus. The very long and slender stalks are the bigness of an ordinary riding wand. Greenish or yellowish bell-shaped flowers are produced on hairless stems.

Where to find it: Both sorts are found in gardens and in the wild. The Garden Asparagus nourisheth more than the wild, yet hath the same medicinal effects.

Flowering time: For the most part they flower in mid to late summer and bear their berries later in the year.

Astrology: Both are under the dominion of Jupiter.

Medicinal virtues: The young buds or branches boiled in ordinary broth, make the belly soluble and open. Boiled in white wine they prevent the urine being stopped. It is good against the strangury or difficulty of making water. It expelleth the gravel and stone out of the kidneys, and helpeth pains in the reins. Boiled in white wine or vinegar it is prevalent for them that have their arteries loosened, or are troubled with the hip-gout or sciatica.

The decoction of the roots boiled in wine and taken, is good to clear the sight and being held in the mouth easeth the toothache. The back and belly bathed with the decoction of the roots in white wine, or sitting therein as a bath, hath been found effectual against pains of the reins and bladder, pains of the mother and colic, and generally against all pains that happen to the lower parts of the body.

It is no less effectual against stiff and benumbed sinews, or those that are shrunk by cramps and convulsions, and helpeth the sciatica.

Modern uses: Besides its use as a vegetable, Asparagus is used by homoeopaths in the treatment of rheumatism and oedema due to heart failure. It is a diuretic and will clear sediment from the bladder. It also has laxative properties.

Asparagus ASPARAGUS OFFICINALIS and SATIVUS

GEUM URBANUM (= G. HERBANUM)

AVENS

It is very safe; you need have no dose prescribed; and is very fit to be kept in every body's house.

A common wayside plant also called Colewort and Herb Bennet. It hath long, rough, dark green winged leaves. On the tops of the branches stand small, pale yellow flowers, consisting of five leaves like the flowers of Cinquefoil.

Where to find it: Under hedges and by pathways in fields. They rather delight to grow in shadowy than in sunny places.

Flowering time: Late spring, early summer. The seed is ripe by midsummer at the latest.

Astrology: It is governed by Jupiter.

Medicinal virtues: It is good for the diseases of the chest or breast, for pains and stitches in the side, and to expel crude and raw humours from the belly and stomach, by the sweet savour and warming quality. It dissolves inward congealed blood happening by falls or bruises, and the spitting of blood, if the roots, either green or dry, be boiled in wine and drunk: as also all manner of inward wounds or outward, if washed or bathed therewith.

The decoction also being drunk, comforts the heart, and strengthens the stomach and a cold brain, and therefore is good in the

Avens GEUM URBANUM (= G. HERBANUM)

springtime to open obstructions of the liver, and helpeth the wind colic. It also helps those that have fluxes, or are bursten, or have a rupture. It taketh away spots or marks in the face being washed therewith. The juice of the fresh root, or powder of the dried root, have the same effect as the decoction. The root in the springtime, steeped in wine, doth give it a delicate flavour and taste, and being drunk fasting every morning, comforteth the heart, and is a good preservative against the plague or any other poison. It helpeth digestion, warmeth a cold stomach and openeth obstructions of the liver and spleen.

Modern uses: Widely used because of its excellent properties as an antiseptic, aromatic, astringent, stomach tonic, febrifuge and styptic. A restorative in debilitating diseases, especially of the intestinal tract. An infusion is made from 1 oz (28 g) of the dried herb or root to 1 pt (568 ml) of boiling water. The dose is 2 fl oz (56 ml). Herbal practitioners find it a useful remedy for colitis.

MELISSA OFFICINALIS

BALM

It is very good to help digestion and open obstructions of the brain, and hath so much purging quality in it (saith Avicen) as to expel those melancholy vapours from the spirits and blood which are in the heart and arteries, although it cannot do so in other parts of the body.

The herb is so well known as to be an inhabitant almost in every garden. It is also known as Sweet Balm or Lemon Balm. The leaves are set in pairs upon the stem, the flowers in whorls above each pair.

Where to find it: A garden plant, but its natural habitat is the mountainous regions in southern Europe.

Flowering time: Midsummer to early autumn.

Astrology: It is an herb of Jupiter and under Cancer and strengthens the body in all its actions.

Medicinal virtues: Let a syrup made with the juice of it and sugar be kept in every gentlewoman's house to relieve the weak stomachs and sick bodies of their poor and sickly neighbours. Also keep the dried herb in the house so that with other convenient simples you may make it into an electuary with honey. The Arabian physicians have extolled the virtues thereof to the skies, although the Greeks thought it not worth mentioning. Seraphio saith, it causeth the mind and heart to become merry and reviveth the heart, faintings and swoonings, especially of such who are overtaken in sleep and driveth away all troublesome cares and thoughts out of the mind, arising from melancholy and black choler, which Avicen also confirmeth.

Dioscorides saith that the leaves steeped in wine, and the wine drank, and the leaves externally applied, is a remedy against the sting of a scorpion, and the biting of mad dogs; and commendeth the decoction for women to bathe or sit in to procure their courses. It is good to wash aching teeth therewith, and profitable for those that have the bloody flux. The leaves also, with a little nitre taken in drink, are good against the surfeit of mushrooms, and help the griping pains of the belly; and being made into an electuary, it is good for them that cannot fetch their breath. Used with salt it takes away the wens, kernels or hard swellings in the flesh or throat. It cleanseth foul sores and easeth the pains of the gout. It is good for the liver and spleen. A tansy or caudle made with eggs and juice thereof, while it is young putting to some sugar and Rose-water, is good for woman in child-bed, when the afterbirth is not thoroughly voided, and for their faintings upon or in their sore travail. The herb bruised and boiled in a little white wine and oil, and laid warm on a boil, will ripen and break it.

Modern uses: It is commonly prescribed as an infusion to induce mild perspiration in feverish patients. It is also used in medicines for the menopause, and for painful or suppressed menstruation, poor digestion, nausea and vomiting. The infusion can be taken freely.

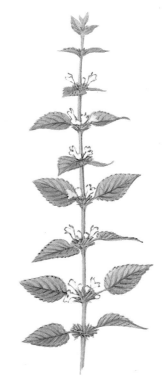

Balm MELISSA OFFICINALIS

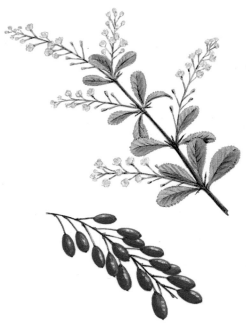

Barberry BERBERIS VULGARIS

BARBERRY

The shrub is so well known by every boy and girl that has but attained the age of seven years, that it needs no description.

It is indeed a common garden bush, but also grows wild in Europe and parts of Asia and Africa. It is a large plant with fearsome spiny stems, oval, sharp-toothed leaves and yellow flowers.

Where to find it: Scrubland, copses and hedges.

Flowering time: Late spring, early summer.

Astrology: Mars owns the shrub and presents it to the use of my countrymen to purge their bodies of choler.

Medicinal virtues: The inner rind of the Barberry tree boiled in white wine, and a quarter of a pint (142 ml) drunk every morning, is an excellent remedy to cleanse the body of choleric humours, and free it from such diseases as choler causeth, such as scabs, itch, tetters, ringworms, yellow jaundice and biles.

It is excellent for hot agues, burnings, scaldings, heat of the blood, heat of the liver, bloody flux, for the berries are as good as the bark, and more pleasing. They get a man a good stomach to his victuals. The hair washed with the lye made of ashes of the tree and water, will make it turn yellow. The fruit and rind of the shrub, the flowers of Broom and Heath, or Furze, cleanse the body of choler by sympathy, as the flowers, leaves and bark of the Peach tree do by antipathy.

Modern uses: *Berberis* has antiseptic, tonic and purgative properties. It is used in only small doses. The dosage of the herbal tincture would be no more than a few drops three or four times a day. Herbalists today prescribe it for jaundice, biliousness, diarrhoea, dyspepsia and general liver conditions.

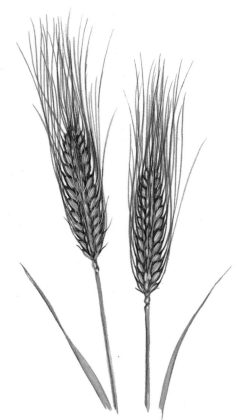

Barley HORDEUM VULGARE

HORDEUM VULGARE

BARLEY

A plaister made thereof with tar, wax and oil, helpeth the king's-evil in the throat.

Where to find it: This is the cereal that is grown all over the world, being yearly sown.

Flowering time: It does not flower, being a cereal it ripens in summer.

Astrology: It is a notable plant of Saturn. If you view diligently its effects by sympathy and antipathy, you may easily perceive a reason of them; as also why Barley-bread is so unwholesome for melancholy people.

Medicinal virtues: Barley is more cooling than Wheat and a little cleansing. All the preparations thereof, as Barley-water, do give great nourishment to persons troubled with fevers, agues and heats in the stomach.

A poultice made of Barley-meal or flour boiled in vinegar and honey, and a few dried figs put in them, dissolveth all hard imposthumes, and assuageth inflammations. Boiled with Melilot and Chamomile flowers, and some Linseed, Fenugreek and Rue in powder and applied warm, it easeth pains in the side and stomach and windiness of the spleen.

The meal of Barley and Flea-worts boiled in water and made into a poultice with honey and Oil of Lilies, and applied warm, cureth swellings under the ears, throat, neck and such like. Boiled with sharp vinegar, made into a poultice and laid on hot, helpeth the leprosy; boiled in red wine with Pomegranate rind, and Myrtles, stayeth the lax or other flux of the belly; boiled with vinegar and Quince, it easeth the pains of the gout. Barley-flour, white salt, honey and vinegar mingled together taketh away the itch speedily and certainly.

The water distilled from the green Barley, in the end of May, is very good for those that have defluxions of humours fallen into their eyes, and easeth the pain being dropped into them. White bread steeped therein, and bound on the eyes, doth the same.

Modern uses: Barley is nutritional and demulcent. It is rich in vitamins B and E and is recommended for those convalescing. It is given as Barley-water or as an extract of malt. Barley-water is soothing to the bowel where there is inflammation or diarrhoea. Hordenine, an alkaloid with properties similar to ephedrine, is produced in the root of the germinating grain, and is therefore of value in the treatment of asthma and bronchitis.

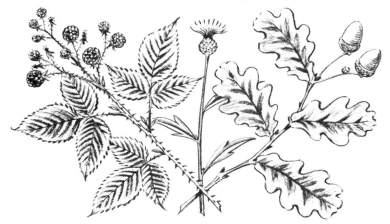

OCYMUM BASILICUM

BASIL

This is the herb which all authors are together by the ears about, and rail at one another, like lawyers. Galen and Dioscorides hold it not fitting to be taken inwardly, and Chrysippus rails at it with downright Billingsgate rhetoric: Pliny and the Arabian physicians defend it.

This is the Garden or Sweet Basil. It has one upright stalk, branching on all sides with two leaves at every joint, a little snipped about the edges. The flowers are small and whitish.

Where to find it: It grows in gardens.

Flowering time: Mid to late summer.

Astrology: A herb of Mars and under the Scorpion, and therefore called Basilicon. It is no marvel if it carry a kind of virulent quality with it.

Medicinal virtues: Applied to the place bitten by venomous beasts, or stung by a wasp or hornet, it speedily draws the poison to it. Every like draws its like. This herb and Rue will never grow together, nor near one another; and we know Rue is as great an enemy to poison as any that grows.

It expelleth both birth and afterbirth and as it helps the deficiency of Venus in one kind, so it spoils all her actions in another. I dare write no more of it.

Modern uses: Basil is a popular culinary herb. It is aromatic, and carminative. It will expel flatulence and help to ease griping pains in the abdomen. The essential oil obtained from the plant contains camphor. As a medicine Basil is taken in the form of an infusion.

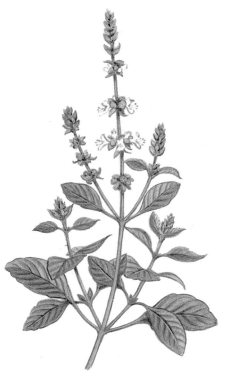

Basil OCYMUM BASILICUM

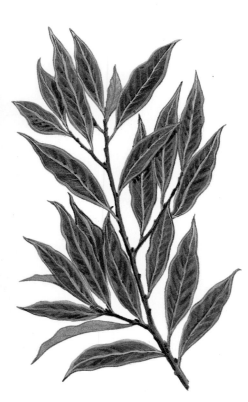

Bay Tree LAURUS NOBILIS

LAURUS NOBILIS
BAY TREE

The berries mightily expel the wind, and provoke urine, help the mother, and kill the worms. The leaves also work the like effects.

Where to find it: It grows in woodland, and prefers warm climates like the Mediterranean.

Flowering time: Mid to late spring.

Astrology: It is a tree of the Sun and under the celestial sign Leo, and resisteth witchcraft very potently, as also all the evils old Saturn can do the body of man, and they are not a few.

Medicinal virtues: Galen said that the leaves or bark do dry and heal very much, and the berries more than the leaves. The bark of the root is effectual to break the stone and to open obstructions of the liver, spleen, and other inward parts which bring the jaundice, dropsy, etc. The berries are effectual against all poisons of venomous creatures, and the sting of wasps and bees, as also against the pestilence, or other infectious diseases and therefore put into sundry treacles for that purpose.

They procure women's courses, and seven of them given to a woman in sore travail of childbirth do cause a speedy delivery, and expel the afterbirth. The berries should not therefore be taken by such as have not gone out of their time, lest they procure abortion, or cause labour too soon.

They wonderfully help all cold and rheumatic distillations from the brain to the eyes, lungs or other parts; and being made into an electuary with honey, do help the consumption, old coughs, shortness of breath, and thin rheums, as also the megrim.

A bath of the decoction of the leaves and berries is singularly good for women to sit in that are troubled with the mother, or the diseases thereof, or the stoppings of their courses, or for the diseases of the bladder, pains in the bowels by wind and stopping of urine.

A decoction of equal parts of Bay berries, Cumin seed, Hyssop, Origanum and Euphorbium, with some honey, and the head bathed therewith, doth wonderfully help distillations and rheums, and settleth the palate of the mouth into its place.

The oil made of the berries is very comfortable in all cold griefs of the joints, nerves, arteries, stomach, belly or womb; and helpeth palsies, convulsions, cramp, aches, trembling and numbness in any part, weariness also, and pains that come by sore travailing.

All griefs and pains proceeding from wind, either in the head, stomach, back, belly or womb, by anointing the parts affected therewith; and pains of the ears are also cured by dropping in some of the oil, or by receiving into the ears the fume of the decoction of the berries through a funnel.

The oil takes away the marks of the skin and flesh by bruises, falls, etc. and dissolveth the congealed blood in them. It helpeth also the itch, scabs and wheals in the skin.

Modern uses: Not widely used medicinally. Herbalists use the oil only for external application in the treatment of rheumatism.

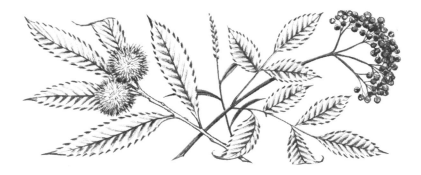

BEANS (Broad)

If a bean be parted in two, the skin being taken away, and laid on the place where the leech hath been set that bleedeth too much, it stayeth the bleeding.

Where to find it: The Broad Bean is one of the hardiest vegetables grown in British gardens.

Flowering time: Spring and summer.

Astrology: They are plants of Venus.

Medicinal virtues: The distilled water of the flowers is good to clean the face and skin from spots and wrinkles. The water distilled from the green husks is held to be effectual against the stone, and to provoke urine.

Bean flour is used in poultices to assuage inflammations rising upon wounds, and the swelling of women's breasts caused by curding of their milk, and represseth their milk.

The flour and Fenugreek mixed with honey, and applied to felons, biles, bruises, or blue marks by blows, or the imposthumes in the kernels of the ears, helpeth them all, and with Rose leaves, frankincense, and the white of an egg, being applied to the eyes, helpeth them that are swollen or do water, or have received any blows upon them, if used in wine.

Bean flour boiled to a poultice with wine and vinegar, and some oil put thereto, easeth both pains and swelling of the testicles. The husks boiled in water to the consumption of a third part thereof stayeth a lax, and the ashes of the husks, made up with hog's grease, helpeth the old pains, contusions and wounds of the sinews, the sciatica and gout.

Modern uses: Broad Beans are not used medicinally in the form of extracts, but they do play an important role in dietetics, particularly in the treatment of conditions which require a vegetarian diet. They are an important source of protein.

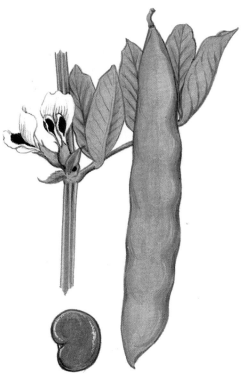

Beans VICIA FABA

BEANS (French)

Dried and beat to a powder they are great strengtheners of the kidneys.

It grows weakly, and its shoots must be sustained on poles. The blossom is of many colours: red, white, yellow, blackish or purple.

Where to find it: French Beans or Kidney Beans, are a common garden vegetable, having been cultivated since ancient times. The natural habitat, however, is central and tropical America.

Flowering time: From late spring to early autumn.

Astrology: They belong to Dame Venus.

Medicinal virtues: A dram (1.7 g) at a time of the powder taken in white wine, prevents the stone, or will cleanse the kidneys of gravel or stoppage. The ordinary French Beans move the belly, provoke urine, enlarge the breast that is straitened with shortness of breath, engender sperm, and incite to venery.

Modern uses: A homoeopathic tincture is used for rheumatism and urinary tract disorders. The pods have a diuretic action and are used as a remedy for diabetes. It is dangerous to consume beans uncooked.

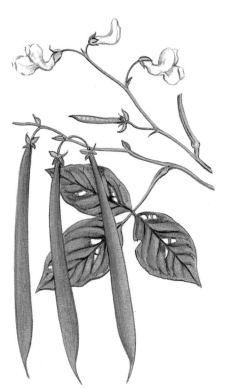

Beans (French) PHASEOLUS VULGARIS

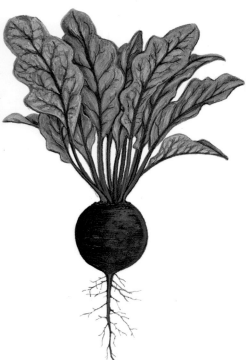

Beets BETA

BEETS

The juice of the Red Beet snuffed up the nose helps a stinking breath, if the cause lies in the nose, as many times it doth.

There are two sorts of Beet, the Common White and the Common Red. The Beets hath many great leaves next the ground. The root is strong and hard, but when it hath given seed it is no use at all.

Where to find it: Beet is extensively cultivated both for its sugar content and as a vegetable. It is derived from *Beta vulgaris* subspecies *maritima* which grows wild along the coasts of Europe.

Flowering time: It should be harvested before it flowers, being a root vegetable.

Astrology: The Red Beet is under Saturn, the White under Jupiter.

Medicinal virtues: The White Beet loosens the belly and is of a cleansing, digesting quality, and provoketh urine. The juice of it openeth obstructions both of the liver and spleen and is good for the headache and swimming therein, and turnings of the brain. It is effectual against all· venomous creatures, and applied upon the temples stayeth inflammations of the eyes. It helpeth burnings, being used without oil. With a little Alum put to it, it is good for St Anthony's fire.

It is good for all wheals, pustules, blisters and blains in the skins. The herb boiled and laid upon chilblains or kibes, helpeth them. The decoction in water and some vinegar healeth the itch if bathed therewith, and cleanseth the head of a dandruff, scurf and dry scabs, and doth much good for fretting and running sores, ulcers and cankers in the head, legs, or other parts, and is much commended against baldness and shedding the hair.

The Red Beet is good to stay the bloody flux, women's courses, and the whites, and to help the yellow jaundice. The juice of the root put into the nostrils purgeth the head, helpeth the noise in the ears, and the toothache.

Modern uses: Beetroot juice is used in combination with other vegetable and fruit juices. For example, the combination of Carrot and Beet juice with Coconut milk gives a potent cleanser of the kidneys and gall bladder. Beet juice is not used on its own.

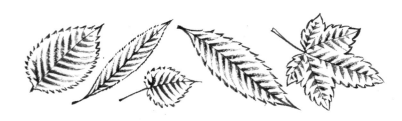

BETONY (Water)

The distilled water of the leaves is used to bathe the face and hands spotted or blemished or discoloured by sun burning.

The Water Betony is also known as Water Figwort with the botanical name of *Scrophularia auriculata*. It is not related to the Wood Betony, although it resembles it. It is also called Brown-wort and, in Yorkshire, Bishop's-leaves. It rises up with square, hard stalks set with dark green leaves. The flowers are many, set at the tops of stalks and branches, and are reddish-purple.

Where to find it: By the sides of ditches, brooks and other water courses.

Flowering time: It flowers in midsummer and the seed is ripe towards the end of the summer.

Astrology: It is a herb of Jupiter in Cancer.

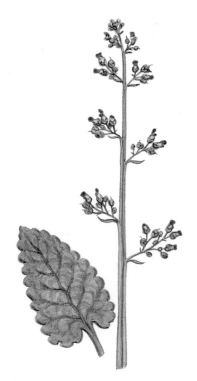

Betony (Water) BETONICA AQUATICA

Medicinal virtues: It is appropriated more to wounds and hurts in breasts than Wood Betony. The leaves bruised and applied are effectual for old and filthy ulcers, especially if the juice of the leaves be boiled with a little honey and dipped therein and sores dressed therewith; also for bruises or hurts, whether inward or outward.

Modern uses: The leaves are used externally in the form of a poultice for haemorrhoids, ulcers and wounds.

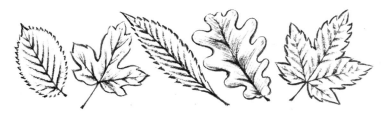

STACHYS OFFICINALIS (= BETONICA OFFICINALIS)

BETONY (Wood)

It is a very precious herb, that is certain, and most fitting to be kept in a man's house, both in syrup, conserve, oil, ointment and plaister. The flowers are usually conserved.

The plant has many leaves rising from the root, which are broad and round at the end and dented at the edges. The stalks are small, square, slender, upright and hairy. It produces several spiked heads of flowers like Lavender but spotted with white spots. The whole plant is somewhat small.

Where to find it: It grows in woods, preferring shady places.

Flowering time: Midsummer.

Astrology: It is appropriated to the planet Jupiter, and the sign of Aries.

Medicinal virtues: According to Antonius Musa, physician to the Roman Emperor Augustus Caesar, Betony preserveth the liver and body of a man from epidemical diseases, and also from witchcraft. It was not the practice of Caesar to keep fools about him.

It helpeth those that cannot digest their meat, those that have weak stomachs, or sour belchings. It helpeth the jaundice, falling-sickness, the palsy, convulsions, shrinking of the sinews, the gout, those that are inclined to dropsy, and those that have continual pains in their heads.

The powder mixed with honey is for all sorts of coughs or colds, wheezing, or shortness of breath, and distillations of thin rheums which causeth consumptions.

The decoction made with mead and a little Pennyroyal is good for those troubled with putrid agues, and to draw down and evacuate the blood and humours, that by falling into the eyes, do hinder the sight. The decoction made in wine killeth the worms in the belly, openeth obstructions of the spleen and liver, cureth stitches and pains in the back or sides, the torments and griping pains of the bowels and the wind colic. It helpeth also to break and expel the stone in the bladder or kidneys.

It stayeth bleeding at the mouth and nose and helpeth those that evacuate blood and those that have a rupture. The fume of the decoction while it is warm received by a funnel into the ears, easeth the pains of them and destroys worms and cures sores in them.

Modern uses: Wood Betony is still used by both herbalists and homoeopaths. The homoeopathic tincture is made from the fresh leaves and used to treat simple diarrhoea. The herb is used for its aromatic, astringent and blood purifying properties. It is available as a tincture or fluid extract from herbalists. The herb is also a sedative and anti-spasmodic and can be used to treat migraine and digestive troubles. For home use an infusion can be made from the dried herb in the ratio of 1 oz (28 g) to 1 pt (568 ml) of boiling water. The dose is 2 fl oz (56 ml) three times a day. The root should not be used.

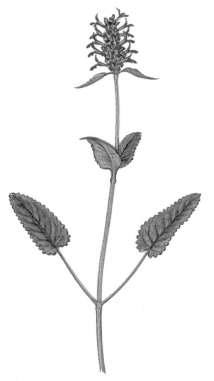

Betony (Wood) STACHYS OFFICINALIS
(= BETONICA OFFICINALIS)

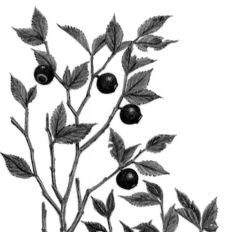

Bilberries VACCINIUM MYRTILLUS

VACCINIUM MYRTILLUS

BILBERRIES

It is a pity they are used no more in physic than they are.

Also known as Whortleberries. There are two sorts – the black and the red berries. The small bush bearing the black berries creeps along the ground and has small dark green leaves with small pinkish coloured flowers. The Whortle-bush has leaves like Box tree leaves, green and round-pointed, which stay on all winter.

Where to find it: In forests and on heathland.

Flowering time: Early to mid spring. The fruit is ripe from mid to late summer.

Astrology: They are under the dominion of Jupiter.

Medicinal virtues: Black Bilberries are good in hot agues, and to cool the heat of the liver and stomach. They bind the belly and stay the vomitings. The juice of the berries made into a syrup, or the pulp made into a conserve with sugar, is good for the aforesaid purposes and for an old cough, or an ulcer in the lungs.

The Red Whorts are more binding and stop women's courses, spitting of blood, or any other flux of blood or humours, and are used both outwardly and inwardly.

Modern uses: Bilberries, when used medicinally, act as an astringent diuretic. The dried berries administered in the form of a decoction are effective in diarrhoea and dysentery. A tincture of the leaves is hypoglycaemic and is indicated as a diabetic remedy. For home use an infusion can be made in the ratio of one teaspoonful of the leaves to a cup of boiling water. Homoeopathic tablets are also available for use by diabetics.

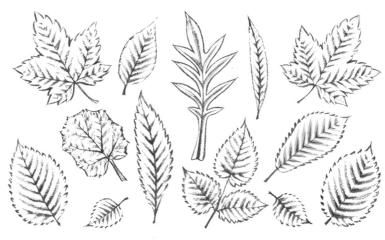

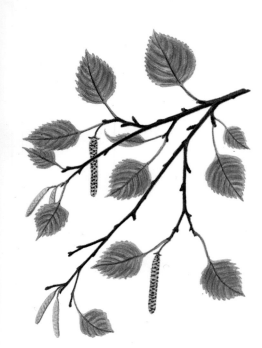

Birch Tree BETULA PENDULA (= B. ALBA)

BETULA PENDULA (=B. ALBA)

BIRCH TREE

The juice of the leaves is good to wash sore mouths.

The Silver Birch or European Birch is a largish tree with many boughs and slender branches which bend downward. The leaves are like Beech leaves but smaller and dented about the edges. It bears catkins like those of the Hazel Nut tree.

Where to find it: It grows in woods.

Flowering time: Spring.

Astrology: It is a tree of Venus.

Medicinal virtues: The juice of the leaves, or the distilled water of them, breaks the stone in the kidneys or bladder, and is good for sore mouths.

Modern uses: The bark and leaves are used in preparations for skin diseases. Distillation of the bark yields Birch tar oil, an astringent ingredient of ointments for eczema and psoriasis. Birch tea is an infusion of the leaves. It is bitter tasting but helpful in gout and rheumatic complaints.

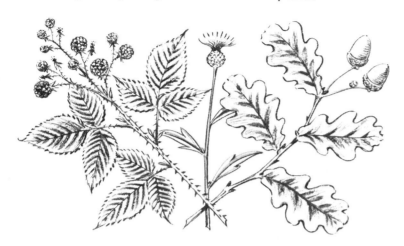

POLYGONUM BISTORTA

BISTORT

The root in powder taken in drink expelleth the venom of the plague, the smallpox, measles, purples, or any other infectious disease, driving it out by sweating.

Also known as Snakeweed, English Serpentary, Dragon-wort, Osterick and Passions, the plant has a thick short knotted root which is blackish on the outside and reddish inside, and shaped like a letter 'S'. The leaves are oval with heart-shaped bases, rather like a Dock leaf. The flowers are a pale flesh colour.

Where to find it: Shadowy moist woods, at the foot of hills and nourished in gardens.

Flowering time: Late spring. The seed is ripe in midsummer.

Astrology: It is a plant of Saturn . . . cold and dry.

Medicinal virtues: Both leaves and roots have a powerful faculty to resist all poisons. A decoction of the powdered root, prepared in wine, stayeth inward bleeding or spitting of blood, fluxes in the body of man or woman, or vomiting. It is also used against ruptures, burstings, bruises or falls, dissolving congealed blood and easing the pains. It also helpeth the jaundice.

The water distilled from leaves and roots is a remedy to wash any place bitten or stung by any venomous creature and for running sores and ulcers. The decoction of the root hinders abortion and miscarriage. The leaves will kill the worms in children. With the juice of the Plantain added to it and applied outwardly, it helpeth the gonorrhoea, or running of the reins.

Modern uses: It is mainly the root that is now used. Rich in tannin, it is one of the strongest astringents available to herbalists. The chief indications are diarrhoea, haemorrhages and mucous discharges when it is prescribed in the form of a medicine, a gargle or an injection. A decoction of the root can be used as an enema, usually in the ratio of 1 oz (28 g) of root to 2 pt (1.1 l) of boiling water. Strain and allow to cool before use. The same preparation can be used as a vaginal injection in leucorrhoea.

Mixing in equal parts with other astringents, such as Cranesbill, and demulcents such as Marsh Mallow, makes it suitable for treating haemorrhoids. A teaspoonful of tincture of Bistort and one of Bloodroot added to half a glass of boiling water is used as a gargle or spray for sore throat and tonsillitis.

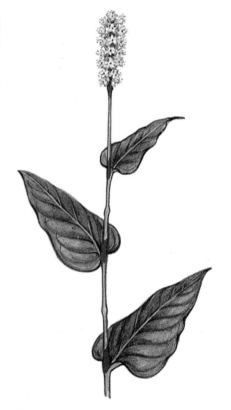

Bistort POLYGONUM BISTORTA

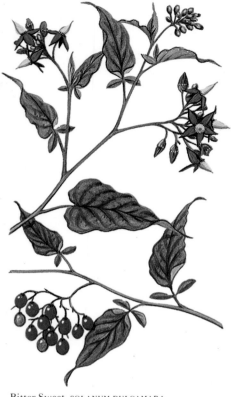

Bitter Sweet SOLANUM DULCAMARA

SOLANUM DULCAMARA
BITTER SWEET
It is good to remove witchcraft both in men and beast, and all sudden diseases whatsoever.

A climbing plant, it grows to a man's height, or even higher. Also known as Mortal, Woody Nightshade, Felon-wort and *Amara Dulcis*, it bears many longish and pointed leaves which fall off at the approach of winter. It produces berries which are toxic.

Where to find it: Moist and shady places. It twines itself around hedgerow plants.

Flowering time: Midsummer. The berries ripen towards the end of the summer.

Astrology: It is under the planet of Mercury.

Medicinal virtues: Being tied about the neck it is a remedy for vertigo or dizziness of the head. The Germans hang it about the necks of their cattle when they fear any evil hath betided them. Country people bruised the berries and applied them to felons, thereby ridding their fingers of such troublesome guests.

Modern uses: This is a narcotic, diuretic, expectorant and depurative. The plant contains toxic alkaloids and in overdosage it will paralyse the central nervous system. It is, therefore, not recommended for domestic use and it is not widely used professionally. The herb was an official medicine until 1907, the twigs and root-bark being the parts used. The action of the medicine is to increase skin and kidney function. It has, therefore, been used for obstinate skin diseases and rheumatism. A decoction is made from the fluid extract. Ten teaspoonfuls of extract are added to 2 pt (1.1 l) of water which is boiled down to 1 pt (568 ml). The dosage is ½–2 fl oz (14–56 ml) in milk two to three times a day. Homoeopathic physicians prepare their own medicine from the leaves, flowers and berries of other species of *Solanum*.

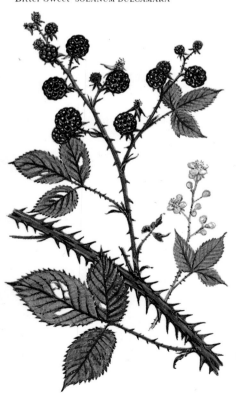

Blackberry RUBUS FRUCTICOSUS

RUBUS FRUCTICOSUS
BLACKBERRY
The berries are a powerful remedy against the poison of the most venomous serpents.

Blackberries are so well known that they need no description.

Where to find it: The Blackberry or Bramble when not being trained to grow up walls and fences in gardens will be found in hedgerows.

Flowering time: The blossoms and the fruits may be seen together in the late summer.

Astrology: It is a plant of Venus in Aries. If any ask why Venus is so prickly, tell them 'tis because she is in the house of Mars.

Medicinal virtues: The buds, leaves and branches, while green, are of good use in ulcers and putrid sores of the mouth and throat and for quinsy, and likewise to heal other fresh wounds and sores. The unripe flowers and fruits are very binding and so profitable for the bloody flux, laxes and for spitting of blood.

The decoction or powder of the root is good to break or drive forth gravel and the stone in the reins and kidneys. The leaves and brambles can be used as a lotion for sores in the mouth or secret parts.

The juice of the berries mixed with the juice of Mulberries bind more effectually and help all fretting and eating sores and ulcers. The distilled water of the branches, leaves and flowers, or of the fruit, is pleasant and effectual in fevers and hot distempers.

Modern uses: The root and leaves are astringent and toning. The root is more potent. An infusion of 1 oz (28 g) of leaves or root to 1 pt (568 ml) of boiling water is taken in doses of 2 fl oz (56 ml) for simple diarrhoea. The American Blackberry (*Rubus villosus*) has similar properties.

BLUE-BOTTLE

It is a remedy against the poison of the scorpion.

We know it now as the Cornflower, a most attractive wild plant, but it was called Cyanus because of its blue colour and also Hurtsickle because its tough stems blunted the edges of the farmer's sickle as he reaped the corn. Another name is Blue-blow. Its leaves spread upon the ground, being of whitish-green colour. The flowers are an innumerable company set in a scaly head.

Where to find it: In cornfields.

Flowering time: From late spring until the corn is harvested.

Astrology: Under the dominion of Saturn . . . cold, dry and binding.

Medicinal virtues: The powder or dried leaves is given with good success to those that are bruised by a fall, or have broken a vein inwardly, and void much blood at the mouth. Taken in the water of Plantain, Horsetail or the Greater Comfrey, it is a remedy against the poison of the scorpion and resisteth all venoms and poison.

The seed or leaves taken in wine is good against the plague and all infectious diseases and in pestilential fevers. The juice put into wounds doth quickly solder up the lips of them together and heals ulcers and sores in the mouth. The juice dropped into the eyes takes away heat and inflammation.

Modern uses: The flowers are occasionally used for their tonic and stimulant properties, but the Blessed Thistle (*Carbenia benedicta*) which has similar properties is now more popular with today's herbalists. The Cornflower gives an infusion a bluish colour. Its main uses are in the treatment of dyspepsia and as an eye lotion.

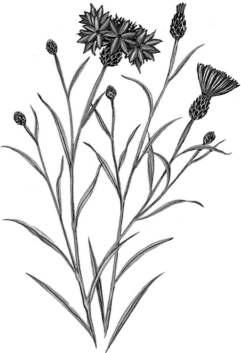

Blue-bottle CENTUAREA CYANUS

BORAGE

The leaves, flowers and seeds are good to expel pensiveness and melancholy.

A hardy annual with prickly hairs, oval leaves and blue flowers. The stems grow to about 18 inches (46 cm) high.

Where to find it: It is grown in gardens to attract bees and may be found wild on rubbish dumps and near houses.

Flowering time: Early to midsummer.

Astrology: Jupiter and Leo, great strengtheners of nature.

Medicinal virtues: The leaves and roots are used to good purpose in putrid and pestilential fevers to defend the heart and to resist and to expel the poison or venom of other creatures. The seed and leaves are good to increase the milk in women's breasts.

The juice made into a syrup is put with other cooling, opening and cleansing herbs to open obstructions and help the yellow jaundice. Mixed with Fumitory it helpeth the itch, ringworms and tetters, or other spreading scabs and sores. The distilled water helpeth the redness and inflammations of the eyes. The dried herb is never used, always the green.

Modern uses: It is now classified as a diuretic with demulcent and emollient properties. French herbalists use it for colds, fevers and lung complaints such as bronchitis and pneumonia. An infusion of the leaves – 1 oz (28 g) to 1 pt (568 ml) of boiling water – is taken in doses of 2 fl oz (56 ml). A poultice is made from the leaves to reduce inflammatory swellings. The diuretic property of the infusion makes Borage useful in rheumatism.

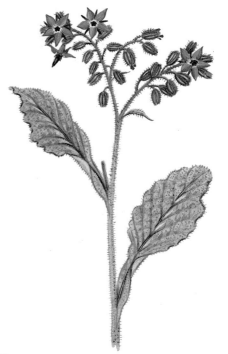

Borage BORAGO OFFICINALIS

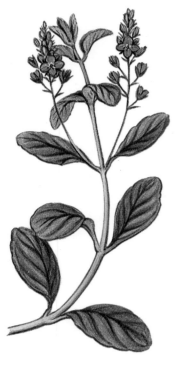

BROOK-LIME

Brook-lime and Watercresses are generally used together in diet drinks with other things serving to purge the blood and body from all ill humours that would destroy health, and are helpful to the scurvy.

Otherwise known as Water Pimpernel, it is an aquatic plant that sends forth a creeping root with strings at every joint. It produces small blue flowers.

Where to find it: It grows in shallow streams and at the edges of ponds and usually near Watercresses.

Flowering time: Early to midsummer.

Astrology: A hot and biting martial plant.

Medicinal virtues: It provokes the urine and helps to break the stone and pass it away. It procures women's courses and expels the dead child. Fried with butter and vinegar and applied warm, it helpeth all manner of tumours, swellings and inflammations.

Modern uses: It is used as a blood purifier. An infusion is made from the leaves and given in doses of 2 fl oz (56 ml) three to four times a day.

Brook-lime VERONICA BECCABUNGA

BRYONIA DIOICA

BRYONY

The root of Bryony purges the belly with great violence, troubling the stomach and burning the liver and therefore not rashly to be taken.

There are several Bryonies and all are poisonous. The Common White Bryony (*Bryonia dioica*) is a rampant twining and climbing plant sending forth long tender branches with rough vine-like leaves and white flowers followed by berries (green, then red) in clusters.

Where to find it: On banks or under hedges. The roots go very deep.

Flowering time: Mid to late summer.

Astrology: They are furious martial plants.

Medicinal virtues: Used correctly it is profitable for diseases of the head, such as falling-sickness, giddiness and swimmings, by drawing away much phlegm and rheumatic humours. Good for palsies, convulsions, cramps and stitches in the side and the dropsy. It provokes the urine and cleanses the reins and kidneys from gravel and stone by opening obstructions of the spleen.

The decoction of the root in wine drunk once a week on going to bed cleanseth the mother and expelleth the dead child. A dram (1.7 g) of the root in powder taken in white wine bringeth down the courses. An electuary made of the roots and honey doth mightily cleanse the chest of rotten phlegm and wonderfully helps any old strong cough, to those that are troubled with shortness of breath.

The root cleanseth the skin from all black and blue spots, freckles, morphew, leprosy, foul scars or other deformity.

The root bruised and applied to any place where bones are broken helpeth to draw them forth, also splinters and thorns in the flesh. Where Bryony must be taken inwardly it purges very violently and needs an abler hand to correct it than most country people have. Therefore it is better for them to leave the simple alone and instead take the compound water of it.

Modern uses: Tincture of *Bryonia dioica* is used by some professional herbalists. It is not recommended for self-medication purposes. In small doses of a few drops it is considered useful in chest complaints, rheumatism and gout. It has similar applications in homoeopathic medicine, being employed in bronchitis, sciatica and arthritis.

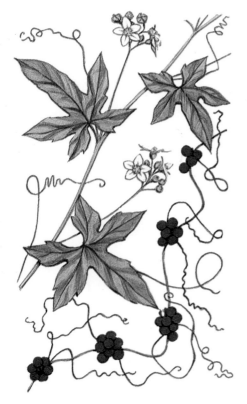

Bryony BRYONIA DIOICA

BUCKTHORN

The herb bruised and applied to warts will make them consume and waste away in a short time.

The botanical name *catharticus* gives an indication of its laxative or purging properties. Buckthorn is also known as Hart's-horn or the Purging Buckthorn. It grows to about six feet (1.8 m) high with straggling branches trailing here and there on the ground. The leaves are small and jagged and the whitish flowers grow in small clusters. The berries are black.

Where to find it: On dry, barren and sandy soils.

Flowering time: Late spring, early summer.

Astrology: Under the dominion of Saturn.

Medicinal virtues: The leaves bruised and applied to a wound will stop the bleeding. The bruised herb is applied to warts to consume them.

Modern uses: The juice of the berries is used to make Buckthorn syrup, a powerful laxative. This medicine was official until 1867 but has fallen into disuse because its action is so severe. It is still used as a laxative for animals. Purging is not a method employed by modern medical herbalists. It can still be used as an ointment to treat warts. The ointment also relieves pruritus.

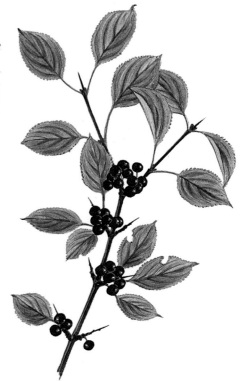

Buckthorn RHAMNUS CATHARTICUS

BUGLE

If the virtues of it make you fall in love with it (as they will if you be wise), keep a syrup of it to take inwardly and an ointment and plaister of it to use outwardly, always by you.

It is also called Middle Confound and Middle Comfrey, Brown Bugle and by some Sickle-wort and Herb-carpenter. The stalk is square and the leaves green or brownish and somewhat hairy. The plant, a perennial, grows about 18 inches (46 cm) high and bears bluish or ash-coloured flowers.

Where to find it: Woods, copses and in fields in damp shady areas.

Flowering time: From late spring until midsummer.

Astrology: This herb belongeth to Dame Venus.

Medicinal virtues: The decoction of the leaves and flowers made in wine and taken will dissolve congealed blood in those that are bruised inwardly by a fall. It is very effectual for any inward wounds, thrusts or stabs in the body or bowels, and wonderful for curing ulcers and sores, whether new and fresh, or old and inveterate. Gangrenes and fistulas are also cured if the leaves are bruised and applied, or the juice be used to wash and bathe the place. Made into a lotion with honey and Alum, it cureth all sores in the mouth and gums, and is no less powerful and effectual for ulcers and sores in the secret parts of men and women.

Many times those that give themselves much to drinking are troubled with strange fancies, strange sights in the night or voices. These I have known cured by taking only two spoonfuls of the syrup of this herb two hours after supper on going to bed.

Modern uses: The whole herb is collected from late spring and dried. It has aromatic and astringent properties, and can be used for arresting internal haemorrhages. It is also regarded as mildly narcotic. An infusion made from 1 oz (28 g) of the dried herb to 1 pt (568 ml) of boiling water may be taken in doses of 2 fl oz (56 ml) at a time quite frequently.

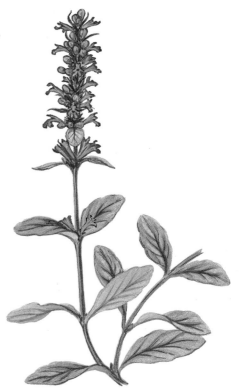

Bugle AJUGA REPTENS

BURDOCK (Greater)

By its leaf or seed you may draw the womb which way you please, either upward by applying it to the crown of the head in case it falls out; or downwards in fits of the mother, by applying it to the soles of the feet: or if you would stay it in its place, apply it to the navel, and that is one good way to stay the child in it.

A biennial, it grows to more than three feet (91 cm). It is well known to little boys who pull off the clinging seed vessels to throw at one another. It is also called Personata, Happy-major and Clot-bur.

Where to find it: It grows by ditches and watersides and by the highways almost every where.

Flowering time: Early to midsummer.

Astrology: Venus challengeth this herb for her own.

Medicinal virtues: The leaves are cooling and moderately drying and can be applied to old ulcers and sores, and also to places troubled with the shrinking in of the sinews or arteries.

The root beaten with a little salt and laid on the place bitten by a snake, will suddenly easeth the pain. The juice of the leaves drunk with honey promotes the flow of urine and eases pain in the bladder. The seed macerated in wine for 40 days provides a wonderfully helpful medicine for sciatica.

Modern uses: Burdock is one of the finest blood purifiers in the herbal system of medicine. It is classified as an alterative, diuretic and diaphoretic. These properties make it of value in the treatment of boils, acne and eczema. It helps the kidneys to filter out impurities from the blood very quickly. The root is mainly used and administered as a decoction in doses of 2 fl oz (56 ml) three or four times a day. The seeds, used alone as a decoction, have similar properties, but are particularly tonic to the kidneys.

Burdock (Greater) ARCTIUM LAPPA

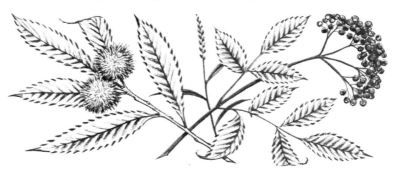

BURNET

A most precious herb, the continual use of it preserves the body in health and the spirit in vigour.

A perennial plant, it is also called Meadow Pimpernel, Sanguisorbia and Solbegrella, and today Salad Burnet. A short, almost hairless plant; the upper flowers bear red styles, and those below have yellow stamens.

Where to find it: Dry pastures and well-drained calcareous soils.

Flowering time: Midsummer to early autumn.

Astrology: A herb the Sun challengeth dominion over. If the Sun be the preserver of life under God, his herbs are the best in the world to do it.

Medicinal virtues: It is a friend to the heart, liver and other principal parts of a man's body. Two or three of the stalks with leaves put into a cup of wine, especially claret, are known to quicken the spirits, refresh and clear the heart and drive away melancholy. It is a special help to defend the heart from noisome vapours and from infection of the pestilence, the juice being taken in some drink.

Burnet SANQUISORBA MINOR

It also has a drying and astringent quality and will staunch inward or outward bleedings, laxes, the bloody flux, and too abundant women's courses, the whites, choleric belchings and castings of the stomach.

It is also a singular herb for all sorts of wounds both of the head and body, running cankers and most sores, using either the juice or decoction of the herb or the powder of the herb or root, or the water of the distilled herb, or the ointment by itself.

Modern uses: The root and herb are used as a diuretic, a stomach tonic and a carminative. An infusion of the whole herb is astringent. A tincture, made from the root, is used to treat infections and inflammation of the throat and upper respiratory tract. The plant is collected for use in May and September. A teaspoonful of the dried powdered herb or root is infused in a cup of boiling water, allowed to cool, strained and swallowed down. One or two cups a day may be taken.

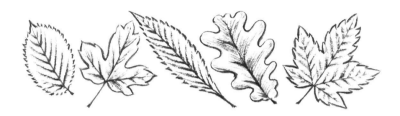

RUSCUS ACULEATUS

BUTCHER'S BROOM

It works no ill effects, yet I hope you have wit enough to give the strongest decoction to the strongest bodies.

Its other names are Ruscus, Bruscus, Kneeholm, Kneehulver and Pettigree. It is also known as Knee-holly because it has prickly leaves and grows to about the height of a man's knee. The first shoots to sprout from the roots resemble Asparagus, but then they spread and form many branches. The shrub produces a small whitish-green flower and a small, round, green berry which turns red when ripe.

Where to find it: It grows in copses, on heathland and waste land and often under or near holly bushes.

Flowering time: Early spring. The berries are ripe in early autumn.

Astrology: It is a plant of Mars, being of a gallant cleansing and opening quality.

Medicinal virtues: The decoction of the root made with wine removes obstructions, provoketh urine, expels gravel and stone, relieves the strangury and helpeth women's courses. It is also useful for the yellow jaundice and headache. With honey or sugar added, it cleanseth the breast of phlegm and the chest of clammy humours gathered therein.

A poultice made of the berries and leaves is effectual in knitting and consolidating broken bones or parts out of joint.

A common way of using it is to boil the root with Parsley, Fennel and Smallage in white wine and drink the decoction, adding a similar quantity of Grass root. The more of the root that is used, the stronger will the decoction be.

Modern uses: A decoction of the dried root is still recommended in the treatment of jaundice, urinary stones and suppression of menstruation – 1 oz (28 g) of the root to 1½ pt (852 ml) of water is used. The water is boiled down to 1 pt (568 ml) and strained. The dose is two teaspoonfuls three times a day. A tea can be made from ½ oz (14 g) of the fresh root or 1 oz (28 g) of the twigs to 1 pt (568 ml) of boiling water. Dose 2 fl oz (56 ml). This acts as a diuretic and diaphoretic.

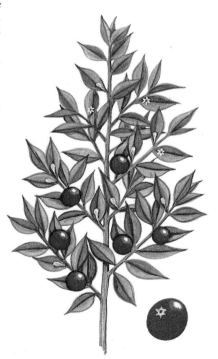

Butcher's Broom RUSCUS ACULEATUS

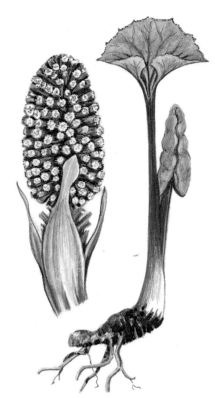

Butter-bur PETASITES HYBRIDUS
(= TUSSILAGO HYBRIDA)

BUTTER-BUR

It were well if gentlewomen would keep this root preserved to help their poor neighbours. It is fit the rich should help the poor, for the poor cannot help themselves.

A perennial plant, Butter-bur has a long root that spreads underground, blackish on the outside, whitish within. The hollow stalk rises to about a foot (30 cm) high bearing flowers of blush or deep red, according to the soil. The leaves appear on the plant after flowering.

Where to find it: By rivers and watersides and muddy soils.

Flowering time: Late winter, early spring. The leaves do not appear until mid spring.

Astrology: It is under the dominion of the Sun and, therefore, a great strengthener of the heart and cheerer of the vital spirits.

Medicinal virtues: The roots are used against the plague and pestilential fevers by provoking sweat. The powder taken in wine resisteth the force of any other poison. The decoction of the root in wine is singularly good for those that wheeze much, or are short-winded. It provoketh the urine and women's courses and killeth flat and broad worms in the belly. The powdered root dries up the moisture of sores and taketh away spots and blemishes of the skin.

Modern uses: The root is used as a heart tonic. It stimulates heart function and is diuretic. It is also used to treat asthmatics, calculi of the urinary tract and colds and fevers. It is prepared in the form of a decoction, 1 oz (28 g) of the root being boiled in 1½ pt (852 ml) of water down to 1 pt (568 ml), allowed to cool, strained and taken in doses of 2 fl oz (56 ml) three or four times a day. Homoeopaths use a tincture of the root for headaches, neuralgia and inflammation of the urethra.

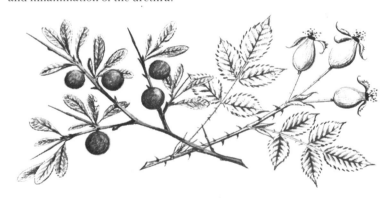

CALAMINT

Let not women be too busy with it, for it works very violently upon the feminine part.

A small herb, it seldom rises above a foot (30 cm) high with square, hairy and woody stalks. The pale blueish flowers are like those of mints and the plant has a minty aroma.

Where to find it: It grows on heaths and uplands and on dry ground.

Flowering time: Midsummer.

Astrology: A herb of Mercury and a strong one, too, therefore excellent in all afflictions of the brain.

Medicinal virtues: The decoction of the herb bringeth down women's courses and provoketh urine. It is profitable for those that have ruptures or troubled with convulsions or cramps, with shortness of breath, or choleric torments and pains in their bellies or stomach. It helpeth those with yellow jaundice and, taken in wine, it stayeth vomiting. It helpeth such as have the leprosy and it hindereth conception in women.

Applied to the buckle-bone, it will by continuance of time spend the humours that causeth the pain of sciatica. The juice dropped into the ears killeth worms in them. The leaves boiled in wine and drank provoke sweat and open obstructions of the liver and spleen. The decoction with some sugar is profitable for those troubled with the overflowing of the gall and that have an old cough or are scarce able to breathe.

Modern uses: The herb is now regarded as an expectorant and is administered as a syrup or decoction. A syrup is made by adding honey or sugar to an infusion or decoction and heating until it thickens, or by adding a fluid extract to syrup made beforehand. A tea made from the dried leaves is helpful in flatulent colic. In this respect it is similar to taking a Mint tea, as the plant contains a camphor-like essential oil.

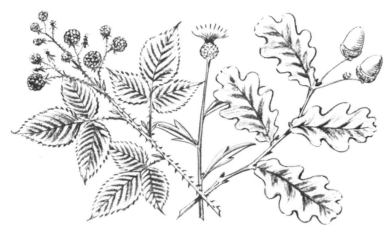

CARUM CARVI

CARAWAY

Caraway confects, once only dipped in sugar, and a spoonful of them eaten in the morning fasting, and as many after each meal, is a most admirable remedy for those that are troubled with wind.

It bears stalks with finely divided leaves, and at the top, tufts of white flowers.

Where to find it: It is a cultivated herb, both in gardens and commercially.

Flowering time: From early to midsummer.

Astrology: This is a mercurial plant.

Medicinal virtues: The seed hath a moderate sharp quality whereby it breaketh the wind and provoketh urine, which also the herb doth. The root makes a better food than Parsnips. It is pleasant and comfortable to the stomach and helpeth digestion.

The seed is conducing to all cold griefs of the head, stomach and bowels, as also the wind in them, and helpeth to sharpen the eyesight. The powdered seed made into a poultice taketh away the black and blue spots of blows and bruises.

The herb itself, or with some of the seed bruised and fried, applied as a hot compress to the lower parts of the belly, easeth colicky pains.

The roots eaten like Parsnips strengthen the stomachs of old people.

Modern uses: Caraway, like Anise, Dill and Fennel, is ideal as a children's medicine when there is flatulence or stomach upset. It also flavours other medicines. The powdered seeds are mostly used and in doses up to half a teaspoonful at a time. The essential oil pressed from the seeds is also used for flatulent dyspepsia, the dose being from one to four drops on sugar. A dose of the powdered seeds can be taken in hot milk when a cold threatens. It forms an ingredient of compound tincture of Cardamom Aromatica, an official medicine.

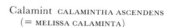
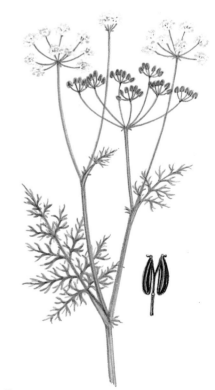

Calamint CALAMINTHA ASCENDENS
(= MELISSA CALAMINTA)

Caraway CARUM CARVI

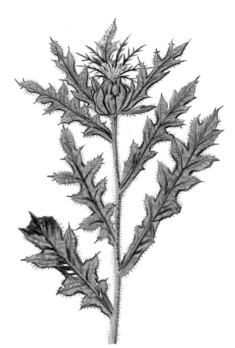

Carduus Benedictus CNICUS BENEDICTUS
(= CARBENIA BENEDICTA)

CNICUS BENEDICTUS (= CARBENIA BENEDICTA)

CARDUUS BENEDICTUS

Every one who can write at all may describe them from his own knowledge.

Better known today as Blessed Thistle or Holy Thistle, it is an annual plant growing to a little over a foot (30 cm) with greyish-green leaves, brittle and spiny. The yellow flowerheads are about an inch (25 mm) long.

Where to find it: It grows in coastal regions, but is also cultivated for pharmaceutical purposes.

Flowering time: From early to late summer.

Astrology: A herb of Mars under the sign of Aries.

Medicinal virtues: It helps giddiness and swimming of the head, or the disease called vertigo. It is an excellent remedy against the yellow jaundice and other infirmities of the gall. It clarifies the blood.

Continually drinking the decoction helps red faces, tetters and ring-worms. It helps the plague, sores, boils and itch, the bitings of mad dogs and venomous beasts.

It cureth the French pox, strengthens the memory and cures deafness. It cures melancholy and provokes urine.

Modern uses: Holy Thistle is still an important medicinal herb. It is mainly used as a tonic, but it also produces sweating and is therefore of use in treating fevers. It stimulates menstruation and is helpful for headaches and migraine. Small doses only are given as the herb is emetic. Overdosing can also cause diarrhoea. An infusion is made from the whole herb – 1 oz (28 g) to 1 pt (568 ml) of boiling water – and administered in doses of 2 fl oz (56 ml). Where there is inflammation, the remedy is used in combination with Elderflowers, and Peppermint with a small amount of Ginger or Capsicum. The cold infusion is best for dyspepsia or anorexia, while the warm infusion is best for colds, fevers and backache. Homoeopaths use a tincture to treat arthritis.

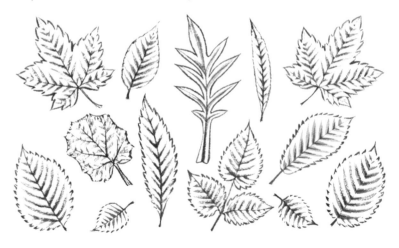

DAUCUS CAROTA

CARROT (Wild)

Galen commended garden Carrots highly to break the wind, yet experience teacheth they breed it first, and we may thank nature for expelling it. The seeds expel wind indeed and so mend what the root marreth.

The Wild Carrot grows altogether like the tame, but the leaves and stalks are somewhat whiter and rougher. The stalks bear large tufts of white flowers with a deep purple flower in the middle of each. The root is small, hard and long and unfit to eat.

Where to find it: By the sides of fields and untilled places and on roadside verges.

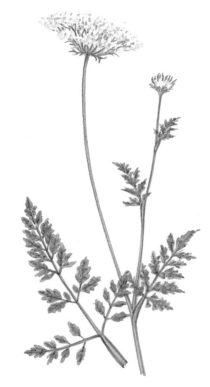

Carrot (Wild) DAUCUS CAROTA

Flowering time: Summer.

Astrology: Wild Carrots belong to Mercury.

Medicinal virtues: They break wind and remove stitches in the side, provoke urine and women's courses and helpeth to break and expel the stone.

The seed is good for the dropsy and for those whose bellies are swollen with wind. It helps the colic, the stone in the kidneys and rising of the mother. Taken in wine, or boiled in wine and taken, the seeds help conception. Applied with honey, the leaves cleanse running sores or ulcers.

Modern uses: Carrots are an important item in the diet of cancer patients. Carrot juice also should be taken. The Wild Carrot is rich in vitamins and carotene, from which the body manufactures vitamin A. The infusion of the herb is used as a treatment for fluid retention. The powdered seeds made into a tea – one teaspoonful to a cup – are taken to relieve colic. The dried flowers are also used as a tea as a remedy for dropsy.

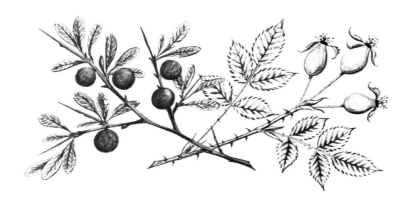

NEPETA CATARIA

CATMINT

It is generally used to procure women's courses.

A perennial growing to about three feet (91 cm), with broad, soft, white, hairy leaves with a dented border. The flowers are produced in long tufts and are purplish-white.

Where to find it: Hedgerows, roadsides, edges of fields, waste ground and in gardens.

Flowering time: Midsummer.

Astrology: A herb of Venus.

Medicinal virtues: To procure women's courses, it is taken outwardly or inwardly, either alone, or with other convenient herbs in a decoction. The women bathe with the decoction or sit over the hot fumes of it. Its frequent use takes away barrenness and the wind and pains of the mother. Use it for pains in the head, catarrhs, rheums and swimming and giddiness, and for wind in the stomach and belly.

It is effectual for cramp or cold aches and for colds, coughs and shortness of breath. The juice drunk in wind is profitable for bruises. The fresh herb, bruised and applied, eases the piles. An ointment for piles is made from the juice.

To take away scabs, wash the head or other parts with the decoction.

Modern uses: The infusion of Catmint – Catnep tea – is used in fevers to promote perspiration, thus reducing temperature. It is a good remedy for children where there is nervousness, pain or flatulence. The tea is given in doses of two to three teaspoonfuls. It can also be injected into the bowel to relieve colic. It is helpful where there is restlessness, and insomnia.

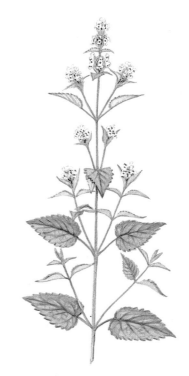

Catmint NEPETA CATARIA

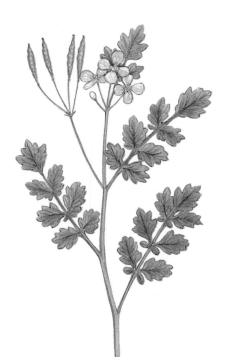

Celandine (The Greater)
CHELIDONIUM MAJUS

CELANDINE (The Greater)

One of the best cures for the eyes. When the Sun is in Leo and the Moon in Aries make it into an oil or ointment to anoint the eyes with. The most desperate sore eyes have been cured by this only medicine; is not this far better than endangering the eyes by the art of the needle?

A perennial with many tender, round, whitish-green stalks and greater joints than usual as if they were knees. The stalks are brittle and easy to break. The leaves are large, tender and broad, dark blueish-green on top and pale blueish-green underneath, and full of yellow sap.

Where to find it: By old walls, hedges and waysides and in untilled places. Once planted in a garden, especially in a shady place, it will remain there.

Flowering time: All summer long.

Astrology: A herb of the Sun and under the celestial lion.

Medicinal virtues: The herb or root boiled in white wine with a few Aniseeds and drunk will open obstructions of the liver and gall. It helpeth the yellow jaundice, the dropsy and the itch and old sores in the legs and other parts.

The juice taken fasting is held to be of singular good use against the pestilence. The distilled water with a little sugar and treacle hath the same effect.

Dropped into the eyes the juice cleanseth them from films and cloudiness that darken the sight, but it is best to allay the sharpness of the juice with a little breast-milk.

It causes old, filthy, corroding, creeping ulcers to heal more speedily and the juice applied to tetters, ringworms or other spreading cankers will quickly heal them too. Rubbed often on warts, it will take them away.

The herb with the root bruised and bathed in Oil of Chamomile applied to the navel taketh away griping pains in the belly and bowels and all the pains of the mother. Applied to women's breasts, it stayeth the overmuch flowing of the courses.

Modern uses: The herb is used as a cholagogue and hepatic tonic. It purifies the blood, increases urine production, but in overdosage it will purge. The fresh juice is still considered to be an effective application for corns and warts. It is used as an eye lotion to remove film on the eyes. Chewing the root relieves toothache. In treating the liver a few drops of the juice are taken in sweetened water. The infusion produces sweating. It is available in tincture or fluid extract form from herbalists.

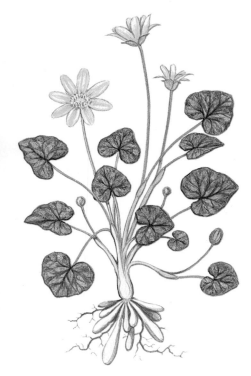

Celandine (The Lesser)
RANUNCULUS FICARIA

CELANDINE (The Lesser)

The virtue of an herb may be known by its signature, as plainly appears in this. For if you dig up the root of it, you shall perceive the perfect image of the disease which they commonly call the piles.

The Lesser Celandine, also known as Pilewort, neither resembles Celandine in nature or in form. It spreads many round pale green leaves on weak and trailing branches, which lie on the ground and are flat, smooth and somewhat shining. The yellow flowers are like Buttercups, but about one inch (25 mm) across.

Where to find it: Moist corners of fields and near watersides, but also in drier ground if it be shady.

Flowering time: It flowers in early spring and is quite gone by late spring, so it cannot be found until the next year.

Astrology: It is under the dominion of Mars.

Medicinal virtues: The decoction of the leaves and root doth wonderfully help piles and haemorrhoids, also kernels by the ears and throat, called the king's-evil, or any other hard wens or tumours. Pilewort made into an oil, ointment or plaister cures piles or haemorrhoids and the king's-evil. I cured my own daughter of the king's-evil, broke the sore, drew out a quarter of a pint of corruption and she was cured without any scar at all in one week's time.

Modern uses: Another herb that is still extensively used. Its astringent properties make it a valuable remedy for haemorrhoids. It can be taken internally as an infusion in doses of 2 fl oz (56 ml), or an ointment can be obtained and applied to the piles.

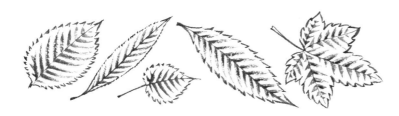

CENTAURIUM ERYTHRAEA (= ERYTHRAEA CENTAURIUM)

CENTAURY

The herb is so safe you cannot fail in the using of it. It is very wholesome, but not very toothsome.

It grows about a foot (30 cm) high, branching at the top into many sprigs. The flowers are of a red colour, consisting of five or six small leaves rather like those of St John's Wort. The whole plant has a bitter taste.

Where to find it: In fields, pastures and woods.

Flowering time: Midsummer.

Astrology: They are under the dominion of the Sun. The flowers open and shut as the Sun either sheweth or hideth his face.

Medicinal virtues: The herb boiled and drunk helpeth the sciatica. It openeth obstructions of the liver, gall and spleen. It helpeth jaundice and easeth pains in the sides and hardness of the spleen. Used outwardly it has very good effect in agues. It helpeth those with the dropsy, or the green sickness, and killeth worms in the belly.

A decoction of the tops with the leaves and flowers is good against the colic, helps bring down women's courses and void the dead birth and also eases the pains of the mother. It is effectual in all pains of the joints, such as the gout, cramps or convulsions.

The juice with a little honey clears the eyes from dimness, mist and clouds that offend or hinder the sight. The decoction dropped into the ears cleanseth them from worms, foul ulcers and spreading scabs of the head. Washing with the decoction taketh away all freckles, spots and marks in the skin.

Modern uses: Centaury is used as a general tonic and as an anti-dyspeptic. The whole herb or just the leaves may be used.

An infusion is the best way to take it as all its properties are soluble in water. The infusion given warm in doses of 2 fl oz (56 ml) before meals will help to allay biliousness. When there is jaundice, Centaury is combined with Dandelion root in equal parts and given by decoction in tablespoonful doses two or three times a day.

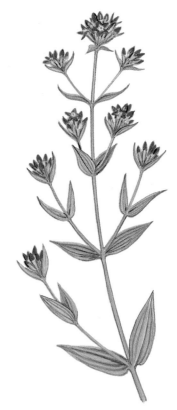

Centaury CENTAURIUM ERYTHRAEA
(= ERYTHRAEA CENTAURIUM)

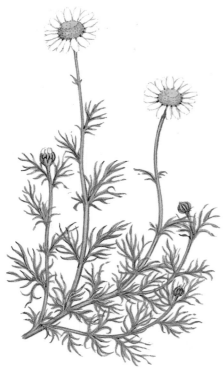

CHAMOMILE

A stone that hath been taken out of the body of a man being wrapped in Chamomile, will in time dissolve, and in a little time, too.

The Common or Roman Chamomile is a low-growing creeping or trailing plant bearing perfumed flowers with yellow centres and white florets rather like a Daisy.

Where to find it: It grows practically everywhere, but it prefers dry sandy soils and grassland.

Flowering time: From midsummer to early autumn.

Astrology: The Egyptians dedicated it to the Sun because it cured agues. They were like enough to do that for they were the arrantest apes in their religion I ever read of.

Medicinal virtues: A decoction of Chamomile takes away stitches and pains in the side. The flowers beaten and made into balls with oil drive away all sorts of agues. If the one grieved be anointed with that oil from the crown of the head to the sole of the foot and afterward laid to bed, he will sweat well.

It is profitable for melancholy or for an inflammation of the bowels and there is nothing more profitable than to apply it to the sides and region of the liver and spleen.

Bathing with a decoction of Chamomile taketh away weariness and easeth pains, particularly of the colic and stone and torments of the belly. It gently provoketh urine.

The syrup made of the juice with the flowers in white wine is a remedy against the jaundice and dropsy. The flowers boiled in lee are good to wash the head and comfort both it and the brain. The oil made from the flowers is much used against all hard swellings, pains or aches, shrinking of the sinews and cramps or pains in the joints or any other part of the body.

Modern uses: Chamomile has been used all down the ages and does not look like falling from favour. It plays an important part in modern herbal practice. The infusion is excellent for migraine and headache due to gastric disturbances. It will also regulate the menstrual periods.

It makes an ideal general tonic for children. It lowers nervous excitability and is useful to relieve toothache, earache and neuralgia if taken internally or used as a poultice. The infusion of the flowers is taken in doses up to 2 fl oz (56 ml) three times a day. A tincture is suitable for highly-strung or hypersensitive individuals. Oil of Chamomile can be taken, three drops on a lump of sugar, as an alternative to the above.

Chamomile CHAMAEMELUM NOBILE
(= ANTHEMIS NOBILIS)

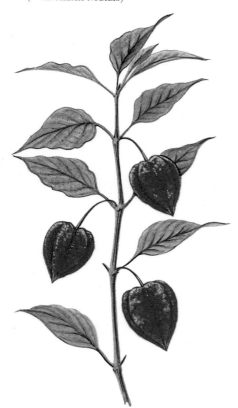

CHERRIES (Winter)

It helpeth those that void a bloody or foul urine.

The Winter Cherry has a creeping root in the ground and quickly spreads over a great compass of ground. The stalk grows no more than 36 inches (91 cm) high with broad and long green leaves, rather like Nightshade, but larger. The whitish flowers are followed by green berries which when ripe turn red and are enclosed in a ribbed covering.

Where to find it: It is cultivated in gardens, but is found wild in many countries. It should not be confused with the pot plant known as 'Winter Cherry'. Gardeners know it as the Chinese Lantern.

Cherries (Winter) PHYSALIS ALKEKENGI

Flowering time: Midsummer. The berries are ripe by late summer or early autumn.

Astrology: A plant of Venus.

Medicinal virtues: The leaves are cooling and may be used in inflammations. The berries draw down the urine when it has grown hot, sharp and painful in the passage. It is good to expel the stone and gravel and to cleanse ulcers in the bladder. Take three or four good handfuls of the berries, fresh or dried, bruise them and put them into beer or ale when it is new and tunned up. Taken daily this drink has been found to ease the pains and expel the stone. A decoction of the berries in wine and water is the most usual way to take them, but the powder of berries taken in a drink is more effectual.

Modern uses: Not used by modern herbalists, but homoeopaths make a tincture from the ripe berries. These are diuretic, laxative, and cooling in fevers. Overdoses cause constipation. The usual dose is about five or six berries. Stoneroot is now more popular as a herbal treatment for urinary tract stones, and Elderflowers for fevers.

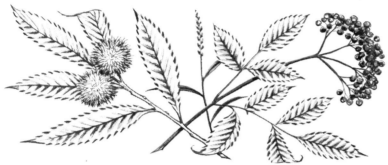

MYRRHIS ODORATA

CHERVIL

It is so harmless you cannot use it amiss.

It grows like the Great Hemlock, having large spreading leaves, but of a fresher green colour and tasting as sweet as Aniseed. At the tops of the branched stalks there are umbels or tufts of white flowers. It is also known as Sweet Cicely.

Where to find it: A common garden plant, but prefers mountain pastures and hilly districts.

Flowering time: Early to midsummer.

Astrology: Under the dominion of Jupiter.

Medicinal virtues: The roots boiled and eaten with oil and vinegar, or without oil, warms old and cold stomachs oppressed with wind and phlegm, or those that have the phthisis or consumption of the lungs. Drunk with wine the same is a preservation from the plague. It provoketh women's courses and expelleth the afterbirth, procureth an appetite and expelleth wind.

The juice is good to heal ulcers of the head and face and the candied roots are held as effectual as Angelica to preserve from infection in the time of a plague and to warm and comfort a cold weak stomach.

Modern uses: Both the root and the herb are used for their anti-flatulent effects. It is also expectorant and therefore of use in productive coughs. The roots are antiseptic which bears out their use in the time of the plague. Some herbalists recommend it for the treatment of high blood pressure. The fresh roots can be eaten. The dried roots are given by decoction in doses of 4–6 fl oz (114–170 ml). The herb is administered as an infusion which is given freely. This has a reputation for preventing and treating anaemia in teenage girls. There are several plants bearing the name Chervil, but with different botanical names, and some are poisonous. The plant may be confused with Hemlock by the unwary.

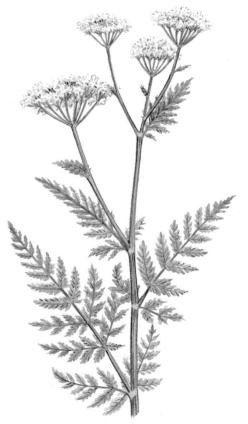

Chervil MYRRHIS ODORATA

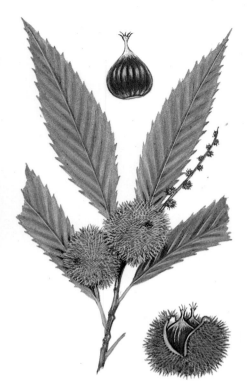

Chestnut Tree CASTANEA SATIVA

CHESTNUT TREE

It were as needless to describe a tree so commonly known as to tell a man he had gotten a mouth.

This is, in fact, the Sweet Chestnut with spreading branches, although it grows more erect when planted in a group.

Where to find it: Originally from sunnier climes, the Chestnut now grows in temperate regions of Britain, Europe and America.

Flowering time: Early summer.

Astrology: Under the dominion of Jupiter.

Medicinal virtues: The fruit breeds good blood and yields commendable nourishment, yet eaten too much makes the blood thick, procures headache and binds the body. The inner skin covering the nut is so binding that a scruple taken by a man, or ten grains (650 mg) by a child soon stops any flux. The powder of the dried nut, taken a dram (1.7 g) at a time, is a good remedy to stop the terms in women. If you dry the kernels, beat them into a powder and make it into an electuary with honey, you have an admirable remedy for the cough and spitting of blood.

Modern uses: The dried leaves are used in the form of an infusion – 1 oz (28 g) to 1 pt (568 ml) of boiling water – for whooping cough and irritation of the respiratory tract. The dosage is 1–2 fl oz (28–56 ml) three or four times a day. The medicine has an expectorant and astringent effect.

The Horse Chestnut (*Aesculus hippocastanum*) is also used in modern practice. An infusion of the bark is used to treat fevers. A tincture of the fruit is recommended for painful haemorrhoids as it improves blood circulation. A few drops are taken internally twice a day. The outer casing of the Horse Chestnut is poisonous.

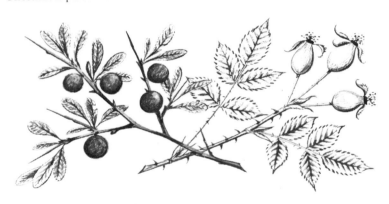

CHICKWEED

Boil a handful of Chickweed and a handful of red Rose leaves dried in a quart (1.1 l) of muscadine until a fourth part be consumed, then put to them a pint (568 ml) of oil of trotters or sheep's feet; let them boil a good while still stirring them well, which being strained, anoint the grieved part therewith, warm against the fire, rubbing it well with one hand; and bind also some of the herb, if you will, to the place, and with God's blessing it will help in three times dressing.

Chickweed is generally known to most people being a common weed, if not the most common, the world over.

Where to find it: It prefers moist places and wood-sides, but seeds readily on cultivated soil.

Flowering time: It flowers throughout the year.

Astrology: A fine, soft pleasing herb under the dominion of the Moon.

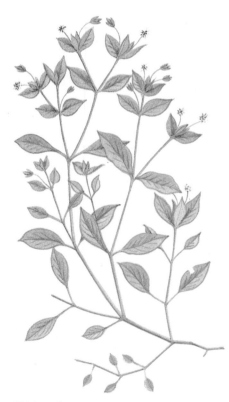

Chickweed STELLARIA MEDIA

Medicinal virtues: The bruised herb or the juice applied with sponges to the region of the liver, doth temperate the heat of the liver, and is effectual for all imposthumes and swellings whatsoever, for all redness in the face, wheals, scabs and the itch. The juice, simply used or boiled with hog's grease and applied, helpeth cramps, convulsions and palsy.

The juice or distilled water is good for all heats and redness in the eyes if some is dropped into them and is good to ease pain from the heat and sharpness of blood in the piles. It is used also in hot and virulent ulcers and sores in the privy parts of men and women, or on the legs or elsewhere.

The leaves boiled with Marsh Mallow and made into a poultice with Fenugreek and Linseed, applied to swellings and imposthumes, ripen and break them, or assuage the swellings and ease the pains. It helpeth the sinews when they are shrunk by cramp or otherwise.

Modern uses: Chickweed is a valuable healing and soothing agent, used in many ways, both internally and externally. The herb digested in oil and made into an ointment is excellent for haemorrhoids and ulcers, or for eczema, psoriasis or other irritating skin diseases. A decoction of the herb is used to wash and bathe swollen and inflamed tissues. The powder is used in poultices to give relief in bronchitis, pleurisy and rheumatism. The tea can be taken internally at the same time – one teaspoonful to a cup of boiling water. Three or four cups a day may be taken.

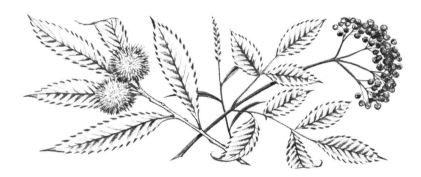

ALLIUM SCHOENOPRASUM

CHIVES

I confess I had not added these had it not been for a country gentleman, who by a letter certified to me that amongst other herbs I had left these out. They are indeed a kind of leeks, hot and dry in the fourth degree.

A hardy perennial, Chives (or Cives) belong to the Onion family which includes Shallots and Garlic. It bears a purple flower.

Where to find it: Not often found growing in the wild, being a cultivated herb, but it prefers the banks of ponds and streams, damp pastures and woodland edges.

Flowering time: Summer.

Astrology: Under the dominion of Mars.

Medicinal virtues: If they be eaten raw they send up very hurtful vapours to the brain, causing troublesome sleep and spoiling the eyesight. Yet when prepared by the alchymist they make an excellent remedy for the stoppage of urine.

Modern uses: The plant is regarded as a culinary herb and is not used medicinally. It contains an essential oil rich in sulphur, similar to that found in Onion and Garlic. As a medicine it would be milder in action to these, both of which are antiseptic and tend to lower the blood pressure. Garlic oil is now obtainable in capsule form.

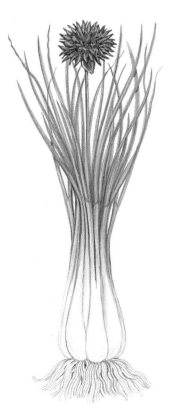

Chives ALLIUM SCHOENOPRASUM

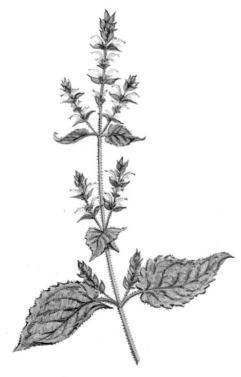

Cinquefoil POTENTILLA REPTANS

POTENTILLA REPTANS

CINQUEFOIL

Some one holds that one leaf cures a quotidian, three a tertian, and four a quartan ague, and a hundred to one if it be not Dioscorides, for he is full of whimsies.

This herb, also called Creeping Cinquefoil, Five-leaved Grass or Five-fingered Grass, spreads and creeps upon the ground with long slender strings like Strawberries, which take root again and shoot forth many leaves made of five parts, sometimes seven. It bears many small yellow flowers.

Where to find it: Meadows, pastures and by hedgerows and woodland edges.

Flowering time: Summer.

Astrology: A herb of Jupiter and therefore strengthens the part of the body it rules.

Medicinal virtues: Give but a scruple (20 grains /1.3 g) at a time in white wine or wine vinegar and you shall seldom miss the cure of an ague. It is used in all inflammations and fevers, whether infectious or pestilential and in lotions, gargles and the like, for sore mouths, ulcers, cancers, fistulas and other corrupt, foul or running sores.

The juice, about four ounces (113 g) at a time for several days cureth the quinsy and yellow jaundice; and for thirty days, cureth the falling-sickness.

The roots boiled in milk and drunk is a most effectual remedy for all fluxes in man or woman, whether the white or red, as also the bloody flux. The juice or decoction of the roots taken with honey helpeth the hoarseness of the throat and is good for a cough of the lungs. Boiled in vinegar, the root helpeth all knots, kernels, hard swellings and lumps in any part of the flesh, and also shingles. Boiled in wine it can be applied to painful joints, and drunk to cure the gout and sciatica and to ease pain in the bowels.

Modern uses: An infusion of 1 oz (28 g) of herb to 1 pt (568 ml) of boiling water is given in doses of 2 fl oz (56 ml) to check loose bowels, and also used as an astringent lotion or gargle for sore throats.

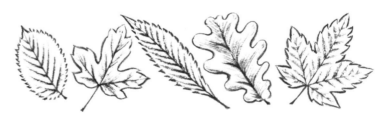

SALVIA SCLAREA

CLARY

It is a usual course with many men, when they have got the running of the reins, or women the whites, to run to the bush of Clary, exclaiming – Maid, bring hither the frying pan, and fetch me some butter quickly. Then they will eat fried Clary just as hogs eat acorns, and this they think will cure their disease, forsooth! Whereas, when they have devoured as much Clary as will grow upon an acre of ground, their backs are as much the better as though they had never touched it – nay, perhaps, very much worse.

The ordinary Garden Clary has four-square stalks with broad, rough wrinkled, whitish-green leaves with a strong sweet scent. The flowers are like those of Sage, but smaller and whitish-blue.

Where to find it: A garden herb. It is seldom seen unless it is sown, although there is a wild sort.

Flowering time: The seed is ripe in late summer.

Astrology: It is under the dominion of the Moon.

Clary SALVIA SCLAREA

Medicinal virtues: The seed put into the eyes clears them from motes and any white and red spots which may be on them. The mucilage of the seed made with water and applied to tumours and swellings disperseth them. It also draweth forth splinters and thorns from the flesh. The leaves used with vinegar, perhaps with a little honey, doth help boils, felons and the hot inflammations that gather, if applied before they grow too great.

The dried root powdered and put into the nose provoketh sneezing and purgeth the head and brain of much rheum and corruption. The seeds or leaves taken in wine provoketh to venery. It is of much use both for men and women that have weak backs and helpeth to strengthen the reins. The juice of the herb put into ale or beer and drunk bringeth down women's courses and expelleth afterbirth.

Yes, Clary strengthens the back, but we do deny that the cause of the running of the reins in men, or the whites in women, lies in the back. It would be as proper for me when my toe is sore to lay a plaster on my nose.

Modern uses: Clary is mostly used for digestive upsets. The herb is pleasantly aromatic and is anti-spasmodic. The leaves can be combined in an infusion with Chamomile flowers and given in doses of 2 fl oz (56 ml). An infusion of Clary alone acts as a tonic to the kidneys. Oil of Clary is used in the manufacture of perfume.

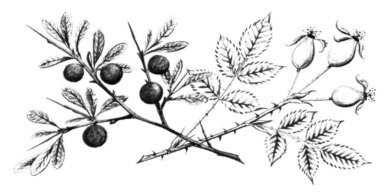

SALVIA VERBENACA

CLARY (Wild)

Wild Clary is most blasphemously called Christ's eye, because it cures diseases of the eyes. I could wish from my soul that blasphemy, ignorance and tyranny were ceased among physicians, that they might be happy and I joyful.

It is like the Garden Clary, but smaller with many stalks about 18 inches (46 cm) high. The stalks are square and hairy and the flowers are a bluish colour.

Where to find it: Dryish pastures, on waste ground and at the roadside.

Flowering time: Summer.

Astrology: It is under the dominion of the Moon.

Medicinal virtues: The seeds beaten to powder and drunk with wine is an admirable help to provoke lust.

A decoction of the leaves warms the stomach, helps digestion and scatters congealed blood in any part of the body.

The distilled water cleanseth the eyes of redness, wateriness and heat. For dimness of sight take one of its seeds, put it into the eye and let it remain until it drops out of itself. The pain will be nothing to speak of. It will cleanse the eyes and in oft repeating it, will take off a film which covereth the sight – a handsome, safer and easier remedy than to tear it off with a needle.

Modern uses: Both the Wild and the Garden Clary are members of the Sage family. Their properties are similar, but the wild variety is considered to be more potent. The seed is mucilaginous, and some herbalists use the mucilage to sooth the eye.

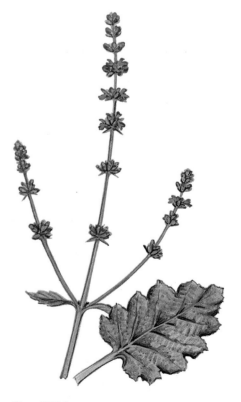

Clary (Wild) SALVIA VERBENACA

47

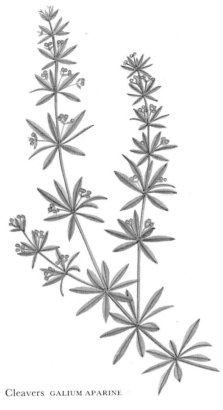

Cleavers GALIUM APARINE

GALIUM APARINE

CLEAVERS

It is familiarly taken in broth, to keep them lean and lank that are apt to grow fat.

An annual herb also known as Goose-grass, Catchweed and Bedstraw, it has prickly stems which grow from two to six feet (0.6 to 1.8 m) high. The flowers are small, white and scattered.

Where to find it: It grows by hedges and ditches and on the edges of woods. It chokes whatever grows near it.

Flowering time: Summer.

Astrology: Under the dominion of the Moon.

Medicinal virtues: The juice of the herb and seed together, taken in wine, helpeth those bitten by an adder by preserving the heart from the venom.

The distilled water drunk twice a day helpeth the yellow jaundice. The decoction of the herb stayeth laxes and bloody fluxes. The juice of the leaves, or the bruised leaves, applied to a wound stayeth the bleeding. Boiled in hog's grease, it helpeth all sorts of hard swellings or kernels in the throat when anointed.

Modern uses: An important remedy in modern practice, *Galium* is a soothing relaxing diuretic and is therefore employed as an infusion in cystitis in doses of two to four tablespoonfuls, three or four times a day. It can also be combined for this purpose with demulcents such as Marsh Mallow in equal parts.

It is extensively used in the internal treatment of skin diseases, such as psoriasis and eczema. It acts on the lymphatic system. The juice is a powerful diuretic and useful in dropsy. Dosage varies from $\frac{1}{6}$–$\frac{1}{2}$ fl oz (5–15 ml). The herb is considered to have anti-tumour properties, but there is as yet insufficient evidence to support this. Tinctures and fluid extracts are usually obtainable from herbalists.

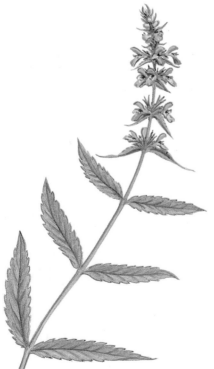

Clown's Woundwort STACHYS PALUSTRIS

STACHYS PALUSTRIS

CLOWN'S WOUNDWORT

The herb deserves commendation, though it has received such a clownish name. Whoever reads this, if he try as I have done, will commend it.

The plant, also called Marsh Woundwort, grows two or three feet (61 or 91 cm) high with square, green, rough stalks and narrow dark green leaves. The flowers are at the top and have reddish-pink hoods. The whole plant has a strong odour.

Where to find it: In or near ditches.

Flowering time: Early to midsummer.

Astrology: Under the dominion of the planet Saturn.

Medicinal virtues: It is effectual in all wounds, for the staunching of blood and to dry up the fluxes in old fretting ulcers.

A syrup is made of the juice for inward wounds, ruptures of veins, or vomiting blood. If any vein or muscle be swollen apply an ointment or plaster of this herb, adding a little Comfrey.

Modern uses: It is antiseptic and anti-spasmodic. The juice is styptic and if the bruised leaves are applied to a wound the bleeding will stop. A similar application relieves painful joints and cramp.

COLT'S FOOT

The dry leaves are best for those who have thin rheums and distillations upon their lungs, causing a cough.

This herb is also called Cough-wort, Foal's-wort, Horse-hoof and Bull's Foot. The small, yellowish flowers appear before the leaves in late winter, being borne on a tender stalk. The leaves are in the shape of a horse's hoof, hence the name Colt's Foot, and the root, small and white, spreads underground. Once planted, it will be difficult to eradicate.

Where to find it: It grows in both wet and dry ground and is often seen near brooks and rivers.

Flowering time: Late winter to mid spring.

Astrology: The plant is under Venus.

Medicinal virtues: The fresh leaves, or juice or syrup made from them, is good for a hot, dry cough, or wheezing and shortness of breath. The dried leaves can be used as a tobacco. The distilled water used alone, or with Elderflowers and Nightshade is a good remedy against all agues. Drink two ounces (56 g) at a time, and apply wet cloths to the head and stomach. This is also good for any hot swellings or inflammations. It helpeth St Anthony's fire and wheals that arise through heat. The burning heat of piles or privy parts are eased also by applying cloths dipped in Colt's Foot water.

Modern uses: Colt's Foot is an important ingredient in many over-the-counter cough mixtures. A diffusive expectorant, it tones the bronchial tubes. Its demulcent properties are also useful when used for tracheitis and bronchitis. Colt's Foot is usually combined in equal parts with other pectoral agents such as Horehound, Marsh Mallow and Ground-ivy. A syrup can be made from the flower stalks by boiling them in water with honey or sugar added. The decoction for colds, flu and asthma is made by placing 1 oz (28 g) of leaves in 2 pt (1.1 l) of water and boiling it down to 1 pt (568 ml) and drinking a cupful at a time. A fluid extract is available from herbalists.

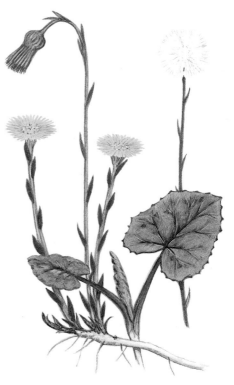

Colt's Foot TUSSILAGO FARFARA

COLUMBINE

The seed taken in wine causeth a speedy delivery of women in childbirth.

A familiar garden plant with flower stems between one and two feet (30 and 61 cm) high and drooping bluish flowers.

Where to find it: A cultivated plant, but occasionally found in the wild growing in woodland clearings.

Flowering time: Late spring, early summer.

Astrology: A herb of Venus.

Medicinal virtues: The leaves of Columbines are generally used in lotions with good success for sore mouths and throats. The Spaniards used to eat a piece of the root in the morning for several days to help them when troubled with stone in the reins or kidneys.

Modern uses: Not used by modern herbalists as Columbine is slightly poisonous. But it has astringent properties, hence its use externally as a lotion.

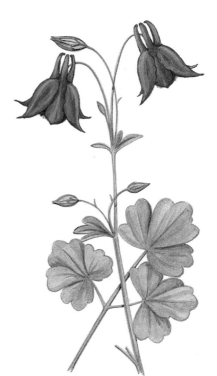

Columbine AQUILEGIA VULGARIS

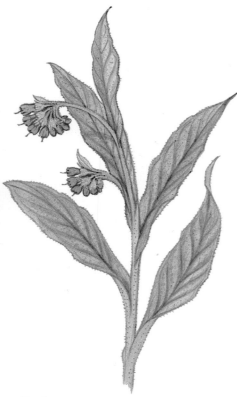

Comfrey SYMPHYTUM OFFICINALE

SYMPHYTUM OFFICINALE

COMFREY

The roots of Comfrey taken fresh, beaten small, and spread upon leather, and laid upon any place troubled with the gout, doth presently give ease of the pains.

A common herb, Comfrey has large hairy green leaves which cause the hands to itch if they touch any tender part. The stalk grows two or three feet (61 or 91 cm) high and is hollow and hairy. The flowers stand in order one above another. They are long and hollow like the finger of a glove and are of pale purplish colour though some bear pale whitish flowers.

Where to find it: It grows by ditches and watersides and in moist fields.

Flowering time: Early to midsummer. The seeds ripen in late summer.

Astrology: A herb of Saturn and under the sign of Capricorn, cold, dry and earthy in quality.

Medicinal virtues: Comfrey helpeth those that spit blood or make a bloody urine. The root boiled in water or wine and the decoction drunk helps all inward hurts, bruises, wounds and ulcers of the lungs and causes the phlegm to be easily spit forth. It helpeth the defluxion of rheum from the head upon the lungs, the fluxes of blood or humours by the belly, women's immoderate courses, the reds and the whites and the running of the reins.

A decoction of the leaves can be used for all the same purposes, but is not so effectual as the roots. The roots outwardly applied help fresh wounds or cuts and are especially good for broken bones and ruptures. It is also good applied to women's breasts that grow sore with an abundance of milk and also to repress bleeding of the haemorrhoids.

Modern uses: A valuable demulcent and healing herb, also known as Knitbone for its power to mend broken bones. Comfrey contains allantoin which is used to encourage wound-healing and is an ingredient of skin preparations to treat psoriasis. A decoction of the root, or tablets made from the powdered root, available from herbalists, are used for peptic ulcers, colitis and hiatus hernia. The root and leaves are still recommended as an external application for wounds, fractures and leg ulcers, although it is more convenient to use an ointment made by digesting the root or leaves in hot paraffin wax, straining and allowing to cool. The decoction of the root – 1 oz (28 g) to 1 pt (568 ml) of boiling water – is useful for the treatment of tonsillitis, bronchitis and irritating coughs.

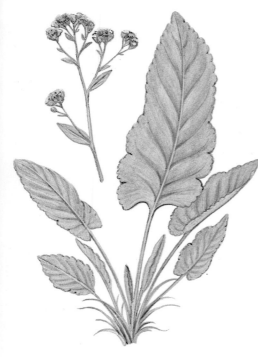

Costmary BALSAMITA MAJOR
(= B. VULGARIS)

BALSAMITA MAJOR (= B. VULGARIS)

COSTMARY

It is an especial friend and help to evil, weak and cold livers.

Once a common garden herb, now a rarity. It is closely allied to the common Tansy. It gives off a pleasanter aroma than Tansy and where it is still grown it is known as Mace. It is also called Alecost and Balsam Herb.

Where to find it: An oriental herb formerly grown in every herb garden. It does well in all soils, but prefers dry.

Flowering time: Early to midsummer.

Astrology: It is under the dominion of Jupiter.

Medicinal virtues: It provoketh urine, gently purgeth choler and phlegm and is a wonderful help to all sorts of dry agues. It is astringent to the stomach, and strengthens the liver and other inward parts. Taken first thing in the morning it is very profitable for pains in the head that are continual. It is helpful to those that have fallen into the continual evil disposition of the body called cachexia, but especially in the beginning of the disease. The seed is given to children for the worms and so is the infusion of flowers in white wine, two ounces (56 g) at a time. It maketh an excellent salve to cleanse and heal old ulcers, being boiled with olive oil and Adder's Tongue with it. After straining a little wax is added to thicken it.

Modern uses: Not used in modern practice, because of its rarity. Tansy is now used, and it has similar properties. See Tansy.

PRIMULA VERIS

COWSLIP

Our city dames know well enough the ointment or distilled water of it adds to beauty, or at least restores it when it is lost.

A well-known perennial belonging to the Primrose family. Also called Peagle.

Where to find it: Dry meadows, hedgerows and in woodland.

Flowering time: Mid to late spring.

Astrology: Venus lays claim to this herb as her own, and it is under the sign of Aries.

Medicinal virtues: An ointment made from the flowers taketh away spots and wrinkles of the skin, sun-burnings and freckles. The flowers remedy vertigo, nightmares, false apparitions, frenzies, falling-sickness, palsies, convulsions, cramps, and nerve pains.

The roots ease pains in the back and bladder and open the urinary passages. The leaves are good to apply to wounds and the flowers take away trembling.

Modern uses: The flowers are used for their sedative and anti-spasmodic properties. A teaspoonful of the dried flowers made into a tea and taken at night will prevent insomnia. An ointment made from the flowers is a good application to relieve sunburn.

A decoction of the root is excellent as a remedy for bronchitis and whooping cough – 1 oz (28 g) of the dried root is boiled in 1 pt (568 ml) of water, strained and taken in doses of 1–2 fl oz (28–56 ml) for its expectorant properties.

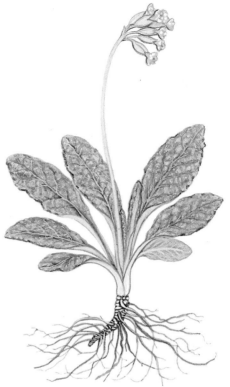

Cowslip PRIMULA VERIS

CRUCIATA LAEVIPES (= GALIUM CRUCIATA)

CROSSWORT

The decoction of the herb in wine helpeth a decayed appetite.

Common Crosswort grows with square, hairy stalks up to about a foot (30 cm) high and has four small and pointed, hairy leaves at every joint. The flowers are small and pale yellow.

Where to find it: Moist meadows and uncultivated ground.

Flowering time: It flowers from late spring and all through the summer.

Astrology: It is under the dominion of Saturn.

Medicinal virtues: A good herb for wounds, used inwardly to stay the bleeding and outwardly to consolidate them. The decoction of the herb in wine helpeth to expectorate phlegm from the chest and remove obstructions in the chest, stomach or bowels. It is also good to wash wounds and sores with, to cleanse and heal them.

The herb bruised, boiled and applied outwardly and renewed often for a few days, while the decoction is taken inwardly, doth certainly cure the rupture.

Modern uses: Its main use is as an ointment to apply to cuts and abrasions, but Comfrey ointment is more popular. An ointment can be made by boiling the herb in oil or wax, straining and pouring into jars before it cools. The amounts of oil or wax depend on the consistency of the ointment required. The amount of herb used will also dictate its strength. The process of boiling in oil and straining can be repeated several times before the ointment is allowed to cool, if a particularly strong ointment is required.

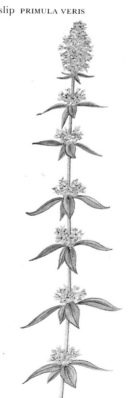

Crosswort CRUCIATA LAEVIPES
(= GALIUM CRUCIATA)

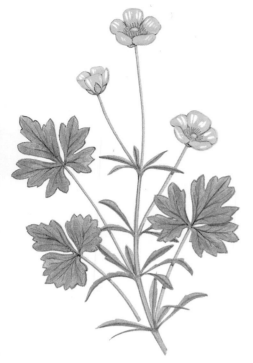

Crowfoot RANUNCULUS AURICOMUS

RANUNCULUS AURICOMUS
CROWFOOT

I do not remember that I ever saw anything yellower. Virgins in ancient times used to make a powder of them to furrow bride-beds.

This furious biting herb has many names – including Frog's-foot, Goldknobs, Gold-cups and Butter-flowers. These days it is also known as Goldilocks. It is a member of the Buttercup family, growing to about 16 inches (40 cm).

Where to find it: Unless you turn your head into a hedge, you cannot but see them as you walk. They are found in woods, on wood edges and hedgebanks.

Flowering time: From mid spring to early summer.

Astrology: A fiery and hot-spirited herb of Mars.

Medicinal virtues: In no way is this herb fit to be given internally. An ointment of the leaves or flowers, however, will draw a blister. It may also be applied to the nape of the neck to draw back rheum from the eyes. The bruised herb mixed with mustard will draw a blister too, as perfectly as cantharides and with far less danger to the vessels of urine which cantharides naturally delights to wrong.

The herb was once applied to a pestilential rising that was fallen down and it saved life even beyond hope, so it were good to keep an ointment and plaster of it, if just for that.

Modern uses: As pointed out, this herb is poisonous and modern herbalists do not use plants with toxic properties. Other members of the Buttercup family are also poisonous. The common Field Buttercup (*Ranunculus acris*) is poisonous, but the juice of the leaves has been used as an application to remove warts. A homoeopathic tincture made from the fresh plant, according to specific pharmaceutical techniques, is also used as a remedy for irritating skin conditions such as eczema, and rheumatic complaints.

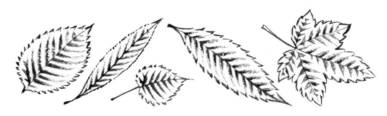

ARUM MACULATUM
CUCKOO-PINT

The berries or roots beaten with hot ox-dung, and applied, easeth the pains of the gout.

A perennial with large leaves. The flowering organs are enveloped in a characteristic sheath-like bract called a spathe. The plant is also known as Lords and Ladies because of its likeness to male and female genitalia. Another name is Wake Robin.

Where to find it: It grows at the foot of hedges in the shade and in open woodland.

Flowering time: Mid to late spring.

Astrology: Under the dominion of Mars.

Medicinal virtues: A dram (1.7 g) or more if need be of the spotted Wake Robin either fresh or dried, being beaten and taken is a sure remedy for the poison and plague. A spoonful of the juice of the herb hath the same effect, but a little vinegar added allayeth the sharp biting taste.

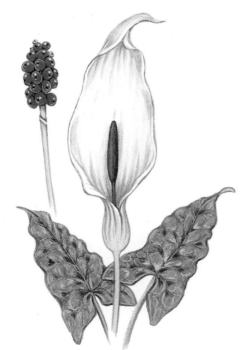

Cuckoo-pint ARUM MACULATUM

The bruised leaves laid upon any boil or plague-sore help draw forth the poison. A dram (1.7 g) of the powdered dried root taken with twice as much sugar in the form of a licking electuary helpeth those that are pursy and short-winded, and those that have a cough. It breaketh, digesteth and riddeth away phlegm from the stomach, chest and lungs. The powder taken in wine provoketh urine and bringeth down women's courses and purgeth them effectually after childbearing to bring away the afterbirth.

Taken with sheep's milk it healeth the inward ulcers of the bowels. The root mixed with Bean flour and applied to the throat or jaws that are inflamed helpeth them.

The juice of the berries boiled in Oil of Roses, or beaten into powder mixed with the oil and dropped into the ears, easeth pains in them. The leaves and roots boiled in wine with a little oil and applied to the piles easeth them.

Modern uses: This plant does contain poisonous and purgative substances and is not recommended for domestic use. The berries have caused poisoning in children. A homoeopathic tincture is prepared from the plant and used for respiratory conditions, such as bronchitis and whooping cough.

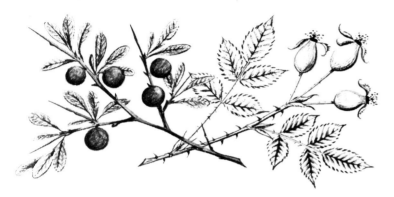

CUCUMIS SATIVUS

CUCUMBER

The face being washed with the distilled water of them cureth the reddest face that is.
A very well-known salad vegetable in use for at least 3,000 years.

Where to find it: Every keen gardener grows it.

Flowering time: Summer.

Astrology: There is no dispute to be made but that they are under the dominion of the Moon, though they are much cried out against for their coldness. If they were one degree colder, they would be poison.

Medicinal virtues: They are excellent for a hot stomach and liver, although the unmeasurable use of them fills the body full of raw humours.

The face being washed with their juice cleanseth the skin and is excellent for hot rheums in the eyes. The seed is excellent to provoke urine and cleanseth the passages thereof when they are stopped. There is not a better remedy than Cucumbers for ulcers in the bladder. The usual method is to use the seed in emulsions, as one makes Almond milk; but a better way is to bruise the Cucumbers and distil the water from them. Those that are troubled with ulcers in the bladder should take no other drink. The distilled water is also excellent for sun-burning, freckles and morphew.

Modern uses: Cucumber juice is an ingredient of many natural beauty creams, cosmetics and lotions. The seeds, like Celery and Pumpkin seeds are diuretic, but also have the ability to expel tapeworms from the body. As a beauty aid, slices of Cucumber can be applied direct to the skin. As a diuretic, the juice is indicated in kidney ailments and rheumatic conditions. It is usually combined with Carrot juice in the ratio of one part Cucumber to three parts Carrot. One or two glasses a day may be taken.

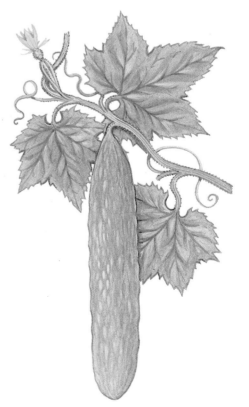

Cucumber CUCUMIS SATIVUS

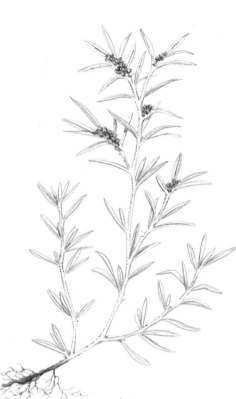

FILAGINELLA ULIGINOSA (= GNAPHALIUM ULIGINOSUM)

CUDWEED

It is drunk or injected for the disease called tenesmus, which is an often provocation to stool without doing anything.

The Cudweed, Marsh Cudweed or Cottonweed has a thick stalk with whitish and woody leaves. The flowers are small and yellowish.

Where to find it: Damp waste ground.

Flowering time: Early to midsummer.

Astrology: Venus is lady of it.

Medicinal virtues: The plants are all astringent, binding or drying and therefore profitable for all defluxions of rheum from the head and to stay fluxes of blood. The decoction is made into red wine or the powder is taken. It stayeth the immoderate courses of women and is also good for inward and outward wounds or bruises and helpeth children with ruptures or worms. The juice of the herb, as Pliny saith, is a sovereign remedy against the mumps and quinsy.

Modern uses: It is an astringent. The infusion made from 1 oz (28 g) of the dried herb to 1 pt (568 ml) of boiling water is taken internally in doses of 2 fl oz (56 ml) or used as a gargle for peritonsillar abscess.

Cudweed FILAGINELLA ULIGINOSA
(= GNAPHALIUM ULIGINOSUM)

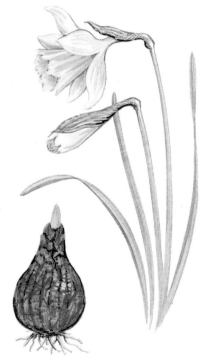

NARCISSUS PSEUDONARCISSUS

DAFFODIL

The juice, mingled with honey, frankincense, wine and myrrh, and dropped into the ears, is good against all the corrupt filth and running matter in these parts.

There are several kinds of Daffodils, but the Common or Wild Daffodil grows about a foot (30 cm) high and has a single, large yellow flower. The bulb is round, and white within.

Where to find it: It grows in gardens, but it prefers damp meadows and pastures.

Flowering time: Early to mid spring.

Astrology: Venus governs all the Daffodils, except the Yellow, which belongs to Mars.

Medicinal virtues: The fresh roots are used. Given internally in small quantity, either by decoction or as a powder, they act as an emetic and purgative. Daffodil is mainly used externally. The bruised roots, boiled with parched Barley-meal, will heal wounds and, mixed with honey, strengthen sprains. They are good to apply to aching joints. The juice of the bruised root will allay swellings and inflammations of the breast.

Modern uses: Not recommended for domestic use. There have been cases of poisoning when the bulbs have been eaten in mistake for Onions. A homoeopathic medicine is made from the bulb and used for respiratory disease, particularly bronchitis and whooping cough.

LEUCANTHEMUM VULGARE (= CHRYSANTHEMUM LEUCANTHEMUM)

DAISY

The leaves bruised and applied to the testicles or any other part that is swollen and hot, doth dissolve it and temper the heat.

This is not the little Daisy that grows in the lawn, but the Ox-eye Daisy, or what some know as Marguerite. It grows to 26 inches (66 cm).

Daffodil NARCISSUS PSEUDONARCISSUS

Where to find it: A common perennial of grassland roadsides.

Flowering time: From late spring to late summer.

Astrology: It is under the sign of Cancer and under the dominion of Venus and therefore excellent for wounds in the breast and very fitting to be kept in oils, ointments, plasters and syrups.

Medicinal virtues: The Greater Wild Daisy is a wound herb of good respect, often used in those drinks and salves that are for wounds, either inward or outward.

The juice or distilled water of these, or the Small Daisy, doth much temper the heat of choler, and refresh the liver and other inward parts. A decoction made of them and drank, helpeth to cure the wounds made in the hollowness of the breast. The same cureth also all ulcers and pustules in the mouth or tongue, or in the secret parts. A decoction made of the Daisy leaves, Agrimony and Wall-wort (Dwarf Elder) and used as a fomentation giveth great ease to those troubled with the palsy, sciatica or gout. It will also disperseth and dissolveth the knots or kernels that grow in the flesh of any part of the body, or bruises due to falls or blows. An ointment made from Daisies helps all inflammatory wounds or where there is delayed healing. The juice dropped into the running eyes of any doth much help them.

Modern uses: The Ox-eye Daisy is a member of the Compositae family of plants which provides many valuable herbs. It is similar in action to Chamomile which, today, is a more popular herb. The Daisy has diuretic, anti-spasmodic and tonic properties, but is emetic if more than the recommended dose is taken. Its main uses are in the treatment of whooping cough and asthma. It is taken as a decoction – 1 oz (28 g) of the whole dried herb being boiled in 1½ pt (852 ml) of water until the mixture measures 1 pt (568 ml). It is then strained and administered in doses of 2 fl oz (56 ml) three times a day.

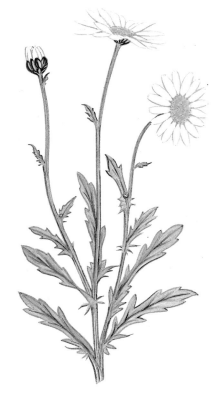

Daisy LEUCANTHEMUM VULGARE
(= CHRYSANTHEMUM LEUCANTHEMUM)

BELLIS PERENNIS

DAISY (Little)

This is another herb which nature has made common, because it may be useful.

The common Little Daisy is the one that grows in lawns. The roots are a thick bush of fibres and the leaves grow in a circle close to the ground. The flowers seldom grow to more than four inches (10 cm) high.

Where to find it: Lawns, fields and meadows.

Flowering time: All the year round.

Astrology: This Daisy is governed by Venus in the sign of Cancer.

Medicinal virtues: The leaves, and sometimes the roots, are used. They are among the traumatic and vulnerary herbs, being used in wound-drinks, and are accounted good to dissolve congealed and coagulated blood. They also help the pleurisy and peripneumonia. In the king's-evil the decoction given inwardly and a cataplasm of the leaves applied outwardly, are esteemed by some. The leaves taste like Colt's Foot, but are more mucilaginous and not bitter. An infusion boiled in asses' milk is effectual in consumption of the lungs.

Modern uses: The crushed fresh leaves will still soothe wounds and help healing as in former days. It is still known as Bruisewort in some places. In medicine it is mainly used by homoeopaths who make a fresh plant tincture as a remedy for lumps and swellings as a result of injury, and also for chronic skin diseases due to impure blood, such as boils. An infusion of 1 oz (28 g) of the herb to 1 pt (568 ml) of water is used cold in an eye bath for minor eye troubles. An ointment is also used for this purpose being applied to the eyelids.

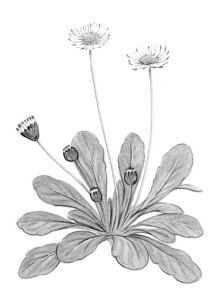

Daisy (Little) BELLIS PERENNIS

DANDELION

This herb helps one to see farther without a pair of spectacles. This is known by foreign physicians who are not so selfish as ours, but more communicative of the virtues of plants to people.

A well-known plant which barely requires description. It is known to the vulgar as Piss-a-Beds, which is due no doubt to its diuretic property. The root grows down exceedingly deep and if broken off within the ground it will shoot forth again.

Where to find it: A troublesome weed all over the world in meadows, pastures and gardens.

Flowering time: Throughout the year.

Astrology: It is under the dominion of Jupiter.

Medicinal virtues: It has an opening and cleansing quality and, therefore, very effectual for removing obstructions of the liver, gall bladder and spleen and diseases arising from them, such as jaundice.

It openeth the passages of the urine both in young and old and will cleanse ulcers in the urinary tract. For this purpose the decoction of the roots or leaves in white wine, or the leaves used as pot herbs are very effectual. It is of wonderful help in cachexia, the severe wasting condition in severe illness. It also procures rest and sleep in those with fever. The distilled water can be drunk in pestilential fever and be used as a wash for the sores. This common herb hath many virtues, which is why the French and Dutch eat them so often in the spring.

Modern uses: Bile production by the liver and urinary output from the kidneys is increased with the use of this herb. As a diuretic, it is superior to many produced synthetically by pharmaceutical companies. The leaves are particularly strong, being equivalent to frusemide, a drug used to treat hypertension. The dried herb contains significant amounts of potassium, which people on long-term diuretic therapy need. Modern herbalists, therefore, have a safe, but powerful remedy, not only for hypertension but also for cardiac oedema, hepatogenic dropsy and water retention, due to stasis or congestion in the blood vessels serving the liver.

The diuretic effect of Dandelion is helpful in the treatment of a number of other conditions, particularly chronic disorders like rheumatism, gout and eczema. A fluid extract is available from herbalists and the recommended dose is between one and two teaspoonfuls three times a day. The dried root taken in the form of a decoction is a powerful liver tonic – 1 oz (28 g) of the root is boiled in 2 pt (1.1 l) of water until the mixture is reduced to 1 pt (568 ml). The dose is two to four teaspoonfuls three or four times a day. A Dandelion coffee made from the roasted roots is available from health stores. The fresh, clean young leaves can be added to salads in spring.

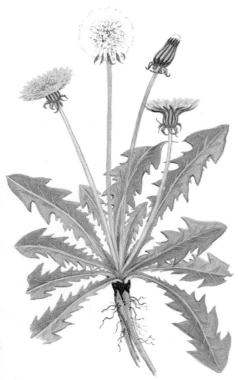

Dandelion' TARAXACUM OFFICINALE

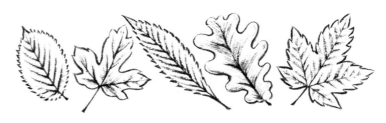

DARNEL

As it is not without some vices, so hath it also many virtues.

A common weed in cornfields. It has a long spike composed of many heads set one above the other, containing two or three husks with sharp beards or awns at the ends. It is also called Jura and Wary.

Where to find it: It grows in cornfields and along the borders and pathways of fields that are fallow.

Flowering time: Summer.

Astrology: It is a malicious part of sullen Saturn.

Medicinal virtues: The meal of Darnel is used to stay gangrenes and putrid sores. It also cleanseth the skin of leprosies, morphews and ringworms, if it be used with salt and Radish roots. With brimstone and vinegar it is used to dissolveth knots and kernels. A decoction made with water and honey can be used to bathe the parts affected by sciatica. Darnel-meal applied in a poultice draweth forth splinters.

Modern uses: Darnel is considered poisonous, although this may be due to the seeds being affected by a fungus. Because of its unpredictable effects it is not used by modern herbalists and is not recommended for domestic use. Other herbalists record that it can cause blindness.

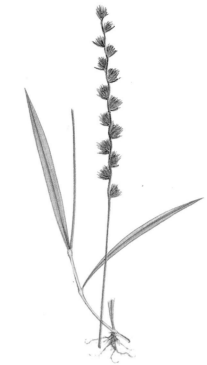

Darnel LOLIUM TEMULENTUM

SUCCISA PRATENSIS (= SCABIOSA SUCCISA)

DEVIL'S BIT

The root was longer, until the devil (as the friars say) bit away the rest of it for spite, envying its usefulness to mankind: for sure he was not troubled with any disease for which it is proper.

It grows about two feet (61 cm) high with narrow, smooth, dark green leaves nipped about the edges. At the end of each branch there is a round head of many flowers of a blueish-purple colour.

Where to find it: Dry meadows and heathland.

Flowering time: Late summer.

Astrology: The herb is not ascribed a planet or astrological sign.

Medicinal virtues: The herb or the root (all that the devil hath left of it) being boiled in wine and drank, is very powerful against the plague and all pestilential diseases or fevers and poisons. It also helpeth all that are inwardly bruised by any casualty, or outwardly by falls or blows, dissolving the clotted blood. The herb or root beaten and outwardly applied taketh away the black and blue marks that remain in the skin.

The decoction of the herb, with Honey of Roses, helpeth inveterate tumours and swellings of the throat if used as a gargle. It helpeth also to procure women's courses and easeth all pains of the mother and to break wind therein. The powder of the root taken in drink driveth forth worms from the body.

The juice or distilled water of the herb is effectual for wounds or old sores and cleanseth the body inwardly.

Modern uses: Still recommended in the treatment of fevers and inflammatory disease. The infusion is soothing, helps to reduce temperature naturally and to excrete toxic substances through the skin. It is made by adding 1 oz (28 g) of the dried herb to 1 pt (568 ml) of boiling water. Doses of 2 fl oz (56 ml) can be taken frequently to produce perspiration.

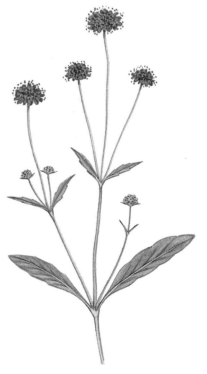

Devil's Bit SUCCISA PRATENSIS
(= SCABIOSA SUCCISA)

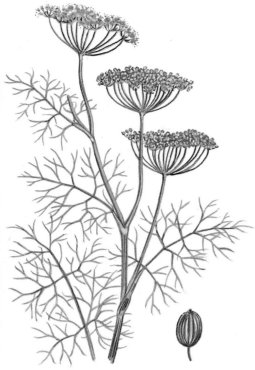

Dill ANETHUM GRAVEOLENS

DILL

The decoction of Dill is a gallant expeller of wind.

The common Dill has feathery leaves and looks like Fennel, although the plant does not grow so large. The seed is flatter and thinner than Fennel seed.

Where to find it: It is usually grown in herb gardens or cultivated commercially because of the large demand for it, but its natural habitat is the Mediterranean countries, where it grows wild in cornfields.

Flowering time: Mid to late summer.

Astrology: Mercury has dominion over this plant and therefore it strengthens the brain.

Medicinal virtues: It is the seeds that are used. Boiled and drank they ease both swellings and pains. They stayeth the belly and stomach from casting. Women with pains and windiness will be helped if they sit in the decoction. Boiled in wine and tied in a cloth the seeds will stayeth hiccough if they are smelled. The roasted or fried seeds used in oils or plaisters drieth moist ulcers in the fundament. An oil made of Dill is effectual to warm or dissolve humours or imposthumes, to ease pains and to procure rest.

Modern uses: An excellent remedy for children with flatulence or digestive upsets. Oil of Dill is used in many over-the-counter medicines for digestive problems. A few drops can be taken on a lump of sugar, or Dill water can be made by adding eight drops to 1 pt (568 ml) of distilled water. The dose of the water is from one to eight teaspoonfuls. The seeds are used for flavouring cakes.

DITTANDER (Karse)

The women in Suffolk give the leaves boiled in ale to hasten the birth.

The common Dittander has a small, white, slender, creeping root, which is difficult to remove from a garden once it is planted there. It grows about 18 inches (46 cm) high with small, white flowers. It is also known as Pepper-wort because of its hot, biting taste, and Garden Cress.

Where to find it: It is grown as a cress for salads, but it likes moist places and grows near rivers.

Flowering time: Early to midsummer.

Astrology: A herb of Venus.

Medicinal virtues: The bruised leaves mixed with hog's lard and applied as a cataplasm to the hip, easeth sciatica. Chewed in the mouth they cause a great flux of rheum to run out of it and by that means are said to help scrofulous tumours in the throat.

Modern uses: The Cress, eaten in salads, does contain a natural antibiotic, but it has not found a place in medicine. The antibiotic is similar to one found in the Nasturtium (*Tropaeolum majus*), which is used. An infusion of fresh Nasturtium leaves – ½ oz (14 g) to 1 pt (568 ml) of boiling water – is a useful remedy for bronchitis, catarrh and emphysema. The dose is 2 fl oz (56 ml) two or three times a day.

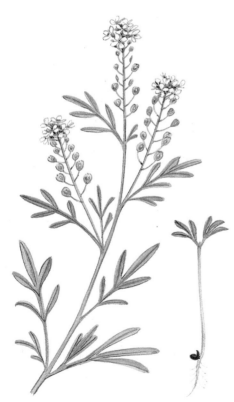

Dittander (Karse) LEPIDIUM SATIVUM

DITTANY OF CRETE

It is an excellent wound herb and in much reputation among the ancients.

A pretty plant, Dittany of Crete grows six or eight inches (15 or 20 cm) high with square stalks and short round leaves covered with a white downy matter. The flowers are small and purple.

Where to find it: It grows in gardens and is cultivated as an ornamental plant for the window sill. It originally grew wild in Crete.

Flowering time: Mid to late summer.

Astrology: It is an herb of Venus.

Medicinal virtues: Made as a decoction in wine, it procures a speedy and easy delivery, or can be used together with Vervain, Hyssop and Pennyroyal. The decoction made by boiling the herb in ale is more effectual.

Dittany and milk are good for spitting of blood. The roots are cordial and cephalic, resist putrefaction and poison, and are useful in malignant and pestilential distempers. The whole herb is good for diseases of the head, and to open all manner of obstructions.

Modern uses: This herb has given way to Sweet Marjoram (*Origanum marjorana*) and Wild Marjoram (*Origanum vulgare*). They are members of the Labiatae family of plants, and are described later in this book.

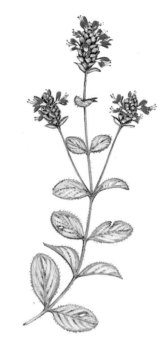

Dittany of Crete ORIGANUM DICTAMNUS

DITTANY (White)

In the summer months, the whole plant is covered with a kind of inflammable substance, which is glutinous to the touch, and of very fragrant smell; but if it takes fire, it goes off with a flash all over the plant. This does it no harm, and may be repeated after three or four days, a new quantity of the inflammable matter being produced in that time.

Its leaves resemble those of an Ash tree, and it bears large elegant flowers of various colours: red, white, striped or blue.

Where to find it: It grows in gardens and in warm places. It can be found in woodland where it is sheltered.

Flowering time: Early to midsummer.

Astrology: Under the dominion of Venus.

Medicinal virtues: The roots are mainly used. Like Dittany of Crete they are cordial, cephalic, resist poison and putrefaction, and are useful in malignant and pestilential fevers. They are also used for cases of hysteria.

An infusion of the tops of the plant are a pleasant and efficacious medicine in the gravel. It works powerfully by provoking urine and eases colicky pains which frequently accompany that disorder. The root is a sure remedy for epilepsies, and other diseases of the head, opening obstructions of the womb and procuring the discharges of the uterus.

Modern uses: The plant is more commonly known today as the Burning Bush. It is the essential oil, which has a lemon-like smell, that is inflammable. The herb is not much used these days, but is classified as a stomach tonic. A simple infusion of the leaves can be used as a substitute for tea and as a remedy for nervous complaints. The powdered root combined in equal parts with Peppermint has been administered in doses of 2 drams (4 g) for epilepsy.

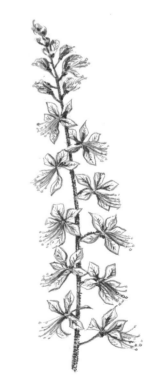

Dittany (White) DICTAMNUS ALBUS

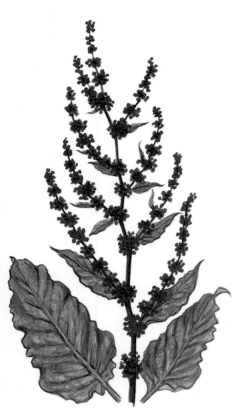

Dock (Common) RUMEX OBTUSIFOLIUS

DOCK (Common)

All docks being boiled with meat, make it boil the sooner.

This is the Round-leaved or Common Wayside Dock which produces large spreading leaves about a foot (30 cm) long, the whole plant reaching two or three feet (61 or 91 cm) in height. Also called the Broad-leaved Dock.

Where to find it: A common weed, but it likes rich soil. It grows at the roadside, by hedges, in fields and on waste land.

Flowering time: From late spring to mid autumn.

Astrology: All Docks are under Jupiter.

Medicinal virtues: The Red Dock, also known as Bloodwort, cleanseth the blood and strengthens the liver, but the Yellow Dock root is best used when either the blood or liver is affected by choler.

All the docks have a cooling, drying quality, Sorrel being most cold and the Bloodworts most drying. The Burdock has been dealt with already. The seed of the Dock doth stay laxes and fluxes of all sorts, and is helpful for those that spit blood.

The roots boiled in vinegar helpeth the itch, scabs and breaking out of the skin, if it be bathed therewith. The distilled water of the herb and roots cleanseth the skin from freckles, morphews and other spots and discolourings.

Modern uses: It is the Yellow Dock or Curled Dock (*Rumex crispus*) that is used in modern practice. It is widely employed as a blood purifier, a gentle laxative and as a tonic. All parts of the plant are used – root, leaves, seeds or the whole herb. It has many uses, but is mainly used in the treatment of eczema and psoriasis. It does, indeed, improve the quality of the blood, because it acts as an iron carrier.

An infusion of the dried powdered root is the best way to secure its properties as these are fully soluble in water. Use 1 oz (28 g) to 1 pt (568 ml) of boiling water and administer in doses of 2 fl oz (56 ml). A syrup can be made by using about 8 oz (227 g) of the crushed root to 1 pint (568 ml) of boiling water to which sugar or honey is added to thicken it. The medicine is also valuable in the treatment of rheumatism and gout. A fluid extract is available from herbalists.

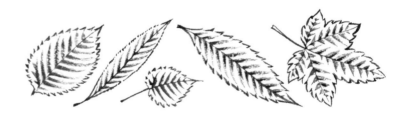

DODDER OF THYME

He is a physician indeed that hath wit enough to choose his Dodder according to the nature of the disease and humour peccant. We confess Thyme is the hottest herb it usually grows upon and therefore that which grows upon Thyme is hotter than that which grows upon colder herbs; for it draws nourishment from what it grows upon, as well as from the earth where its root is.

Dodder is a parasitic plant and a member of the Convolvulus family. Its stems are like threads, and it bears clusters of white or pinkish flowers but has no leaves. There are many Dodders, but Dodder of Thyme, also called Flax Dodder, is best.

Where to find it: Heaths and grassy places in most parts of the world.

Flowering time: Early summer to early autumn.

Astrology: All Dodders are under Saturn who is wise enough to have two strings to his bow.

Medicinal virtues: It is most effectual for melancholy diseases and to purge black or burnt choler, which is the cause of many diseases of the head and brain, as well as for the trembling of the heart, faintings and swoonings.

It is helpful in all diseases and griefs of the spleen and the melancholy that arises from the windiness of the hypochondrium. It purgeth also the reins or kidneys by urine. It openeth obstructions of the gall and profiteth them that have jaundice.

Dodders found growing upon Nettles hath by experience been found very effectual to procure plenty of urine, where it hath been stopped or hindered.

All the diseases that Saturn causes Dodder helps by sympathy, and strengthens the parts that Saturn rules.

Modern uses: Dodder is a laxative and a liver tonic. It can be used for jaundice and sciatica. The whole plant is very bitter to the taste and an infusion acts as a purge. It is better to add a little ginger and pimento to the infusion of the stems. This acts as a tonic when the kidneys, spleen or liver are affected by any condition. Half an ounce (14 g) of the dried plant is boiled in 1 pt (568 ml) of water, strained and taken in doses of 1 fl oz (28 ml). The dose of the fluid extract when available is 30 drops.

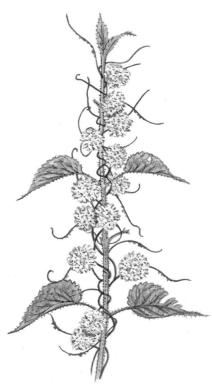

Dodder of Thyme CUSCUTA EPITHYMUM

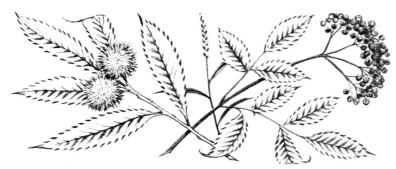

ROSA CANINA

DOG ROSE

The flowers of the Wild Briar are accounted more restringent than the Garden Roses and by some are reckoned as a specific for the excess of the catamenia.

The leaves of the Dog Rose are smoother and greener than are Garden Roses. The flowers are white or pale red. The seed vessels are round and red and full of pulp and the white seeds are cornered.

Where to find it: In hedges.

Flowering time: Late spring, early summer. The seed is ripe in early autumn.

Astrology: It is under the dominion of the Moon.

Medicinal virtues: The pulp of the hips has a pleasant acidity. It strengthens the stomach, cools the heat of fevers, is good for coughs and the spitting of blood and for scurvy.

The seed has been known to do great things against the stone and gravel. The best way of preserving its virtues is by keeping it conserved.

Modern uses: The leaves have been used as a substitute for tea. Rose hip tea may be purchased from health stores. The 'pleasant acidity' is due to the hips containing citric acid, malic acid and ascorbic acid (vitamin C) which explains why it is 'good for the scurvy'. The hips can be eaten or made into a jam, or syrup. Rose hip syrup is especially good for infants and young children as a nutritional supplement. The seeds are diuretic, and when dried and powdered they can be used as a remedy for urinary stones. Use about a teaspoonful in water.

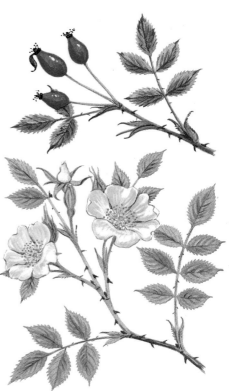

Dog Rose ROSA CANINA

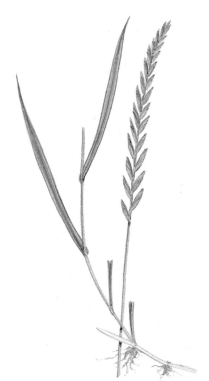

Dog's Grass
ELYMUS (= AGROPYRUM) REPENS

ELYMUS (= AGROPYRUM) REPENS
DOG'S GRASS

Watch the dogs when they are sick and they will quickly lead you to it . . . and although a gardener be of another opinion, yet a physician holds that an acre (0.4 hectare) of them be worth five acres (1.6 hectares) of Carrots twice told over.

Grasses provide food as cereals, as well as medicines. This is better known as Couchgrass, or Twitch, and formerly had the botanical name of *Triticum repens*. It has a creeping underground stem with small fibres at every joint and is very sweet to taste.

Where to find it: It grows in fields and on waste ground and is a menace to the farmer as it prefers ploughed ground.

Flowering time: Early summer to early autumn.

Astrology: It is under the dominion of Jupiter.

Medicinal virtues: The roots boiled and drunk openeth obstructions of the liver and gall, and the stopping of the urine. It easeth griping pains in the belly and inflammations. The seed expels the urine more powerfully, and stayeth laxes and vomiting. The distilled water alone, or with a little worm-seed, killeth worms in children.

The way to use it is to bruise the roots and, having well boiled them in wine, drink the decoction. It is opening, but not purging, very safe.

Modern uses: A popular and widely used herb in modern medical practice. It increases production of urine, but it is also soothing to the urinary tract. It contains an antibiotic substance and these properties together make it an ideal remedy for cystitis or other inflammatory disease of the urinary tract. It has also been found helpful to those with gout or rheumatism.

A decoction using about 1 oz (28 g) of the root to 1½ pt (852 ml) of water and boiling down to 1 pt (568 ml), can be taken in doses from ½–2 fl oz (14–56 ml), depending on the severity of the disease. The tincture or fluid extract is available from herbalists.

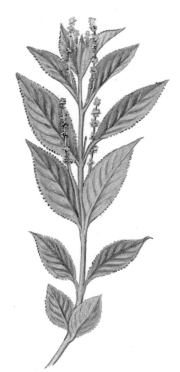

Dog's Mercury MERCURIALIS PERENNIS

MERCURIALIS PERENNIS
DOG'S MERCURY

This is a rank poisonous plant.

This plant grows about a foot (30 cm) high and its leaves are large. The stalk is round, thick and a little hairy.

Where to find it: It is commonly found under hedges.

Flowering time: Spring.

Astrology: It belongs to Mercury.

Medicinal virtues: This species has been confused with others of the same name, with which it has been thought to agree in nature. But there is not a more fatal plant than this.

The common herbals, as Gerard's and Parkinson's, instead of cautioning their readers against the use of this plant, after some trifling, idle observations upon the qualities of Mercury in general, dismiss the article without noticing its baneful effects.

Other writers have done this, but they have written in Latin, a language not very likely to inform those who stand most in need of this caution.

Modern uses: Dog's Mercury is certainly poisonous if used fresh, and has proved fatal to animals and humans. Its action on the body is purgative and diuretic. Homoeopaths make a tincture from the fresh plant which they use for rheumatism and gastro-intestinal upsets. It is not used by herbalists and not recommended for domestic use.

DOG'S TOOTH VIOLET

A very powerful remedy, and a small dose will take effect.

A very pretty plant with two broad leaves and a drooping flower. It grows five or six inches (13 or 15 cm) high. The leaves enclose a round, slender, weak stalk, green at the top and often white at the bottom. The flower is large and white with a tinge of red. It is long and hollow and hangs down. A very elegant plant.

Where to find it: A garden plant, but is also found in damp, open woodlands.

Flowering time: Early summer.

Astrology: It is governed by the Moon.

Medicinal virtues: The freshly gathered roots are good against the worms in children and quickly ease the pains of the belly which the worms produce. The expressed juice is best; but if children will not take it, the roots should be boiled in milk. It is best to begin with a very small dose; and if that is well borne, to increase the quantity.

Modern uses: *Erythronium americanum* is the variety now used. This is commonly known as American Adder's Tongue as well as Dog's Tooth Violet. English Adder's Tongue (*Ophioglossum vulgatum*) is dealt with separately in this book under Adder's Tongue. The American herb has a yellow flower. It is emetic, emollient and anti-scrofulous. The herb is mainly used externally as small internal doses cause vomiting. A poultice is made from the fresh leaves and applied to tumours, swellings and ulcers to stimulate healing. It is not recommended for internal use domestically.

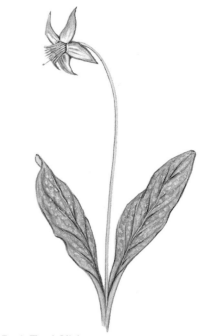

Dog's Tooth Violet
ERYTHRONIUM DENS CANIS

DOVE'S-FOOT

The decoction in wine fomented to any place pained with gout, or to joint-ache, or pains of the sinews, giveth much ease.

This has several small, round, pale green leaves, cut about the edges like Mallows, standing upon long reddish, hairy stalks. The small, bright red flowers are followed by seed pods shaped like small, short beaks, just like other sorts of this herb which we now known as Cranesbill.

Where to find it: In pastures and by the sides of paths. It also grows in gardens.

Flowering time: From mid spring to early autumn.

Astrology: A very gentle, though martial plant.

Medicinal virtues: It is found by experience to be singularly good for colicky wind and to expel the stone and gravel in the kidneys. The decoction in wine is excellent for those that have inward wounds, hurts or bruises, to stay the bleeding, to dissolve and expel the congealed blood, and to heal the parts. It is also used to cleanse and heal outward sores, ulcers and fistulas. For small wounds many just bruise the herb and apply it to the place.

The powder or decoction of the herb taken for some time is good for ruptures and burstings in either young or old.

Modern uses: Medical herbalists now prefer to use the American Wild Cranesbill (*Geranium maculatum*), which is also known as Dove's-foot. The root and herb are both styptic and therefore excellent for internal haemorrhage. Use the fluid extract of the root when available. The root is more astringent but for simple diarrhoea an infusion of the herb, 1 oz (28 g) to 1 pt (568 ml) of boiling water, can be used. For leucorrhoea, a vaginal injection or douche is prepared from an infusion of 1 oz (28 g) of the root. This can be combined in equal parts with an infusion of Beth root (*Trillium pendulum*), which is also indicated for this condition. The treatment is given night and morning. The fluid extract can be taken internally as well. The dose varies between 30 and 60 drops, according to the severity of the condition.

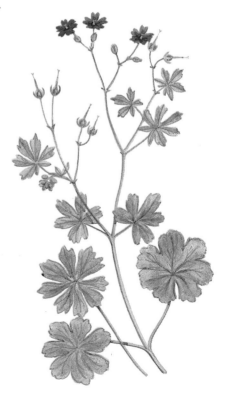

Dove's-foot GERANIUM MOLLE

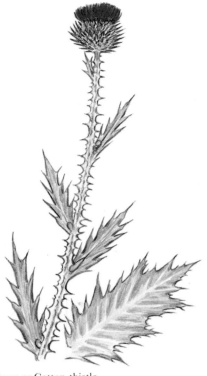

Down or Cotton-thistle
ONOPORDUM ACANTHIUM

ONOPORDUM ACANTHIUM

DOWN or COTTON-THISTLE

Though it may hurt your finger, it will help your body.

This has large leaves covered with a white cotton down and purplish flowers. The prickles are sharp and cruel. It has become known as the Scotch Thistle, although it is not the one depicted on the badge of the Stuart kings.

Where to find it: Roadside, waste ground and fields.

Flowering time: Midsummer to early autumn.

Astrology: Mars owns the plant.

Medicinal virtues: Pliny and Dioscorides say the leaves and roots taken in drink help those that have a crick in their neck, such that they cannot turn their neck without turning their whole body (surely they do not mean those that have a crick in their neck by being under the hangman's hand).

Galen said the roots and leaves are of a healing quality and good for those that have their bodies drawn together by some spasm or convulsion, as it is with children that have rickets – or, as the College of Physicians will have it, rachites. It is the name of the disease they have set forth lately in a particular treatise for public view. The world may now see that they have taken much pains to little purpose.

Modern uses: The juice has been used by some practitioners as an application for tumours and ulcers with some success, but there is insufficient evidence of its efficacy. The juice was, however, specific in ancient times for cancerous complaints.

The decoction of the root – 1 oz (28 g) to 1½ pts (852 ml) of water boiled down to 1 pt (568 ml) and strained – is used as an astringent in doses of 2 fl oz (56 ml) to reduce catarrhal discharges.

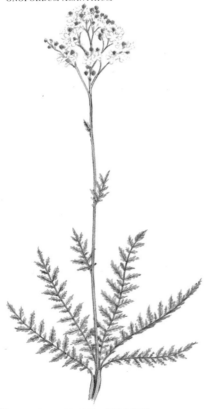

Dropwort FILIPENDULA VULGARIS

FILIPENDULA VULGARIS

DROPWORT

Good for the stone, gravel, and stoppage of urine.

The roots of the Dropwort resemble Dahlia tubers. The stalks grow to about a foot (30 cm) high and bear many pretty flowers in the shape of an umbel. They are white on the inside and red on the outside.

Where to find it: A perennial of calcareous grassland.

Flowering time: It flowers in early summer.

Astrology: It is accounted under Venus.

Medicinal virtues: The root is used to provoke the urine and therefore is good for those with the stone.

Modern uses: There are several plants bearing the name of Dropwort and most of them are poisonous. The root of *Filipendula vulgaris* contains a slightly poisonous glycoside. The Water Hemlock (*Oenanthe crocata*) is also known as Dropwort. It grows in ditches and in stagnant water, and is one of the most poisonous plants, causing death within three hours. The Water Dropwort (*Oenanthe aquatica*) is less poisonous. A homoeopathic tincture of the seeds is used in doses of a few drops for the treatment of coughs, flatulence and urinary tract disorders. The common Tubular Water Dropwort is known botanically as *Oenanthe fistulosa*. Because of the confusion that can arise in discerning the poisonous varieties from the innocuous, it is recommended that they are not used as herbal medicines domestically.

ROSA RUBIGINOSA

EGLANTINE

Excellent for alopecia or falling of the hair.

This is one of the wild Roses, better known today as the Sweet Briar. The flowers are smaller than those of the Dog Rose, previously described.

Where to find it: It grows wild in woodland, on the edges of fields and is also cultivated in gardens.

Flowering time: It buds in early spring and flowers during summer.

Astrology: It is under the dominion of Jupiter.

Medicinal virtues: It is the spongy apples found upon the Eglantine that are used for alopecia. They are pounded to a paste and mixed with honey and wood-ashes and applied to the scalp. Dried, powdered and taken in white wine, they will remove strangury and strengthen the kidneys. Boiled in a strong decoction of the roots, they are good for venomous bites.

The hips, made into a conserve and eaten occasionally, gently bind the belly, stop defluxions of the head and stomach, help digestion, sharpen the appetite, and dry up the moisture of cold rheum and phlegm upon the stomach. The powder of the dried pulp of the hips is good for leucorrhoea and if mixed with the powder of the spongy apples, and given in small quantities, will be found good for colic and to destroy worms.

Modern uses: The Sweet Briar is often mistaken by collectors for the Dog Rose and is used for the same purposes. See Dog Rose.

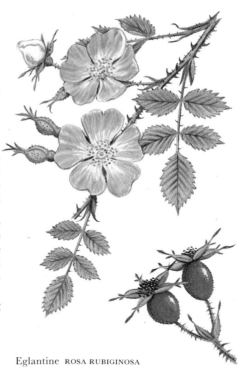

Eglantine ROSA RUBIGINOSA

SAMBUCUS NIGRA

ELDER

The juice of the leaves snuffed up into the nostrils, purges the tunicles of the brain.

A common tree with spreading branches and oval, sharp-pointed leaves serrated about the edges. The flowers grow in large flat umbels and are followed by small, round, deep purple berries, full of juice.

Where to find it: In hedgerows and moist places.

Flowering time: Late spring. The berries are ripe in early autumn.

Astrology: It is under the dominion of Venus.

Medicinal virtues: The bark, leaves, flowers and berries all have medicinal properties. The first shoots to appear, boiled like Asparagus, and also the young leaves and stalks boiled in fat broth, carry forth phlegm and choler.

The middle or inward bark boiled in water and given in drink works much more violently. The berries, either green or dry, expel the same humour. They are also often given with good success to help the dropsy. The bark of the root boiled in wine, or the juice thereof drank, is more powerful than the leaves or fruit.

The juice of the root causes vomiting and purges the watery humours of the dropsy. A decoction of the root mollifies the hardness of the mother, if women sit thereon, and opens their veins and brings down their courses. The berries boiled in wine perform the same effect. The juice of the green leaves applied to hot inflammations of the eyes assuages them. The decoction of the berries in wine provokes urine.

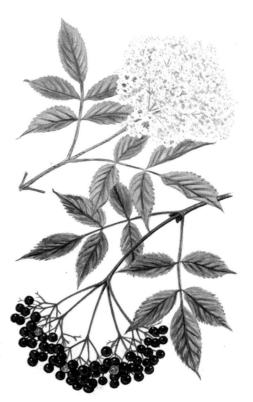

Elder SAMBUCUS NIGRA

65

The leaves or flowers distilled in the month of May and the legs washed with it takes away ulcers and sores. The hands washed with it helps the shaking of them and the palsy.

Modern uses: A valuable remedy in modern herbal medicine. The bark, flowers and berries are all used and are available from herbalists. The berries, rich in vitamin C, are used to make wine or juice; either taken hot is a traditional remedy for colds. Elderflowers mixed with Peppermint herb and made into an infusion – 1 oz (28 g) to 1 pt (568 ml) of water – is taken in doses of 2 fl oz (56 ml) for 'flu. Elderflower water, which can be made by adding eight drops of the essential oil to 1 pt (568 ml) of distilled water, is used in eye and skin lotions. It keeps the complexion clear of freckles and other blemishes.

The leaves are used to make a soothing ointment. They are combined in equal parts with red Poppy flowers and 6 oz (170 g) of this mixture is simmered in 15 fl oz (426 ml) of olive oil. This is then strained and 5 oz (142 g) of melted white paraffin wax is added. The ointment is then allowed to cool. It is suitable for bruises, sprains and chilblains.

An infusion of the bark is laxative and diuretic. It is given in small doses over a period of time to purify the blood.

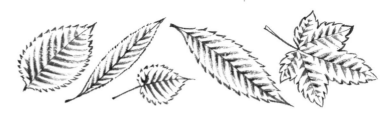

SAMBUCUS EBULUS

ELDER (Dwarf)

The berries are of admirable use in recent colds, and beginning of feverish heats, in which cases nothing is so proper as the juice, without any addition, boiled over a very gentle fire to the consistence of an extract; this is commonly called the Rob of Elder, but is rarely made by apothecaries, though vastly superior to the syrup which is constantly kept in the shops.

The Dwarf Elder is a pretty looking plant which produces umbels of white flowers followed by round black berries.

Where to find it: Waste places and roadsides. Not so frequently found in hedges as the Elder.

Flowering time: Mid to late summer. The berry ripens in the autumn.

Astrology: Under the dominion of Venus.

Medicinal virtues: A more powerful remedy than the Common Elder in opening and purging choler, phlegm and water. It helps the gout, piles and women's diseases, colours the hair black, helps inflammation of the eyes and pain in the ears, bites, burns and scaldings, wind, colic and stone and difficulty in producing urine, and cures old sores and fistulous ulcers.

The bark and seeds are in most repute for jaundice and dropsy. A decoction of the root and seeds is commended, but proper correctors should be added as otherwise it will be very violent in its operation. The expressed oil of the seed is used outwardly to assuage the pain of gout.

The flowers are sudorific and anodyne. Infused in sharp vinegar, with the addition of some spices, they make a more reviving liquor to smell and to rub the temples with in faintings of women in labour and after delivery, than all the volatile salts put together.

Take half a pound (227 g) of Elderflowers, four ounces (113 g) each of red Roses, Rosemary and Lavender, three drams (5 g) of Cinnamon and two drams (3.5 g) each of Nutmeg and Cloves. Pour on five pints (2.8 l) of the sharpest white wine vinegar and infuse a month or six weeks. Press it out well, let the liquor settle and put it into well-stoppered bottles for use.

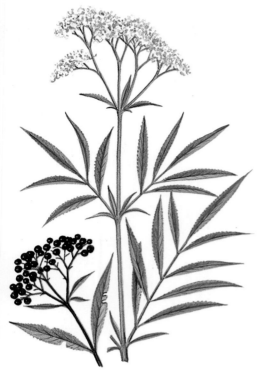

Elder (Dwarf) SAMBUCUS EBULUS

The juice of the berries mixed with a third by weight of genuine liquorice powder, with a few drops of Oil of Aniseeds, and boiled to a proper consistence, is a far better remedy on account of its acidity, for cutting the phlegm, and taking off the irritation to cough, than the juice of our liquorice, or the Spanish juice alone.

Modern uses: Because of its drastic action only the leaves are used. The berries are toxic and should not be confused by amateur collectors with those of the Common Elder. The root is also a drastic purgative.

A decoction of the leaves induces sweating, steps up urine production, clears mucus from the respiratory tract, but is also purgative. Herbalists have used it with success in cardiac oedema, but it is not recommended for domestic use. The Common Elder is far more suitable.

Note: The plant known as Dwarf Elder in the United States is an entirely different plant, *Aralia hispida*.

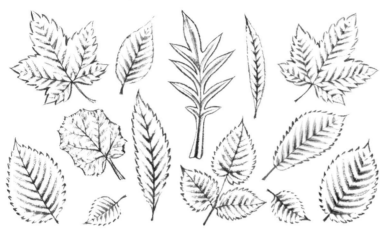

INULA HELENIUM

ELECAMPANE
One of the most beneficial roots nature affords for the help of the consumptive.

A robust and stately perennial plant, commonly known as the Wild Sunflower and also called Elfwort. The root, which is long and large, contains the virtues of the plant.

Where to find it: Moist grounds and shadowy places. It is also grown in herbaceous borders.

Flowering time: Early to midsummer. The seed is ripe in late summer.

Astrology: It is under Mercury.

Medicinal virtues: It is good for all diseases of the chest and has great virtues in malignant fevers. It strengthens the stomach and assists digestion as it is a warm, invigorating medicine. It has not its equal in the cure of whooping cough when all other medicines fail.

The fresh roots preserved with sugar, or made into a syrup, help the cough, shortness of breath and wheezing in the lungs. The powdered root taken with sugar is profitable for those who have their urine stopped, for stone in the reins, kidneys or bladder, for the stopping of women's courses and pains of the mother. It resists poison and stays the spreading of putrid, pestilential fevers and the plague itself.

Modern uses: The root contains inulin, otherwise known as diabetic sugar. The root is used as an expectorant, diuretic and diaphoretic. It is taken as a decoction – 1 oz (28 g) of root to 1 pt (568 ml) of boiling water – in doses of 2 fl oz (56 ml) It can be combined in equal parts with other remedies indicated for coughs, asthma and bronchitis, such as Colt's Foot and Horehound. A liquid extract of the root is available from herbalists.

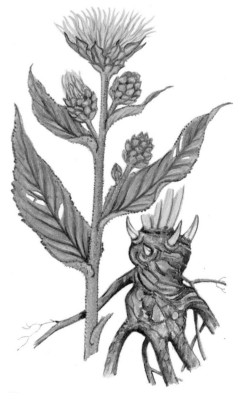

Elecampane INULA HELENIUM

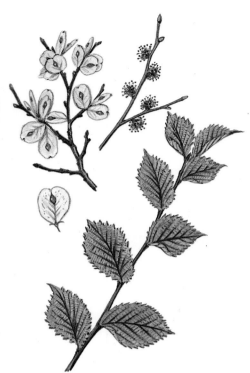

Elm Tree ULMUS MINOR

ULMUS MINOR
ELM TREE
The leaves thereof bruised and applied heal wounds.

This Elm has a rough thick bark and the branches are clothed with rough, crenated green leaves.

Where to find it: Woods and hedgerows. Dutch Elm disease has depleted the numbers of this tree in recent years.

Flowering time: The small flowers appear in early spring before the leaves.

Astrology: A cold and saturnine plant.

Medicinal virtues: The leaves or the bark used with vinegar cure scurf and leprosy very effectually. Bathing with a decoction of the leaves, bark or root, heals broken bones. The decoction of the bark of the root mollifies hard tumours and the shrinking of the sinews.

Modern uses: The bark is soothing and diuretic and is mainly used to treat dropsy. A decoction is made by using 1 oz (28 g) of bark to 8 fl oz (227 ml) of water and boiling for 10 minutes. Add water to make up to the original 8 fl oz (227 ml). The dose is 1 fl oz (28 ml). The decoction is slightly astringent and can be used as a lotion for skin diseases, such as ringworm. Homoeopaths make a tincture from the bark which they use for skin eruptions and ulcerated conditions.

One of the most important remedies in herbal medicine is the Slippery Elm (*Ulmus fulva*), an American tree. The bark has similar properties to the Common Elm, but is superior. The powdered bark is used as a nutritious drink for those with inflammatory bowel disease, or for bronchitis. It is healing and soothing to mucous membranes. A teaspoonful of the powder is added to 1 pt (568 ml) of boiling water, infused for a few minutes and strained. It can be taken freely. Slippery Elm tablets and commercial versions of the gruel are generally available from health stores.

Because it is nutritious, Slippery Elm infusion – 1 oz (28 g) of powdered bark to 1 pt (568 ml) of water – has been injected into the bowel in serious cases of diarrhoea and dysentery where other treatments have failed.

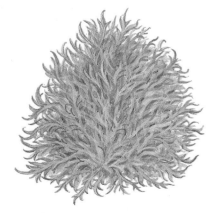

Endive CICHORIUM ENDIVIA

CICHORIUM ENDIVIA
ENDIVE
For faintings, swoonings, and the passions of the heart.

A well-known plant which is used as a vegetable. It bears a longer and larger leaf than Succory (*Cichorium intybus*), but it has similar blue flowers.

Where to find it: It is cultivated in gardens in the West, having originated in Asia. Succory or Wild Chicory is found growing on light, sandy soils, waste land, open borders of fields and roadsides.

Flowering time: Midsummer to early autumn.

Astrology: It is a herb of Jupiter.

Medicinal virtues: A fine, cooling, cleansing plant. The decoction of the leaves, or the juice, or the distilled water of Endive cools the excessive heat of the liver and stomach, and other inflammations. It cools the heat and sharpness of the urine and excoriations. The seeds are rather more powerful. Outwardly applied they serve to temper the sharp humours of fretting ulcers, hot tumours and swellings and pestilential sores. They greatly assist redness and inflammation of the eyes, dimness of the sight and pains of the gout.

Modern uses: The cultivated Endive is not regarded as being of much therapeutic value and the Wild Chicory is preferred. It is, however, a useful salad food. See Succory.

ERYNGO

The roots bruised and applied outwardly, helps the kernels of the throat, commonly called the king's-evil.

Eryngo, or Sea Holly, has large white and long roots. The leaves terminate in prickles and the flowers are blue.

Where to find it: It grows in coastal areas and in sandy places.

Flowering time: Mid to late summer.

Astrology: It is hot and moist and under the Celestial balance.

Medicinal virtues: The plant is venereal and breeds seed exceedingly. It strengthens the procreative spirit. The decoction of the root in wine opens obstructions of the spleen and liver, helps yellow jaundice, dropsy, pain in the loins, wind and colic, and provokes urine, expels the stone and procures women's courses.

Taking the decoction for 15 days, morning and night, helps the strangury, the voiding of urine by drops, the stopping of urine and stone, and all defects of the reins and kidneys. Taken for longer it cures the stone. The juice of the leaves dropped into the ears, help imposthumes therein.

Modern uses: Eryngo root is mainly used for urethritis, cystitis and strangury, but it is also an expectorant and diaphoretic, and can be used for chronic coughs and pulmonary complaints. The fluid extract available from herbalists is taken in doses of 15 to 30 drops. The decoction is made by boiling 1 oz (28 g) of the root in 1 pt (568 ml) of water. The dose is 1–2 fl oz (28–56 ml).

The Field Eryngo (*Eryngium campestre*) has similar properties and may be supplied as Eryngo root if ordered from a herbalist.

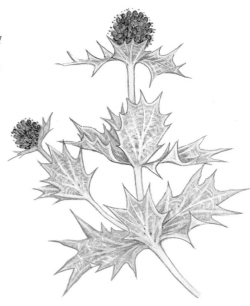

Eryngo ERYNGIUM MARITIMUM

EVEWEED or DOUBLE ROCKET

Some eat it with bread and butter on account of its taste, which resembles Garlick.

Better known these days as Dame's Violet, this plant grows with a round, upright firm stalk, but the top of it usually droops. The leaves are dented along the edges and sharp at the point. The flowers are large, sometimes white and blue, or pinkish-purple.

Where to find it: In scattered places where it has escaped from the garden. It naturalises itself in meadows and hedgerows.

Flowering time: Late spring to midsummer.

Astrology: A plant of Mars.

Medicinal virtues: It is accounted a good wound herb. Its juice, taken a spoonful at a time, is excellent against obstructions of the viscera. It works by the urine. In some places it is a constant ingredient in clysters.

Modern uses: The plant is edible and should be used before flowering. For medicinal purposes the whole plant is collected when it is in flower, dried and powdered. Doses of 15–30 grains (0.98–2 g) were administered in water to prevent scurvy. A larger dose is emetic and can be used to replace Ipecacuanha. One of the reasons for including emetics in medicines is to prevent the patient from taking an overdose. Another is to clear the stomach of mucus by inducing vomiting.

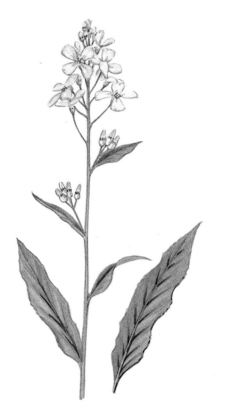

Eveweed or Double Rocket
HESPERIS MATRONALIS

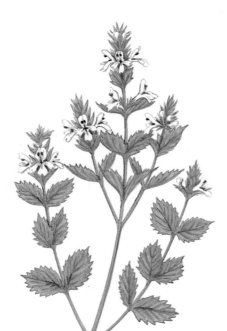

Eyebright EUPHRASIA OFFICINALIS

EUPHRASIA OFFICINALIS

EYEBRIGHT

Helps restore the sight decayed through age. Arnoldus de Villa Nova says it has restored the sight to them that have been blind a long time before. If the herb was as much used as it is neglected, it would half spoil the spectacle maker's trade.

The common Eyebright is a small low herb, usually with one blackish-green stalk, but with many branches spreading from the bottom. The flowers are small and white, steeped with purple and yellow spots or stripes.

Where to find it: In meadows and grassy places and in mountainous regions.

Flowering time: Summer.

Astrology: Under the sign of the Lion, and Sol claims dominion over it.

Medicinal virtues: The juice or distilled water of Eyebright, taken inwardly in white wine or broth, or dropped into the eyes, helps all infirmities of the eyes that cause dimness of the sight. A conserve of the flowers has the same effect. It also helps a weak brain or memory.

Modern uses: Eyebright is probably more popular today than at any previous time. No herbal dispensary is likely to be without it. It is the remedy of choice for inflammatory eye disease. An infusion is made by adding one teaspoonful of the herb to a cup of boiling water for 30 minutes. This is strained and used as an eye lotion. Compresses soaked in the lotion when cold can be applied to the eyes. Some herbalists recommend combining Eyebright with Fennel in equal parts for eye conditions. Tinctures and fluid extracts are available. The infusion of Eyebright is also useful for hay fever, catarrh and nasal congestion. The homoeopathic tincture made from the fresh flowering plant is used for conjunctivitis and other eye infections. A few drops of the tincture are mixed with 2 fl oz (56 ml) Rose-water and used as a lotion.

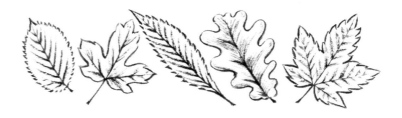

DRABA INCANA

FAVEREL (Wooly)

Commended by the ancients against the sciatica.

An annual, or biennial, growing to about 18 inches (46 cm). The leaves grow in tufts at the bottom of the stem. They are pointed, rough and harsh to touch. The flowers are star-like, white with tiny yellow centres.

Where to find it: Cliffs, rocks and screes.

Flowering time: Mid spring to early summer.

Astrology: Under the dominion of the Moon.

Medicinal virtues: The leaves and roots are beaten into a cataplasm with hog's lard and applied to painful parts caused by sciatica. Men should keep the cataplasm in place for four hours, women for two. After removing it, the place should be washed with wine and oil.

Modern uses: A rare plant and therefore not available for medical use. Plasters made from Comfrey root, or from Capsicum and Lobelia, are now more popular in the treatment of sciatica. Plasters are made by digesting the powdered herbs in oil and wax, dipping strips of linen into the molten mass, and allowing to cool. Internal treatment could include infusions of Couch-grass, Broom, Burdock and Tansy.

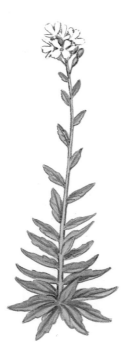

Faverel (Wooly) DRABA INCANA

FOENICULUM VULGARE

FENNEL

The leaves or seed, boiled in Barley-water, and drunk, are good for nurses to increase their milk, and make it more wholesome for the child.

Fennel has a distinctive smell rather like Aniseed. The roots are large, thick and white, the leaves are winged and the small, yellow flowers at the top of the four-foot (1.2-m) stem are in flat umbels.

Where to find it: Waste places, roadsides and sea cliffs. It is also cultivated in gardens.

Flowering time: Early to midsummer.

Astrology: An herb of Mercury under Virgo and bearing antipathy to Pisces.

Medicinal virtues: Fennel is good to break wind, provoke urine, ease the pains of the stone and to help break it. The leaves, or rather the seeds, boiled in water, stays the hiccough and soothes the stomach of sick and feverish persons. The seed boiled in wine is good for those that have eaten poisonous herbs or mushrooms. The seed, or roots, help to open obstructions of the liver, spleen and gall, and ease painful and windy swellings and help the yellow jaundice, the gout and cramps.

The seed helps shortness of the breath and wheezing, by stopping the lungs. The leaves, seeds and roots are much used in drink or broth to make people lean that are too fat.

The distilled water of the whole herb dropped into the eyes cleanses them from mists and films that hinder the sight.

Modern uses: The seeds are mainly used as a flavouring agent in medicines and to disperse flatulence. It is an ingredient of the official compound powder of liquorice. Added to a laxative, it prevents griping. A gripe water can be made by adding eight drops of Oil of Fennel to 1 pt (568 ml) of distilled water and shaking. The dose ranges from one to eight teaspoonfuls. Fennel tea, also for flatulence, is made by pouring ½ pt (284 ml) of boiling water on to one teaspoonful of the seeds and allowed to infuse. This tea will also help produce milk for nursing mothers.

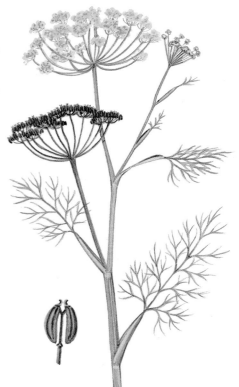

Fennel FOENICULUM VULGARE

PEUCEDANUM OFFICINALE

FENNEL (Sow or Hog's)

A little of the juice dissolved in wine, and dropped into the ears, eases much of the pains in them, and put into a hollow tooth, easeth the pains thereof.

It grows to about three feet (91 cm), with somewhat long leaves and tufts of yellow flowers. The seed is larger than Fennel seed. It is also called Hoar-strange, Hoar-strong, Sulphur-wort and Brimstone-wort.

Where to find it: On banks by the sea.

Flowering time: Mid to late summer.

Astrology: A herb of Mercury.

Medicinal virtues: The juice, say Dioscorides and Galen, used with vinegar and Rose-water, put to the nose, helps those that are troubled with lethargy, frenzy, giddiness of the head, the falling-sickness, long and inveterate headache, palsy, sciatica and the cramp.

The juice dissolved in wine, or put into an egg, is good for a cough, or shortness of breath and for those that are troubled with wind in the body. It purges the belly gently, expels the hardness of the spleen, gives ease to women that have sore travail in childbirth and easeth the pains of the reins and bladder, and also the womb.

Modern uses: A fairly rare plant and, therefore, not in general use. It resembles Dill more than Fennel, and either can be used as a substitute. Russian herbalists have used the powdered herbs as a remedy for epilepsy.

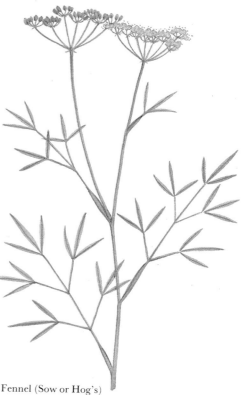

Fennel (Sow or Hog's)
PEUCEDANUM OFFICINALE

FENNEL FLOWER

It helps the tertian and quartan agues.

An annual plant, known commonly nowadays as Love in a Mist. It is not related to Fennel. The flowers are blue.

Where to find it: It is grown in gardens, but originated in Syria.

Flowering time: Early to midsummer.

Astrology: This is also under Mercury.

Medicinal virtues: Only the seed is used. It is accounted heating and drying and said to provoke the urine. But it is seldom used.

Modern uses: The seeds are diuretic, carminative and anti-parasitical, but are more in use as a spice than a herbal medicine. They are used as a pepper and for seasoning curries. Homoeopaths make a tincture from the seed for digestive and bowel complaints.

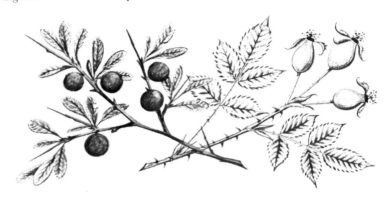

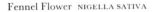

Fennel Flower NIGELLA SATIVA

TRIGONELLA FOENUM-GRAECUM

FENUGREEK

The decoction, or broth of the seed, drank with a little vinegar, expels and purges all superfluous humours which cleave to the bowels.

An annual herb, about two feet (61 cm) high, with tender stalks, yellow or pale whitish flowers and yellowish seeds. Also called Greek Hayes.

Where to find it: It is grown in gardens, but is mainly found in the Middle East and Mediterranean.

Flowering time: Midsummer.

Astrology: It is under the influence of Mercury.

Medicinal virtues: The decoction, made with dates, and afterwards made into a syrup with honey, cleanses the breast, chest and lungs and may be taken with success for any complaint thereof, except a fever or a headache, as it will increase rather than alleviate those disorders.

It is good for women afflicted with an imposthume, ulcer, or stoppage in the matrix, to sit in a decoction of the seeds. A suppository made of the juice, and conveyed to the neck of the matrix, will mollify and soften all hardness thereof.

Modern uses: One of the oldest medicinal plants and still a very useful article in herbal practice. Fenugreek tea made from the seeds is used as a gargle in sore throats and for fevers. The drink is mucilaginous, nutritious, and soothing to the intestinal canal. It is made by pouring 1 pt (568 ml) of boiling water on to 1 oz (28 g) of the seeds, and allowing them to infuse for a few minutes.

Poultices are made from the powdered seeds to which powdered charcoal can be added. They are effective for wounds, ulcers and boils.

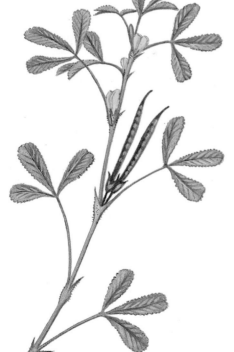

Fenugreek TRIGONELLA FOENUM-GRAECUM

FERN (Brake or Bracken)

The leaves are dangerous for women with child to meddle with by reason they cause abortions.

Bracken issues forth its stems and leaves from an underground rhizome.

Where to find it: All over the world on commons, moors and heathland.

Flowering time: It flowers not, being a fern, but is green all summer.

Astrology: Under the dominion of Mercury.

Medicinal virtues: The roots bruised and boiled in mead, or honeyed water, and drunk, kills both the broad and long worms in the body, and abates the swelling and hardness of the spleen.

The green leaves eaten, purge the belly, and expel choleric and waterish humours that trouble the stomach. The roots, bruised and boiled in oil, make an ointment to heal wounds or pricks in the flesh. The powdered roots dry up malignant moisture in foul ulcers, and cause a speedier healing.

Modern uses: Because use of the plant can induce abortion, it is not recommended for domestic use. It is also purgative. Herbalists have many other safer remedies at their disposal for gently stimulating bowel action and for clearing up ulcers. An agent which is suitable for both conditions is Goldenseal (*Hydrastis canadensis*) which is available in powder or tincture form from herbalists. A few drops of the tincture is taken internally for constipation, or added to distilled water to make a lotion for external ulcers.

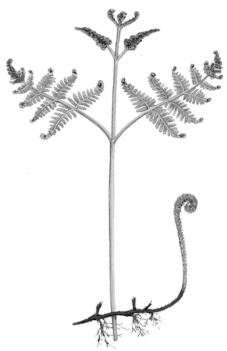

Fern (Brake or Bracken) PTERIDIUM AQUILINUM (= PTERIS AQUILINA)

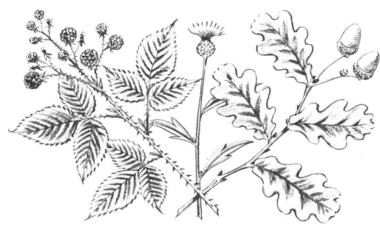

OSMUNDA REGALIS

FERN (Royal)

Singularly good in wounds, bruises, or the like.

This is the largest of the English ferns. It has several large, branched leaves with light yellowish-green pinnulae.

Where to find it: Moors, bogs and watery places.

Flowering time: It flowers not, being a fern, but is green all summer.

Astrology: Saturn owns the plant.

Medicinal virtues: It is much more effectual than other ferns, both for inward and outward uses. The decoction may be drunk or boiled into an ointment with oil, as a balsam or balm. It is good against bruises and bones broken or out of joint. It also gives much ease to the colic and splenetic diseases, ruptures and burstings.

Modern uses: The powdered roots may be made into an ointment by boiling in wax and straining and used for cuts and bruises. This is also a useful application for lumbago. Ointments made from Comfrey or Marigold are generally more popular at present.

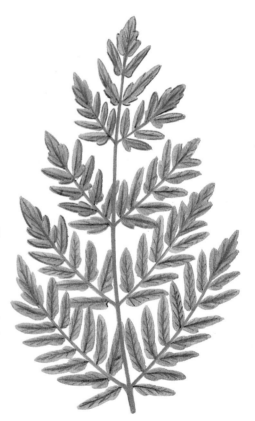

Fern (Royal) OSMUNDA REGALIS

FEVERFEW

Venus has commended this herb to succour her sisters, to be a general strengthener of their wombs, and to remedy such infirmities as a careless midwife has there caused.

Feverfew, also called Featherfew, is a perennial growing to about 18 inches (46 cm) high with many small white flowers, each with many yellow florets in the centre, rather like a Daisy.

Where to find it: A cultivated plant, but can be found wild near gardens and old walls.

Flowering time: Throughout the summer.

Astrology: Venus commands this herb.

Medicinal virtues: The herb boiled in white wine and drunk cleanses the womb, expels the afterbirth and does a woman all the good she can desire of any herb.

If anyone should grumble that they cannot get the herb in winter, tell them to make a syrup of it in the summer. It is chiefly used for the diseases of the mother, such as hardness or inflammations for which the syrup may be applied externally.

A decoction of the flowers in wine, with a little Nutmeg or Mace added, and drunk frequently during the day, is an approved method to bring down women's courses speedily.

The decoction of the herb made with sugar or honey helps the cough or stuffing of the chest due to colds. It also cleanses the reins and bladder and helps to expel the stone.

The powder of the herb taken in wine, with some Oxymel, purges both choler and phlegm, and is available for those that are short-winded, and are troubled with melancholy and heaviness, or sadness of spirits.

It is very effectual for all pains in the head coming of a cold cause, the herb being bruised and applied to the crown of the head. It will also relieve vertigo. The decoction drank warm, and the herb bruised, with a few corns of bay-salt, and applied to the wrists before the coming of the ague fits, does take them away.

Modern uses: Although the benefits of Feverfew have been known to herbalists for centuries, it is only recently that this herb has caught the imagination of people in general as an effective remedy for headaches and migraine. It is suggested that one or two leaves of Feverfew be included in a sandwich and eaten. Some people may be sensitive to Feverfew leaves and develop blisters in the mouth. The herbalists' method of using the herb in combination with other indicated herbs, like Chamomile which it strongly resembles, is to be recommended, rather than to isolate and remove the 'active' principles as has been suggested by some pharmacologists.

Feverfew is a febrifuge and will induce perspiration, thus lowering temperature in fevers. A hot infusion of 1 oz (28 g) of the flowers to 1 pt (568 ml) of boiling water is taken in teaspoonful doses, or a dose of the tincture available from herbalists is taken in hot water. It is recommended during labour as it regulates the contractions, and is indicated in cases of suppressed menstruation.

The tincture applied locally relieves the pain and irritation of insect bites. Made into a lotion by adding the tincture to distilled water and applying to the body, it protects against attack by flying insects. The dosage of the tincture for internal use is 10 to 30 drops.

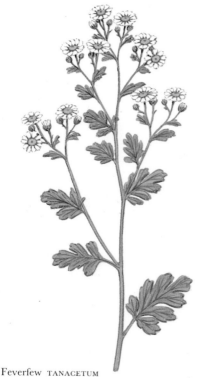

Feverfew TANACETUM
(= CHRYSANTHEMUM) PARTHENIUM

FEVERFEW (Corn)

This is a hateful weed to farmers; but yet it possesses virtues that may recompense all the damage it can do among the corn.

An annual herb, strongly aromatic, it often grows to 18 inches (46 cm) high. The flowers are large and white with a yellow disc in the centre. It is more commonly known today as the Wild Chamomile, because it so closely resembles Chamomile, previously described. It is also known as German Chamomile and Scented Mayweed.

Where to find it: Cornfields, gardens, waste ground and on banks.

Flowering time: Midsummer.

Astrology: A herb of the Sun.

Medicinal virtues: Similar to the flowers of the Chamomile, but with more cordial warmth. For those that have cold and weak stomachs, scarcely any thing equals them. They are best taken by infusion, like tea.

Modern uses: More widely used today than at any previous time, the Wild Chamomile has many important properties. It is a nerve relaxant, gastrointestinal tonic, carminative, anti-allergic, anti-spasmodic, and soothing and healing. It is still best taken as an infusion using ½ oz (14 g) of the dried flowers to 1 pt (568 ml) of boiling water. It is a useful remedy for teething troubles in infants and the infusion can be administered to children in teaspoonful doses. The infusion is also used as an enema and douche, and as a lotion or wash for cuts and bruises. It reduces inflammation and nerve pain. The herb infused in olive oil makes a useful massage oil. A tincture is available from herbalists.

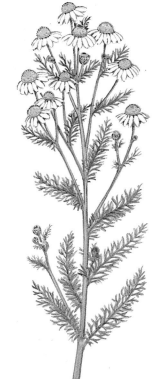

Feverfew (Corn) CHAMOMILLA RECUCITA
(= MATRICARIA CHAMOMILLA)

FICUS CARICA

FIG TREE

Figs are fitter for medicine than any other profit that is gotten by the fruit of them.

The trees may grow to 18 feet (5.5 m) and bear a fleshy inflorescence, which is neither flower nor fruit, and called a fig. The leaves are deeply lobed and deciduous.

Where to find it: A native of the Middle East, but grows wild throughout the Mediterranean. It is cultivated in gardens in milder regions, but the figs do not always ripen.

Flowering time: The fig ripens towards the end of the summer.

Astrology: The tree is under the dominion of Jupiter.

Medicinal virtues: The milk from the leaves or branches dropped upon warts takes them away. The decoction of the leaves clears the face of morphew and the body of white scurf, scabs and running sores. Dropped into old fretting ulcers, it cleanses them and brings up the flesh. Made into a syrup, a decoction of the leaves taken inwardly dissolves congealed blood caused by bruises or falls and helps the bloody flux. The juice dropped into a hollow tooth eases pain, and dropped into the ears relieves deafness and pain and noises in them. A syrup made of the leaves or green fruits is excellent for coughs, hoarseness or shortness of breath and all diseases of the chest and lungs. It is also very good for dropsy and falling-sickness.

Modern uses: The fig is laxative, but also soothing and nutritious. Syrup of Figs is a mild laxative which can be given to children. The stronger Compound Syrup of Figs contains Figs, Senna and Rhubarb, and is more suitable for adults. These preparations are official and obtainable from pharmacies. The milky juice will remove warts if applied to them. The soft, pulp interior of roasted figs can be applied as a poultice to boils and carbuncles.

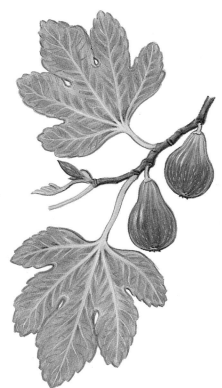

Fig Tree FICUS CARICA

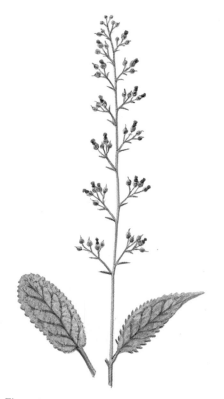

SCROPHULARIA NODOSA
FIGWORT

A better remedy cannot be for the king's-evil, because the Moon that rules the disease is exalted there.

A perennial woodland plant with square stems, oval leaves and purple flowers. Also known as Throatwort.

Where to find it: Moist and shadowy woods and in the lower parts of fields and meadows.

Flowering time: Midsummer.

Astrology: Venus owns the herb.

Medicinal virtues: The decoction of the herb taken inwardly, and the bruised herb applied outwardly, dissolved clotted and congealed blood coming from wounds, bruises and falls; and is no less effectual for the king's-evil, or any other knobs, kernels, bunches or wens growing in the flesh. It is also useful for haemorrhoids.

Modern uses: An important remedy in modern herbal practice, its main action is diuretic. The whole herb is used as a tonic for the kidneys and pelvic organs. Large doses are purgative and emetic. An infusion can be used as a fomentation for sprains, swellings, and abscesses, such as boils and carbuncles. An ointment made by digesting the herb in hot wax and straining is excellent for skin eruptions and irritating conditions such as eczema, piles and pruritus vulvae. Taken internally the infusion – 1 oz (28 g) of the herb to 1 pt (568 ml) of boiling water – or tincture purifies the blood and regulates menstruation. It is a rich source of manganese. Dose of the infusion is 1 fl oz (28 ml) two or three times a day.

The fresh plant tincture used by homoeopaths is recommended for conjunctivitis, mastitis and piles.

Figwort SCROPHULARIA NODOSA

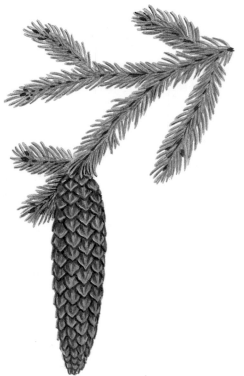

PICEA ABIES (= PINUS PICEA)
FIR TREE

From this tree is gotten the Strasbourg turpentine, . . . a good diuretic, and of great use in gonorrhoea and the fluor albus.

This is the Spruce Fir or Norway Spruce, and one of a large number of species of pine valuable to medicine.

Where to find it: It is planted in gardens, but grows wild in European forests. It has small, sharp leaves encompassing the stalk without any order. The cones hang downwards.

Flowering time: Early summer.

Astrology: Jupiter owns this tree.

Medicinal virtues: The leaves are used in diet-drinks for the scurvy, for which they are highly commended. The turpentine is mollifying, healing and cleansing and is used outwardly in wounds and ulcers. Given in clysters mixed with the yolk of an egg, it is serviceable against the stone and gravel. It is also a good pectoral, and often given in affections of the chest and lungs. Tar, another product of the tree, is by some accounted a good pectoral medicine and used for obstructions of the lungs and shortness of breath.

The young tops of *Picea abies* make an excellent anti-scorbutic, either infused or boiled in beer or wine. Experience has sufficiently confirmed their efficacy in that distemper on our American plantations, where the inhabitants used to be severely afflicted with it. Since brewing a kind of liquor or molasses, in which they boil the young Fir-tops, they are very little troubled with the scurvy.

Modern uses: Pines yield a resin from which is made oil of turpentine. Pine oil and oil of tar is also produced commercially. Stockholm tar is obtained from the Scots Pine (*Pinus sylvestris*).

Fir Tree PICEA ABIES (= PINUS PICEA)

Oil of turpentine is antiseptic, rubefacient and vesicant. It is mainly used in rheumatic liniments and plasters for its counter-irritant effects. Tar is used to combat itching and is an ingredient of ointments for psoriasis and eczema. Internally it is sometimes used as an expectorant for obstinate bronchial coughs. The tar is mixed with water and allowed to settle. The clear fluid is poured off and taken in doses of 2 fl oz (56 ml).

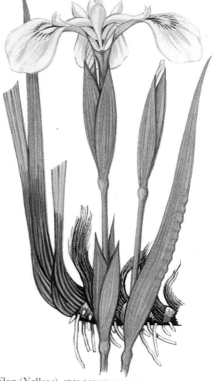

IRIS PSEUDACORUS

FLAG (Yellow)

It has a strong smell, not so pleasant while green, but growing more grateful and aromatic as it dries.

This is the commonest of the wild Irises and is distinguished from the others because of its longer and narrower leaves. It sometimes grows to more than seven feet (2.1 m). It is also called Myrtle Flag, Myrtle Grass and Fleur-de-lys.

Where to find it: Marshes, wet woods and wet ground by rivers, lakes and ditches.

Flowering time: Midsummer.

Astrology: Flags are under lunar domination.

Medicinal virtues: The roots, which only are used, are hot and dry, opening and attenuating, and good for the obstructions of the liver and spleen. They provoke the urine and the menses, help the colic, resist putrefaction, are useful against pestilential contagions and noxious air. They are an ingredient in theriaca and mithridate, and are also used in sweet bags and perfumes.

Modern uses: The infusion of the dried root has been used to check diarrhoea and leucorrhoea and to ease menstrual pains. The sap itself is purgative and emetic and very bitter. It is toxic in large doses. Applied to the skin it can cause blisters. Because of its acrid nature it is little used nowadays and not recommended for domestic use. It is also an example of a herb whose properties differ in the fresh and dried states.

Flag (Yellow) IRIS PSEUDACORUS

LINUM USITATISSIMUM

FLAX

It is of great use against inflammations, tumours and imposthumes.

Flax is an annual cultivated herb bearing blue flowers. The seeds are commonly known as linseeds.

Where to find it: In temperate and tropical regions. Flax is both cultivated and found wild on waste ground.

Flowering time: Early summer.

Astrology: Mercury owns this useful plant.

Medicinal virtues: The seed is emollient, digesting and ripening, and is frequently put into fomentations and cataplasms for use against inflammations and tumours. Cold-drawn linseed oil is of great service in all diseases of the chest and lungs, such as pleurisies, peripneumonia, coughs, asthma and consumption. It likewise helps the colic and stone, both taken at the mouth and given in clysters. The oil, by expression, is the only officinal preparation.

Modern uses: An important article in modern botanic practice. Its use goes back to earliest times. Flax seeds were found in Egyptian tombs. The seeds are soothing and laxative, because of the oil and mucilage that they contain. In bronchitis a poultice is made from the powdered seeds, to which a little mustard can be added. For boils powdered Lobelia seed is added instead.

The infusion of the seeds – 1 oz (28 g) to 1 pt (568 ml) of boiling water – is taken in doses of 2 fl oz (56 ml) for inflammatory bowel disease, such as colitis, and urinary tract inflammation, such as cystitis. Linseed oil can be applied to burns and scalds. It is a rich source of unsaturated fatty acids.

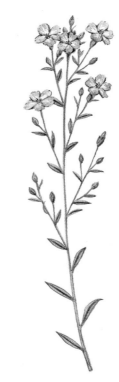

Flax LINUM USITATISSIMUM

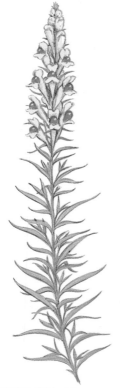

Flaxweed LINARIA VULGARIS

LINARIA VULGARIS

FLAXWEED

This is frequently used to spend the abundance of those watery humours by urine, which cause the dropsy.

A perennial commonly known as Toadflax, it has several stems with ash-coloured leaves and pale yellow flowers, which have a strong unpleasant scent.

Where to find it: Meadows, borders of fields, waysides and on banks.

Flowering time: Summer.

Astrology: Mars owns this herb.

Medicinal virtues: In Sussex we call it Gallwort, and lay it in our chickens' water to cure them of the gall. It relieves them when they are drooping.

The decoction of the herb, both leaves and flowers, in wine, does somewhat move the belly downwards, opens obstructions of the liver, and helps the yellow jaundice. It expels poison, provokes women's courses, drives forth the dead child, and afterbirth.

The distilled water of the herb and flowers is effectual for all the same purposes. Drunk with a dram (1.7 g) of the powder of the seeds, bark or roots of Wall-wort, and a little cinnamon, it is held a singular remedy for the dropsy.

The juice of the herb, or the distilled water, dropped into the eyes, is a certain remedy for all heat, inflammation and redness in them. Put into foul cancerous or fistulous ulcers the juice or water cleanses them thoroughly and heals them up safely. The juice or water also cleanses the skin of morphew, scurf, wheals, pimples and spots and also deformities as in leprosy.

Modern uses: The plant is collected when in flower. An infusion of the dried herb – 1 oz (28 g) to 1 pt (568 ml) of boiling water – is taken in teaspoonful doses of 1–2 fl oz (28–56 ml). It is an astringing diuretic, liver tonic and blood purifier. The remedy is, therefore, indicated in jaundice, skin diseases and dropsy, but has a bitter, unpleasant taste. It should be used with caution as the bitter principle is reputed to be toxic in overdosage. An ointment made from the flowers is a useful application for piles.

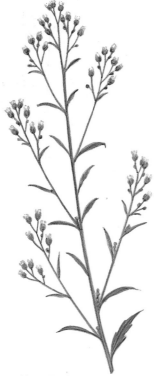

Fleabane (Canadian) CONYZA CANADENSIS
(= ERIGERON CANADENSE)

CONYZA CANADENSIS (= ERIGERON CANADENSE)

FLEABANE (Canadian)

An excellent pectoral; but being unpleasant is not often used.

An annual with a dusky green stalk tinged with brown, broad lower leaves, narrow upper leaves, and white flowers, with a yellow disc. Also called Simson.

Where to find it: Dry banks and waste ground. In the United States it is a stubborn weed, seeding itself in mint fields.

Flowering time: Summer.

Astrology: It is under Venus.

Medicinal virtues: The juice makes an excellent pectoral tonic, although unpleasant to take. The decoction, or infusion, may be sweetened and used with success in consumptive cases.

Modern uses: The whole herb or seeds are used, the plant being gathered when in flower and dried. The leaves contain an essential oil. An infusion of the herb, prepared in the usual way and given in doses of 2 fl oz (56 ml), has an astringing diuretic action. It is therefore useful in checking simple diarrhoea, and in treating kidney disease, particularly urinary stones. The oil is haemostatic and will stop bleeding from the lungs or colon. A few drops are given on a lump of sugar.

PULICARIA DYSENTERICA
FLEABANE (Small)

The smell is supposed delightful to insects, and the juice destructive to them.

Another ill-looking annual weed, also known as the Common Fleabane. It grows to eight inches (20 cm) high. The rays of the flower are very short and waved. The flowers are a dirty yellow.

Where to find it: Marshes, wet meadows, ditches and hedgerows.

Flowering time: Late summer.

Astrology: Under Venus.

Medicinal virtues: Decoctions and infusions of the dried herb have an astringent action, and are used against dysentery; but its main use is to kill fleas, for which the juice is used.

Modern uses: This plant has never been popular with English herbalists, being used against dysentery and ulcers by the ancient Arabian physicians. Because there is inadequate information regarding dosages and modern observation on its use, the Common Fleabane is not one that should be used domestically. Animals do not eat the plant. The leaves have a soapy smell when crushed.

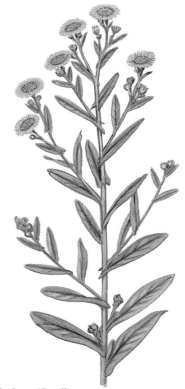

Fleabane (Small) PULICARIA DYSENTERICA

IRIS GERMANICA
FLEUR-DE-LYS (Garden or Blue)

It purges the head and clears the brain.

The Garden Iris, or Common Blue Flag as it is otherwise known, grows in clumps. The leaves are broad and flat with thin edges like a sword. The flowers are purplish-blue and the roots, which spread themselves on the surface of the ground, are reddish brown on the outside and whitish on the inside.

Where to find it: It grows in gardens, but originates in the Mediterranean.

Flowering time: Late spring and early summer.

Astrology: The herb is lunar.

Medicinal virtues: The juice of the root is a strong errhine; being snuffed up the nostrils, it purges the head, and clears the brain of thin, serious, phlegmatic humours. Given internally, the juice or a strong decoction of the root, is a strong vomit, and good for the dropsy, jaundice and agues. It is rarely used without honey and Spikenard as it vellicates and offends the stomach; but prepared as such it does ease the pains and torments of the belly, the shaking of the agues, diseases of the liver and spleen, worms of the belly, stone in the reins, convulsions and cramps, and those whose seed passes from them unawares.

The juice of the root applied to piles gives much ease. A decoction of the roots, gargled, eases toothache and helps a stinking breath. The powdered root helps cleanse and heal wounds, ulcers, fistulas and cankers.

Modern uses: The root is collected in autumn. It is used mainly as an aromatic to improve the taste of other medicines. The violet-like aroma intensifies on storing the dried root. The fresh root is purgative, mainly because of the juice it contains. Compare this with the medicinal virtues of Yellow Flag (*Iris pseudacorus*). It should be noted that *Iris versicolor* is also known as Blue Flag, and is the Iris mainly used by herbalists. This grows in swamps in the United States and Canada and is a useful remedy for non-malignant enlargements of the thyroid. It is available as a tincture of which the dose is 10–25 drops in water, three times a day. It also acts on the liver and will correct pale-coloured stools. In larger doses it is laxative.

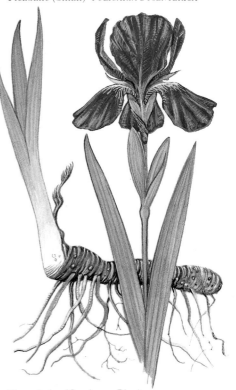

Fleur-de-lys (Garden or Blue)
IRIS GERMANICA

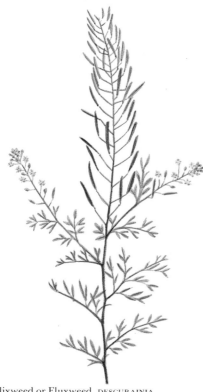

Flixweed or Fluxweed DESCURAINIA
(= SISYMBRIUM) SOPHIA

DESCURAINIA (= SISYMBRIUM) SOPHIA

FLIXWEED or FLUXWEED

It is called Fluxweed because it cures the flux.

It has a white woody root, long, winged and finely divided leaves, small yellow flowers which bear a reddish seed; and it grows to about two feet (61 cm).

Where to find it: Sandy ground and waste places.

Flowering time: Early summer.

Astrology: The herb is saturnine.

Medicinal virtues: Both herb and seed are excellent to stay the flux and lax of the belly and are no less effectual than Plantain and Comfrey. It is also used to consolidate bones that are broken or out of joint. A decoction of the herb kills worms in the stomach. A salve made from the herb quickly heals all old sores, however foul and malignant they may be. Paracelsus extols it to the skies. It is fitting that the syrup, ointment and plasters of it, were kept in all houses.

Modern uses: The juice mixed in equal parts with honey is used a teaspoonful at a time for chronic coughs or ulcerated throat. A strong infusion of the dried herb relieves asthma. Use one teaspoonful to one cup of boiling water and allow to infuse for 30 minutes, then sip. The plant is related to Hedge Mustard (*Sisymbrium officinale*), which is dealt with later in this book. See Mustard.

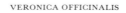

VERONICA OFFICINALIS

FLUELLEIN, LLUELLIN, SPEEDWELL or PAUL'S BETONY

Fluellein is a vulnerary plant, and accounted good for fluxes and haemorrhages of all sorts.

A common, wild perennial plant with a creeping stem. The flowers, somewhat like Snapdragons, have an upper jaw of yellow and the lower of purple. Commonly known as Heath Speedwell.

Where to find it: Woodland, pastures, heaths and moors.

Flowering time: Early to midsummer.

Astrology: It is a lunar herb.

Medicinal virtues: The bruised leaves applied with Barley-meal to watering eyes does help them. It also helps fluxes of blood, or humours, as the lax, bloody flux, women's courses, and stay all manner of bleeding at nose or mouth. It cleanses and heals all foul or old ulcers and fretting or spreading cankers.

Modern uses: Speedwell is an expectorant and will relieve bronchitis, whooping cough and catarrh. An infusion of the dried plant is taken in wineglassful doses. It was once used as a substitute for ordinary tea, but its popularity has waned over the years.

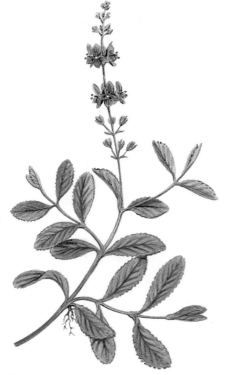

Fluellein, Lluellin, Speedwell or Paul's
Betony VERONICA OFFICINALIS

DIGITALIS PURPUREA

FOXGLOVE

It has a gentle, cleansing quality, and withal very friendly to nature.

A tall plant with reddish-purple flowers, with some black on white spots within them, the Foxglove has many long and broad leaves, dented upon the edges. The leaves have a hot and bitter taste.

Where to find it: It grows on dry sandy ground and under hedge-sides and is also cultivated in gardens.

Flowering time: It seldom flowers before midsummer.

Astrology: Under the dominion of Venus.

Medicinal virtues: It is used by the Italians to heal fresh wounds, the leaves being bound thereon. The juice is used to cleanse, dry and heal old sores. The decoction with some sugar or honey cleanses and purges the body both upwards and downwards and opens obstructions of the liver and spleen.

Modern uses: For the past 200 years Digitalis has been the leading cardiac drug for heart failure. The dried leaf is listed as an official drug in the British Pharmacopoeia. Pharmaceutical companies make synthetic versions of it for use by the orthodox medical profession. Recent evidence, however, suggests that the synthetic versions are more toxic than the dried leaf. Herbalists do not use Foxglove because of its reputed toxic effects. They have several other remedies to choose from, including Hawthorn and Lily of the Valley.

The cardiotonic properties were reported to the medical profession by Dr William Withering in 1775. He learned of its use from a medical herbalist of that time who cured a patient of heart failure when the college physicians had failed. Whereas modern physicians use Digitalis as a specific heart tonic, the herbal method would be to include it in a prescription aimed at treating the whole person. Used in this traditional way, the dosage would be such that toxicity is unlikely. This is not to say that Digitalis is recommended for domestic use. It is not. The drug is available only on a doctor's prescription.

An infusion of one teaspoonful of the dried leaves to 1 pt (568 ml) boiling water should not be taken in more than teaspoonful doses. The toxicity tends to be cumulative.

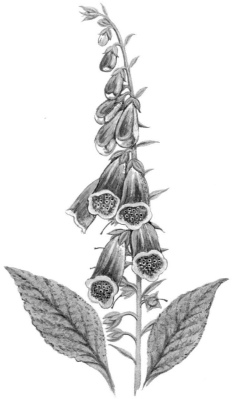

Foxglove DIGITALIS PURPUREA

FUMARIA OFFICINALIS

FUMITORY

The juice of the Fumitory and Docks mingled with vinegar, and the places gently washed or wet therewith, cures all sorts of scabs, pimples, blotches and wheals.

A tender sappy herb with a slender weak stalk and straggling branches two or three feet (61 or 91 cm) long. The many small flowers are in spikes, of a reddish-purple colour.

Where to find it: Cornfields and gardens.

Flowering time: Spring.

Astrology: Saturn owns the herb and presents it to the world as a cure for his own disease, and strengthener of the parts of the body he rules.

Medicinal virtues: The juice or syrup made of it, opens obstructions of the liver and spleen. It clarifies the blood from saltish, choleric and other humours which cause leprosy, scabs, tetters and itches and other outbreaks of the skin.

It eradicates the yellow jaundice through the urine which it produces in abundance. The powdered herb cures melancholy if given for some time. The distilled water taken with treacle is good against the plague and pestilence. With Honey of Roses, it is gargled to help sores of the mouth and throat.

Dropped into the eyes, the juice takes away redness and other defects in them, although it causes pain and tears in the process.

Modern uses: The dried herb is used in infusions as a tonic, diuretic and aperient. It is indicated in eczematous skin conditions, stomach upsets and liver derangements. Dosage of the warm infusion is 2 fl oz (56 ml) three times a day.

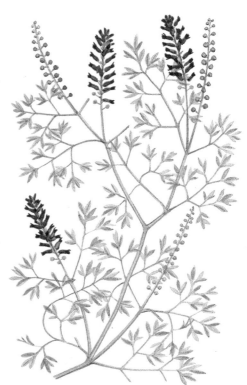

Fumitory FUMARIA OFFICINALIS

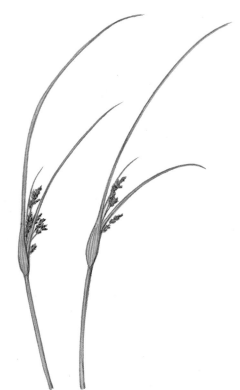

Galingale CYPERUS LONGUS

GALINGALE

Good for the swimming of the head.

A hardy perennial, also known as the Sweet Cyperus or Umbrella Plant, growing to about four feet (1.2 m). It has a triangular stem on top of which grows a tuft of grass-like flowers.

Where to find it: Marshland in Brazil, Palestine, South Africa and Europe.

Flowering time: Early in midsummer.

Astrology: A plant of Mars.

Medicinal virtues: It expels wind and strengthens the bowels. It eases colic, provokes urine and the terms and prevents dropsy. Good for giddiness. Sometimes it is used in gargles for mouth ulcers.

Modern uses: The roots are the part used. A decoction is employed as a gastro-intestinal tonic and for treating water retention. This variety is not widely available and has fallen from popularity. Several other varieties of *Cyperus* are in use. *C. esculentus* produces underground tubers, known as tiger nuts, which are used in southern Europe in making iced drinks. The root of *C. odoratus* is used by Indian doctors for its stomachic properties.

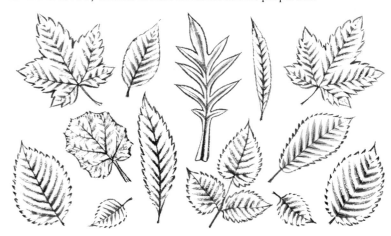

GALL-OAK

It is effectual in drawing together and fastening loose and faint parts.

The strong Gall-oak, so-called from the fruit it bears, does not grow so large or high as other oaks. It flowers and bears acorns and also the round woody substances known as galls. These are caused by a gall-wasp puncturing the bark and laying eggs inside.

Where to find it: The Gall-oak is a native of Asia, but grows in other warm climates. Galls do occur on the Common Oak.

Flowering time: The tree blossoms in early spring. The acorns are ripe in mid autumn.

Astrology: The Gall-oak is saturnine.

Medicinal virtues: The small gall expels and dries up rheums and other fluxes, especially those of the gums, mouth and throat. The white gall binds and dries, but not so much, yet is good against the dysentery and bloody flux. The galls boiled and bruised and applied to any swelling or inflammation will prove a certain cure.

The oak apple is much of the nature of galls, though inferior, and may be substituted for them with success to help rheums, fluxes and other painful distempers.

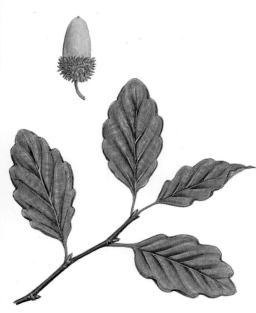

Gall-oak QUERCUS INFECTORIA

Modern uses: The galls are powdered, or made into a tincture or an ointment. They are powerfully astringent and are used to check dysentery, diarrhoea and cholera. An infusion made from the powder makes an excellent mouthwash in relaxed throat or can be injected in cases of leucorrhoea. The ointment is still an official preparation listed in the British Pharmacopoeia, but an impromptu version can be made by digesting one part of the powder in four parts of wax. This is used as an application for bleeding piles.

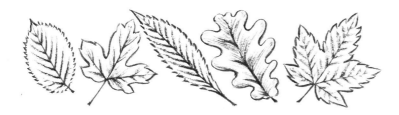

ALLIUM SATIVUM

GARLIC

This was anciently accounted the poor man's treacle, it being a remedy for all diseases and hurts (except those which itself breeds).

The Garlic bulb is a member of the Onion family with Chives, Leeks and Shallots. The root is several reddish-white bulbs together enclosed in one whitish skin. The leaves are long, like Leeks; on top of the stalk, which grows two or three feet (61 or 91 cm) high, stands an umbel of small, pink or whitish flowers.

Where to find it: Garlic is cultivated everywhere, but originates in India or central Asia.

Flowering time: Summer.

Astrology: Mars owns this herb.

Medicinal virtues: It provokes urine and women's courses, helps the biting of mad dogs, and other venomous creatures; kills the worms in children, cuts and voids tough phlegm, purges the head, helps the lethargy, is a good preservative against, and a remedy for, any plague, sore or foul ulcer.

It takes away spots and blemishes in the skin, eases pains in the ears, and ripens and breaks imposthumes or other swellings. Onions are equally as effectual for all those diseases. But Garlic has some more peculiar virtues. It has a special quality to discuss inconveniences, coming by corrupt agues or mineral vapours; by drinking corrupt and stinking waters; or by taking Wolf'sbane, Henbane, Hemlock or other poisonous and dangerous herbs. Garlic is also good in hydropic diseases, jaundice, falling-sickness, cramps, convulsions, piles or other cold diseases.

However, its heat is vehement; and in choleric men it will add fuel to the fire. In men oppressed by melancholy, it will attenuate the humour. Therefore, let it be taken inwardly with great moderation; outwardly you may make more bold with it.

Modern uses: Garlic is antiseptic and the juice diluted with water can be applied direct to wounds. It may also be used as a lotion or in an ointment. The plant contains a natural antibiotic substance and the oil obtained in capsule form is a popular method of taking it internally, although, of course, the bulb is widely used in cooking. It is taken to prevent colds.

The juice made into a syrup is given for coughs, colds and asthma, because of its expectorant properties. Garlic is also diaphoretic and diuretic and helps to prevent the dropsy. The dose of the juice taken on its own is between 10 and 30 drops. The tincture of Garlic, available from herbalists, causes a drop in blood pressure, and is also effective against angina.

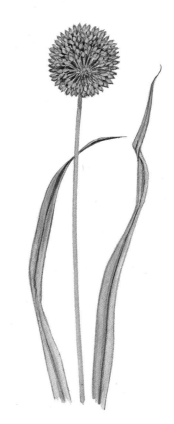

Garlic ALLIUM SATIVUM

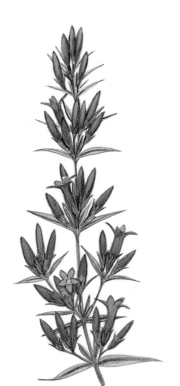

Gentian (Autumn) GENTIANELLA
(= GENTIANA) AMARELLA

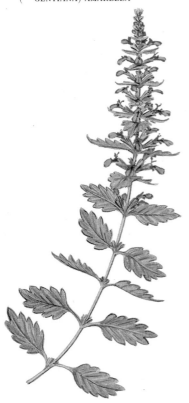

Germander TEUCRIUM CHAMAEDRYS

GENTIANELLA (= GENTIANA) AMARELLA

GENTIAN (Autumn)

It is confessed that Gentian, which is most used among us, was brought from beyond the sea, yet we have several sorts of it growing frequently in this country, which, besides the reasons so often alleged, why English herbs should be fittest for English bodies, has been proved, by the experience of divers physicians, not to be a whit inferior in virtue to that which comes from beyond the sea.

There are two sorts of Gentian commonly found, known also as Gelwort and Balmony. They are the Autumn Gentian and the·Field Gentian (*G. campestris*). The former bears large, bell-shaped, purple flowers, and the latter bears small blue flowers.

Where to find it: Pastures with chalky soils.

Flowering time: Midsummer to early autumn.

Astrology: Both are under the dominion of Mars.

Medicinal virtues: The virtues of both are similar. They resist putrefactions and poison and a more sure remedy to prevent the pestilence cannot be found. It strengthens the stomach, helps digestion, comforts the heart, and preserves it against faintings and swoonings. The powdered dried root opens obstructions of the liver and restores the appetite.

The herb provokes urine and the terms exceedingly, and therefore should not be given to women with child. But it is profitable for those troubled with cramps and convulsions, to drink the decoction. This also breaks the stone and helps ruptures. To kill the worms, take half a dram (890 mg) of the powder in the morning in any convenient liquor. It will also instantly heal lites on cattle's udders.

Modern uses: Herbalists prefer to use the Yellow Gentian (*Gentiana lutea*), which they regard as one of the finest of all tonic medicines. It has a very bitter taste even when greatly diluted.

It is used for all cases of general debility, anorexia, dyspepsia and jaundice. There are several official preparations listed in the British Pharmacopoeia; but as the root yields all of its medicinal properties in water, it can be used domestically in the form of an infusion. It is better to combine the powdered root with an aromatic herb, like Cardamoms, to reduce the bitterness. One-fifth to one-half a teaspoonful of the powder is infused in a cupful of boiling water, and sweetened with honey.

TEUCRIUM CHAMAEDRYS

GERMANDER

It is commended by some as a specific for the gout.

Commonly known as Wall Germander, it has a spreading creeping root, square hairy branches, with leaves resembling that of the Oak, and labiated flowers of a purplish-red.

Where to find it: Cultivated in gardens, but also found growing on ruins of old buildings.

Flowering time: Early to midsummer.

Astrology: Germander is a herb of warm thin parts, under Mars.

Medicinal virtues: It opens obstructions of the liver, spleen and kidneys, and is used for jaundice, dropsy and stoppage of urine. It is also a good emmenagogue. A specific for gout, rheumatism and pains in the limbs, it is also undoubtedly a good vulnerary and a useful ingredient in pectoral medicines.

The juice is justly recommended among the rest of the anti-scorbutic juices to be taken in the spring for some time.

Modern uses: The whole herb is used. It is collected in July and dried. It is a stimulating tonic with diuretic and diaphoretic properties. It can be used in the form of an infusion for rheumatism, gout, fevers and suppressed menstruation. It can also be used instead of Horehound for coughs and asthma. One ounce (28 g) of the dried herb is steeped in 1 pt (568 ml) of boiling water and taken in doses of 1–2 fl oz (28–56 ml) two or three times a day.

BUTOMUS UMBELLATUS

GLADIOLE (Water)

The flowers are good for inflammations.

This is a beautiful, hardy, aquatic, perennial plant, perhaps one of the most attractive plants found growing wild in Britain. Also known as the Flowering Rush, it grows to about three feet (91 cm). It has long, sharp-edged leaves, tall stems and rose-coloured flowers.

Where to find it: The margins of ponds and pools, sides of ditches and in marshland.

Flowering time: Midsummer to early autumn.

Astrology: It is under Saturn.

Medicinal virtues: It is seldom used in medicine except for the cooling nature of the flowers which are applied to fresh wounds, imposthumes and other hot humours.

Modern uses: A rare plant in the wild, but it is popular in gardens. It has never been of much interest to physicians or herbalists. For treating wounds, herbalists prefer to use a common herb such as Comfrey. Homoeopaths use Arnica.

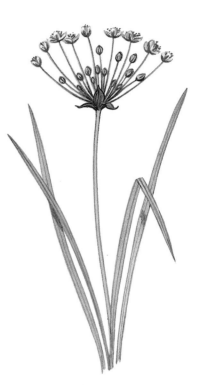

Gladiole (Water) BUTOMUS UMBELLATUS

IRIS FOETIDISSIMA

GLADWIN

The root boiled in wine procures women's courses; and used as a pessary, works the same effect, but causes abortion to women with child.

This is one of the iris family, also known as the Stinking Iris; but it is smaller than the Common Iris. The flowers are a dead purplish ash-colour; the seeds are bright orange.

Where to find it: Woods and shady places, particularly near the sea.

Flowering time: Midsummer.

Astrology: Under the dominion of Saturn.

Medicinal virtues: It is used by many country people to purge corrupt phlegm and choler, by drinking a decoction of the roots. The roots and leaves can also be sliced and added to ale for weak stomachs. The powder in wine helps those with cramp and convulsions, or with gout and sciatica, gives ease to the most griping pains of the body and the belly, and helps those that have the strangury. The juice of the root snuffed up the nose causes sneezing and draws corruption from the head.

Half a dram (890 mg) of the seed beaten to powder, and taken in wine, speedily relieves those troubled with a stoppage of the urine.

The root used with a little verdigris and honey and with the addition of Great Centaury root is effectual for wounds of the head and to help draw forth thorns and splinters.

The root boiled in vinegar dissolves and consumes swellings and tumours when applied to them.

Modern uses: It is purgative, but also anti-spasmodic and will relieve stomach cramps. The former action is achieved by administering a decoction of the roots, the latter by infusing a quarter teaspoonful of the powdered root in a cupful of boiling water. The infusion also helps hysterical and nervous complaints. In action, Gladwin is similar to Yellow Flag root. It can be a violent remedy if not used correctly and should not be used domestically.

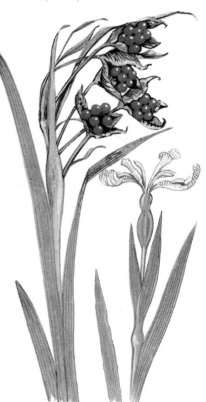

Gladwin IRIS FOETIDISSIMA

GOAT'S BEARD

A large double handful of the entire plant, roots, flowers, and all bruised and boiled, and then strained, with a little sweet oil, is an excellent clyster in the most desperate cases of strangury or suppression of urine, from whatever cause.

This is also known as Noon Flower and Jack-go-to-bed-at-noon, because the large and beautiful yellow flowers close at midday. They grow on firm stalks a foot (30 cm) high, with flat, bluish-green leaves.

Where to find it: Meadows and roadside verges.

Flowering time: Midsummer.

Astrology: Under the dominion of Jupiter.

Medicinal virtues: A decoction of the roots is good for heart-burn, loss of appetite, and liver and chest disorders. It expels sand and gravel, slime and small stones.

The roots cooked like Parsnips, with butter, are good for cold, watery stomachs. They strengthen the lean and the consumptive and the weak after a long illness. The distilled water gives relief to inward imposthumes, pleurisy, stitches or pains in the sides.

Modern uses: The reputation of Goat's Beard as a medicinal plant has not survived although it is commonly available. Meadowsweet is more popular for dyspepsia; Dandelion, which is of the same family as Goat's Beard, is one of the best liver tonics; while for chest disorders there are many good remedies, such as Colt's Foot and Horehound. The fresh juice of Goat's Beard was considered to be better than any antacid in relieving dyspepsia.

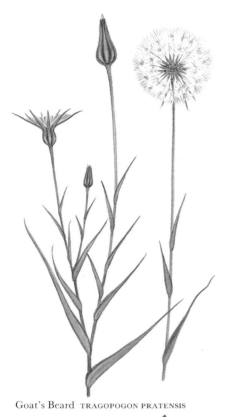

Goat's Beard TRAGOPOGON PRATENSIS

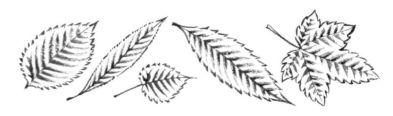

GOAT'S RUE

A bath made of it is very refreshing to wash the feet of persons tired with overwalking.

A perennial plant about three feet (91 cm) high with hollow branches, pinnate leaves, and pale whitish-blue flowers that hang down in long spikes rather like pea blossoms.

Where to find it: Cultivated in gardens, but grows wild in moist fields and meadows.

Flowering time: Early to midsummer.

Astrology: It is under Mercury in Leo.

Medicinal virtues: It is accounted cordial, sudorific and alexipharmic. It is good against pestilential distempers, expelling the venom through the pores of the skin; and is of use in all kinds of fevers, smallpox and measles. It will kill worms and cure the bites of all kinds of venomous creatures. Some commend a decoction of it for the gout.

Modern uses: The herb was official in the United States Pharmacopoeia. The plant is collected while in flower and the flowering tops dried. The seeds are also used. An infusion made from the flowers promotes the flow of milk in nursing mothers and is also anti-diabetic. The dried herb powdered is diuretic and is taken in doses of 5–20 grains (0.33–1.3 g). It also induces perspiration and thus will help to reduce temperature in fevers.

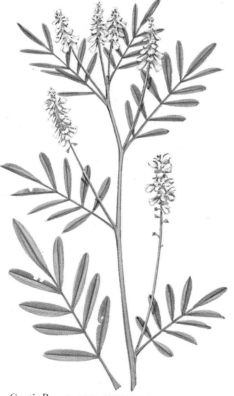

Goat's Rue GALEGA OFFICINALIS

GOAT'S THORN

It is good for tickling coughs, . . . but is far from being a pleasant medicine.

More commonly known as Tragacanth, this herb grows with a woody tough root, a thick stem, and produces clusters of small, white flowers at the tops of its branches. The blossom is butterfly-shaped.

Where to find it: It grows in gardens, but is really a native plant of the East.

Flowering time: Late summer.

Astrology: Under the dominion of Mars.

Medicinal virtues: This little shrub produces a gum which it sweats out at the bottom of the stem during the summer heat. Good for coughs arising from sharp, acrid humours and against the strangury and heat of urine.

Modern uses: Tragacanth is demulcent and mucilaginous. It can be used to soothe coughs, but is not ideal as it does not dissolve completely in water. As an aid to pharmacy, however, it is a very valuable item. The mucilage is used as a suspension agent when making lozenges with insoluble powders to prevent clumping. Mucilage of Tragacanth is an official preparation in both British and United States Pharmacopoeias. It is widely used to make emulsions, i.e. mixtures of oil and water, and as an application to burns. It is therefore of more use to the pharmacist than for domestic use.

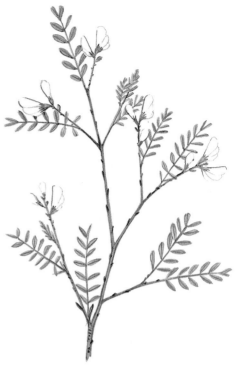

Goat's Thorn ASTRAGALUS GUMMIFER

GOLDEN ROD

Long famous against inward hurts and bruises.

A handsome perennial plant, Golden Rod is about two feet (61 cm) high with numerous small golden yellow flowers.

Where to find it: In woodland and heathland.

Flowering time: Mid to late summer.

Astrology: Venus rules this herb.

Medicinal virtues: A balsamic, vulnerary herb, most effectively used as a distilled water. In this form it is also an excellent diuretic and few remedies exceed it where there is gravel, stone in the reins and kidneys, or strangury. When small stones cause bloody or purulent urine, its balsamic healing virtues co-operate with its diuretic quality so that the parts are cleansed and healed at the same time.

It is a sovereign wound-herb, inferior to none, both for inward and outward use. It is good to stay the immoderate flux of women's courses, the bloody flux, ruptures and mouth and throat ulcers. As a lotion it is used to wash the privy parts in venereal cases. No preparation is better than a tea of the herb made from the young leaves, fresh or dried.

Modern uses: An infusion of 1 oz (28 g) of the leaves to 1 pt (568 ml) of boiling water is taken in doses of 2 fl oz (56 ml) three or four times a day as a treatment for excessive menstruation, arthritis and eczema. An aromatic herb, the warm infusion is also carminative and will remove feelings of nausea due to stomach disorder. The powder of the dried leaves can be applied to ulcers externally to stimulate healing.

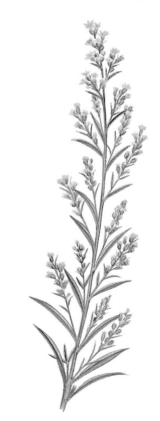

Golden Rod SOLIDAGO VIRGAUREA

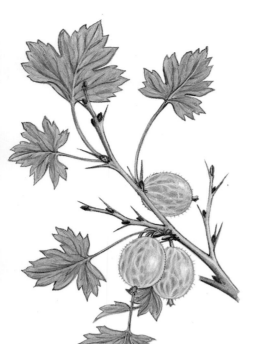

Gooseberry RIBES UVA-CRISPA

RIBES UVA-CRISPA

GOOSEBERRY

They create an appetite and quench the thirst.

A shrub three to four feet (0.9 to 1.2 m) high, which produces the well-known fruit.

Where to find it: Cultivated in gardens.

Flowering time: It blossoms in spring. The berries ripen in midsummer.

Astrology: Under the dominion of Venus.

Medicinal virtues: The berries are cooling and astringent. Baked while still unripe, they stir up a fainting or decayed appetite, especially where the stomach is afflicted by choleric humours. A decoction of the leaves cools hot swellings and inflammations, and St Anthony's fire.

Ripe Gooseberries allay the violent heat of stomach and liver. The young leaves can be used to break the stone and expel gravel from the kidneys and bladder.

Modern uses: An infusion of 1 oz (28 g) of the dried leaves to 1 pt (568 ml) of boiling water if drunk a cupful at a time three times a day will be found useful to those with sediment in the urine and a tonic for adolescent girls, if taken just before the menstrual period.

Gooseberry juice is rich in calcium, sodium and sulphur, and vitamins A, C and B1.

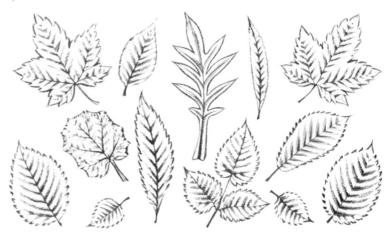

AEGOPODIUM PODAGRARIA

GOUTWEED

It should not be supposed that Goutwort has its name for nothing.

Also known as Goutwort and Goat-herb, because the leaves resemble the shape of a goat's foot, Goutweed is a low-growing herb with umbels of white flowers and blackish seeds.

Where to find it: It grows by hedges and wall-sides and often in the borders and corners of fields. It is also grown in gardens.

Flowering time: It flowers and seeds in midsummer.

Astrology: Saturn rules it.

Medicinal virtues: Upon experiment it is found to heal the gout and sciatica. It is also used for aching joints and other cold pains.

Modern uses: It is a diuretic and a sedative and therefore successful for arthritic and rheumatic pains. An infusion of the herb is used internally or as a fomentation externally. The roots and leaves can be applied directly to a painful hip after boiling them together and making them into a poultice. A liquid extract is used by herbalists for the same purposes.

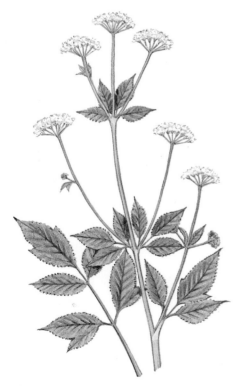

Goutweed AEGOPODIUM PODAGRARIA

GREEN (Winter)

A singularly good wound-herb.

More commonly known as the Chickweed Wintergreen, it is a perennial with leaves resembling those of the Pear tree, and small but very bright white flowers.

Where to find it: It grows in mossy pine woods, but is rare elsewhere.

Flowering time: Midsummer.

Astrology: Under the dominion of Saturn.

Medicinal virtues: It speedily heals fresh wounds, the leaves being bruised and applied. The juice can be used instead. An ointment made by adding the juice to melted wax and cooling or by digesting the herb in wax, is sovereign for wounds. The herb can be boiled in wine and water and given to those with internal ulcers. It stays all fluxes, including women's courses and the bleeding of wounds and takes away inflammations from the heart.

Modern uses: This Wintergreen should not be confused with *Gaultheria procumbens*, the Wintergreen of the United States. It is rare and, therefore, not in common use. However, where available the ointment can be made and used as a treatment for wounds. An infusion of the leaves is taken as a blood purifier and for treating eczema. The root is emetic.

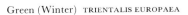

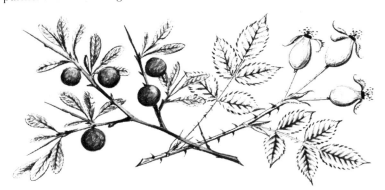

Green (Winter) TRIENTALIS EUROPAEA

GROUND PINE (Common)

It powerfully promotes the menses and ought not to be given to pregnant women.

Although commonly known as the Yellow Bugle and closely related to the Common Bugle (*Ajuga reptans*), the two plants bear little resemblance. Ground Pine has a long, slender root, numerous stems, about four inches (10 cm) high, thickly covered with leaves, and small yellow flowers. The upper lip of the flower is spotted with purple on the inside.

Where to find it: It likes sandy and chalky soils.

Flowering time: Early to midsummer.

Astrology: A martial plant, hot and dry.

Medicinal virtues: It is warming and strengthening to the nerves. It helps the palsy, gout, sciatica and rheumatism, the scurvy and all pains of the limbs. It is a strong diuretic and opens obstructions of the womb.

Modern uses: A stimulating diuretic and emmenagogue, Ground Pine is taken as an infusion. One ounce (28 g) of the dried leaves are infused in 1 pt (568 ml) of boiling water for 20 minutes and taken in doses of ⅓–⅔ fl oz (10–20 ml), which may be repeated three or four times a day. It can be combined with other remedies such as Couchgrass or Broom for gout and rheumatism. Mix the herbs in equal parts and use 1 oz (28 g) of the mixture for an infusion in the usual way. Take heed of the warning about using the herb during pregnancy.

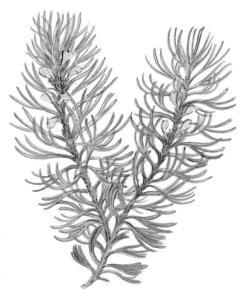

Ground Pine (Common)
AJUGA CHAMAEPITYS

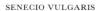

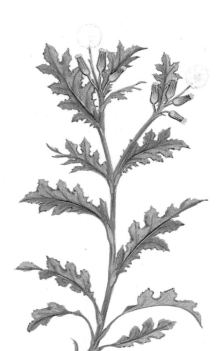

Groundsel (Common) SENECIO VULGARIS

SENECIO VULGARIS

GROUNDSEL (Common)

Taken in ale, it acts against the pains of the stomach, strangury and jaundice.

A very common annual weed, growing to about a foot (30 cm) high. The stalk is tender and juicy. The yellow flowers are poor but numerous.

Where to find it: Fields and gardens, tilled and untilled ground.

Flowering time: All the summer.

Astrology: Under the dominion of Venus.

Medicinal virtues: Although a common plant, it has many virtues. It is cooling and digesting in inflammations and, made like tea, it is an emetic. It will destroy worms and is useful in scrofulous tumours, inflammation of the breasts and scald head.

The juice is purgative and the dose should not exceed two ounces (56 g). The leaves, bruised and applied outwardly to the stomach, produce a similar effect, and there is no better application for the gripes and colic of infants.

For sore breasts, pick a handful of the fresh juicy leaves, bruise them and make a poultice with a little bread boiled in milk. Then lay the poultice on and repeat as often as needed, and an effectual cure will result.

When taken in wine the juice provokes urine and expels the gravel. A dram (1.7 g) of the juice is sufficient taken inwardly and caution should be used so that it may not work mischief.

Modern uses: It is mainly used as a diuretic and diaphoretic. The herb is used as an infusion, but this should not be too strong, otherwise it becomes emetic and purgative. A weak infusion of ½ oz (14 g) of herb to 1 pt (568 ml) of boiling water taken in doses of 1 fl oz (28 ml) will still have a laxative action.

The root contains a toxic substance known as senecionine which irritates the liver and should not be used internally.

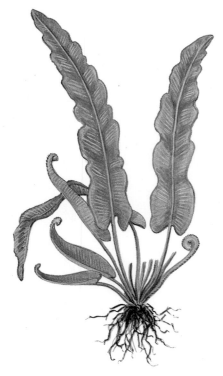

Hart's Tongue PHYLLITIS (= ASPLENIUM)
SCOLOPENDRIUM

PHYLLITIS (= ASPLENIUM) SCOLOPENDRIUM

HART'S TONGUE

A good remedy for the liver, both to strengthen it when weak, and ease it when afflicted.

A perennial fern, the leaves are about a foot (30 cm) long when fully grown.

Where to find it: Shady spots, among rocks, near walls and shady copses.

Flowering time: It flowers not, being a fern, but remains green all winter.

Astrology: Jupiter claims dominion over this herb.

Medicinal virtues: A syrup should be made of it, so that it is always available. It is commended for hardness and stoppings of the liver and spleen, heat from the stomach, lax and the bloody flux. The distilled water is very good against the passions of the heart, to stay the hiccough, to help the falling of the palate, and to stay the bleeding of the gums, by gargling with it.

Modern uses: A soothing diuretic with laxative and pectoral properties. A decoction is made from 2 oz (56 g) of the herb to 1 pt (568 ml) of boiling water and taken in doses of 2 fl oz (56 ml). It is a liver tonic and will also remove sediment from the bladder. Its mucilaginous content is useful in treating bronchial disease.

HIERACIUM MURORUM
HAWKWEED

Good for the heat of the stomach, and gnawings therein.

There are many kinds of Hawkweeds and some are difficult to distinguish. This one has many large leaves lying upon the ground, indented like Dandelion. The hollow stalk rises two or three feet (61 or 91 cm) with pale yellow flowers at the top. Commonly known as the Few-leaved Hawkweed.

Where to find it: The sides of fields and paths in dry grounds in hilly districts.

Flowering time: Late summer.

Astrology: Saturn owns it.

Medicinal virtues: The Hawkweeds all have much the same medicinal properties. They are somewhat drying and binding and used for inflammations and the hot fits of agues.

The juice in wine helps digestion, dispels wind, hinders crudities abiding in the stomach, and helps the difficulty in making water. A scruple of the dry root given in wine and vinegar is profitable for dropsy. The decoction of the herb taken in honey digests phlegm, and with Hyssop helps the cough. The decoction of the herb and Wild Succory with wine eases the colic and hardness of the spleen, procures rest and sleep, hinders venery, cools heat, purges the stomach, increases blood, and helps diseases of the reins and bladder.

Outwardly applied, it is good for the defects and diseases of the eyes, used with some women's milk. It is also good for healing spreading ulcers.

Modern uses: The Hawkweeds are not much used by modern herbalists, but could be used if need be as pectoral tonics for coughs, asthma and bronchial troubles. The Mouse-eared Hawkweed is still employed by some.

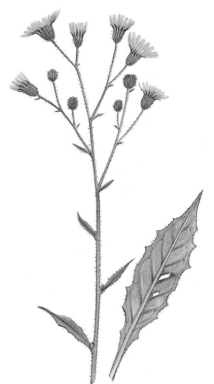

Hawkweed HIERACIUM MURORUM

CRATAEGUS MONOGYNA
HAWTHORN

The seeds in the berries beaten to powder being drunk in wine, are good against the stone and dropsy.

The Hawthorn is known by many names, including May Blossom and Quickthorn. Young twigs are reddish, clothed with small leaves. The flowers grow in clusters, consisting of five white petals, with reddish apices in the middle of each petal.

Where to find it: It will make a tree of 30 feet (9 m) but it is commonly used to provide cheap hedging as it grows fast.

Flowering time: Late spring. The berries are ripe in early autumn.

Astrology: It is a tree of Mars.

Medicinal virtues: The distilled water of the flowers stays the lax. The seeds cleared of the down and bruised, being boiled in wine, are good to relieve inward pains. If the distilled water be applied to any place pierced with thorns or splinters, it will draw them out.

Modern uses: This is a remedy which is more in use today than in former times because of its use as a cardiac tonic. Of course heart disease is at epidemic proportions in western countries and, therefore, remedies for the heart become of more importance. Hawthorn, particularly the berries, increases the muscular action of the heart. It is a remedy that is suitable for most cardiac disorders. Where there is angina, palpitations, irregular pulse or other circulatory disorders, Hawthorn can be tried. A tincture made from the berries is available from herbalists, the dosage being 5–12 drops three times a day. An infusion of the blossoms, made just as the buds are opening, acts as a mild heart tonic. Use two tablespoonfuls of the buds to one cup of boiling

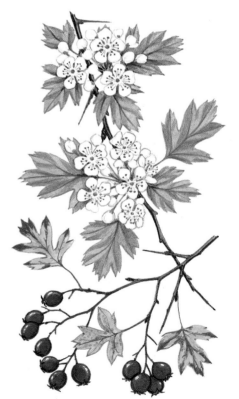

Hawthorn CRATAEGUS MONOGYNA

water, and take a cup twice a day. This can also be taken as a preventive treatment against atherosclerosis, or fatty degeneration of the heart. Cardiac patients are, however, advised to be in the care of a competent practitioner.

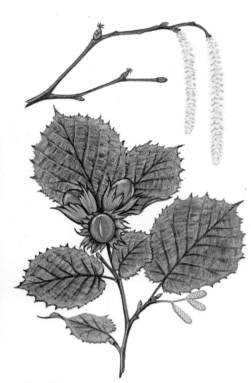

Hazel Nut CORYLUS AVELLANA

CORYLUS AVELLANA

HAZEL NUT

Good to help an old cough.

This variety of Hazel Nut makes a small tree which produces several nuts together on one stalk, covered with a husk. The branches are smooth, tough and pliable and the leaves large and round, but indented at the edges. The male flowers are presented as yellow, drooping catkins.

Where to find it: A common occupant of woods and coppices.

Flowering time: Late spring.

Astrology: Under the dominion of Mercury.

Medicinal virtues: The dried husks and shells are powdered and two drams (3.5 g) taken in red wine to stay the laxness of the bowel and women's courses. The skins have a similar virtue. To help an old cough, the kernels are made into an electuary with mead or honied water. With a little pepper added, rheum is drawn from the head.

Modern uses: Hazel nuts, Cob nuts and Filberts are related. The latter two are selected strains which are grafted on to stocks of the Common Hazel. Nuts are rich in protein and unsaturated fatty acids. Hazel nuts are particularly rich in phosphorus, magnesium, potassium and copper, and are best used as a food.

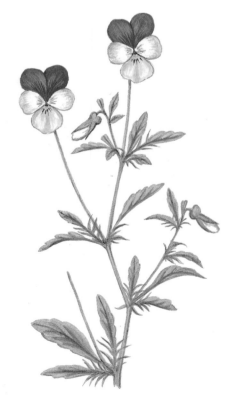

Heart's Ease VIOLA TRICOLOR

VIOLA TRICOLOR

HEART'S EASE

A strong decoction or syrup of the herb and flowers is an excellent cure for the venereal disease.

Also known as the Wild Pansy, the flowers are a beautiful purple variegated with yellow.

Where to find it: Fields and gardens.

Flowering time: Spring and summer.

Astrology: The herb is saturnine, cold, viscous and slimy.

Medicinal virtues: Good for convulsions in children and a remedy for the falling-sickness, inflammation of the lungs and breasts, pleurisy, scabs and the itch.

The flowers are cooling, emollient and cathartic when used on their own, but it is best to make a syrup of them when they are fresh, as their virtues are lost by drying.

Modern uses: The Pansy is mildly laxative, diuretic, diaphoretic and expectorant. It is also considered to be a good blood purifier. An infusion is recommended for skin eruptions in children, catarrh and asthma. The dose is half a teaspoonful of the powdered leaves in a cupful of boiling water.

HELLEBORE (Black)

The roots are very effective in quartan agues and madness.

Also known as the Christmas Rose, it is a perennial plant with leaves arising from the root. It has whitish flowers, which are sometimes purplish towards the edges, with pale yellow centres.

Where to find it: Mainly grown in gardens, but is a native of the alpine regions of Europe.

Flowering time: Winter.

Astrology: It is a herb of Saturn.

Medicinal virtues: It has some sulleness about it and would be better purified by the alchymist than given raw. Goat's milk is an antidote for it, if any one suffers from taking too much.

The roots help the falling-sickness, the leprosy, yellow and black jaundice, gout, sciatica and convulsions. Used as a pessary, the roots provoke the terms exceedingly. Beaten to powder and strewed upon foul ulcers, it eats away the dead flesh, and instantly heals them. It helps gangrenes in the beginning. Twenty grains (1.3 g) taken inwardly is sufficient a dose for one time and that should be given with half as much Cinnamon.

Modern uses: This root is not recommended for domestic use as it contains poisonous constituents which have a similar effect to the Foxglove. It is used in homoeopathic medicine, a tincture being prepared from the fresh root, and used for nervous disorders and epilepsy.

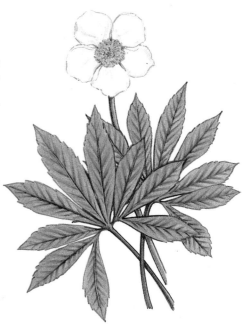

Hellebore (Black) HELLEBORUS NIGER

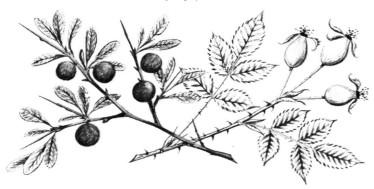

HELLEBORE (White)

A very harsh medicine and should be given with caution.

This is American Hellebore or Indian Poke. It is a perennial with large single flowers, green but paler than the leaves, with white buttons in their centres.

Where to find it: In woods, swamps and moist meadows.

Flowering time: Early spring.

Astrology: A cold, saturnine plant.

Medicinal virtues: It possesses the virtues of Black Hellebore but to an inferior degree. The leaves are given dried and powdered to those of robust habits. It ought not to be given to pregnant women.

Modern uses: This is another poisonous plant which is used medicinally, but must be administered with great caution. It is a cardiac depressant, and has emetic and purgative side-effects. It is not prescribed by herbalists, but orthodox medicine uses the alkaloids from the plant in anti-hypertensive drugs. A homoeopathic tincture is used for the treatment of liver disorders.

A close relative of the American Hellebore is the False Hellebore (*Veratrum album*). This is also an irritant poison.

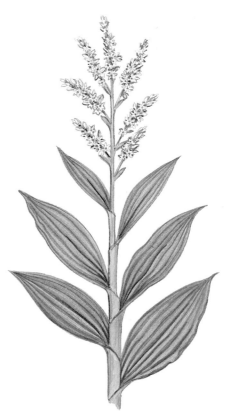

Hellebore (White) VERATRUM VIRIDE

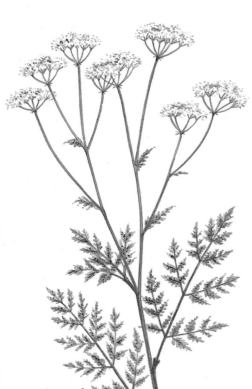

Hemlock CONIUM MACULATUM

CONIUM MACULATUM

HEMLOCK

The root roasted and applied to the hands, helps the gout.

The common Great Hemlock grows four or five feet (1.2 or 1.5 m) high, with very large winged leaves and umbels of white flowers. The whole plant has an ill-favoured scent.

Where to find it: By walls and hedges and by the edges of streams.

Flowering time: Midsummer.

Astrology: Saturn claims dominion over this herb.

Medicinal virtues: Hemlock is very dangerous, especially if taken inwardly. It may be safely applied to inflammations, tumults and swellings, to St Anthony's fire, wheals and creeping ulcers. The bruised leaves on the forehead are good for red and swollen eyes.

Pure wine is the best antidote if too much of this herb is taken.

Modern uses: It is a sedative and pain reliever, but overdosage produces paralysis. It is sometimes used as an ingredient in ointments for haemorrhoids, anal fissure or pruritus ani, but the concentration of herb in the ointment base is critical. It is not recommended for domestic use. An alkaloid from the plant is used as a pain reliever in terminal cancer and the homoeopathic tincture is given for symptoms due to an enlarged prostate gland.

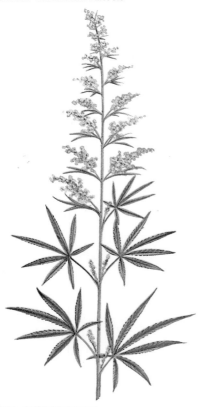

Hemp CANNABIS SATIVA

CANNABIS SATIVA

HEMP

Too much use of it dries up the seed for procreation.

This Indian Hemp is similar to the one that produces the drug known as 'pot', 'grass' or hashish. The stalks grow to five or six feet (1.5 or 1.8 m) and are covered with a strong tough bark. The leaves are shaped like fingers. The green flowers grow toward the top of the stalks.

Where to find it: It is a cultivated plant in India. It is illegal to possess it in most western countries.

Flowering time: Late summer to mid autumn.

Astrology: It is a plant of Saturn.

Medicinal virtues: The seed expels wind. Boiled in milk, and taken, it helps those that have a hot or dry cough. An emulsion made from the seed is good for jaundice, particularly if there be an ague accompanying it, for it opens obstructions of the gall and causes digestion of choler. The emulsion or decoction of the seed stays the lax and continual fluxes, eases the colic, and allays the troublesome humours of the bowels. It also stays bleeding at the mouth, nose or other places. It kills worms in man or beast and if the juice is dropped into the ears, it will kill worms in them and draw forth earwigs or other living creatures.

The decoction of the root allays inflammations of the head, or any other parts. The herb or distilled water of it does the same. A decoction of the root eases gouty pains, hard knots in the joints, and pain in the sinews and hips. The fresh root mixed with a little oil and butter is good for burns.

Modern uses: Cannabis is an analgesic and hallucinatory drug. It is smoked like Opium in many eastern countries and illegally in the West. It is anti-spasmodic and will reduce nerve pain, but it has toxic side-effects.

HENBANE (Common)

The leaves applied as a warm fomentation are good for swellings of the testicles or women's breasts.

Henbane has large, thick, soft, woolly leaves, thick stalks two or three feet (61 or 91 cm) high, and hollow deadish yellow flowers with purplish veins. The root is white and thick, very like Parsnip. The whole plant has an offensive smell.

Where to find it: It can be found in hedgerows, waysides, waste ground and on banks.

Flowering time: Summer.

Astrology: This herb is under the dominion of Saturn.

Medicinal virtues: The leaves cool inflammations of the eyes, and any part of the body, if they be boiled in wine and applied. It also assuages the pain of the gout, the sciatica and other pains in the joints which arise from a cold cause. Applied with vinegar to the temples and forehead, it helps the headache and want of sleep in hot fevers. The juice of the herb or seed does the same.

The oil of the seed is good for deafness, noise and worms in the ears, being dropped there. The decoction of the herb or seed kills lice in man or beast.

This herb must never be taken inwardly. It is altogether an outward medicine. Goat's milk, Honey water and Mustard-seed are among the best antidotes when Henbane has been taken inwardly.

Modern uses: Henbane is a poisonous plant which is listed as an official medicine in the British Pharmacopoeia. It is sedative and analgesic, depressing the brain and producing drowsiness. It has been used in the treatment of Parkinson's disease.

Linctuses and mixtures, prepared pharmaceutically, and containing Henbane, are prescribed for asthma and whooping cough. It is not to be used except on medical prescription.

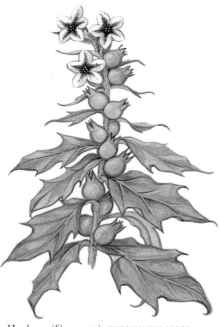

Henbane (Common) HYOSCYAMUS NIGER

HENRY (Good)

It is preferred to Spinach and is much superior in firmness and flavour.

A perennial, known as Good King Henry, Mercury or All-good. The root is thick and yellowish, and the leaves grow on long stalks like Spinach. The flowers are very small and grow in a spike.

Where to find it: Roadsides, waste places, pastures and arable farmland.

Flowering time: Spring.

Astrology: It is under the dominion of Mercury.

Medicinal virtues: Detersive and diuretic, the herb ought to have a place in vulnerary decoctions and fomentations. The young shoots, the succeeding leaves and the flowery tops are fit for kitchen purposes. It is good for scurvy and provokes urine. Outwardly it is much used in clysters, and a cataplasm of the leaves helps the pain of the gout.

Modern uses: The leaves can be used externally in compresses to soothe aching and painful joints, but it is not considered to be of much value internally. Its main use has always been as a vegetable to be used as an alternative to Spinach.

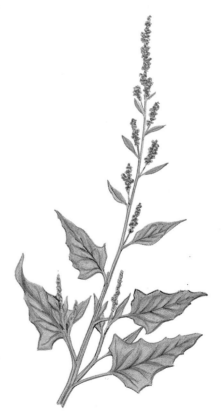

Henry (Good)
CHENOPODIUM BONUS-HENRICUS

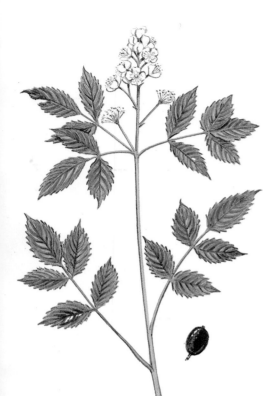

HERB CHRISTOPHER

The leaves may be applied with good success to hard tumours or swellings on the breast.

A perennial, commonly called Banebarry, growing to about two feet (61 cm) high. The root is long and thick, black on the outside, yellow within. The leaves are large and divided and the flowers are small and white. It bears black, shiny berries.

Where to find it: Woods and scrubland.

Flowering time: Midsummer.

Astrology: It is under the dominion of Saturn.

Medicinal virtues: The berries are poisonous; but used externally, the leaves are good for inflammations and can be used in place of Common Nightshade.

Modern uses: The whole plant is poisonous, and is not to be used internally. A homoeopathic medicine is made from the root and is a remedy for rheumatism.

There is an American variety with white berries, known as White Cohosh (*Actaea alba*). This is indicated in the treatment of painful menstruation and pelvic congestion, with emotional upsets and depression. The dosage of the tincture is 2–5 drops only, three times a day.

Herb Christopher ACTAEA SPICATA

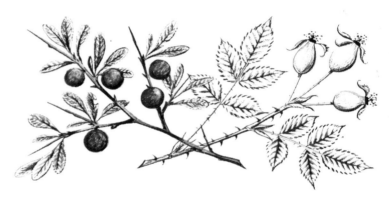

GERANIUM ROBERTIANUM

HERB ROBERT

All Geraniums are vulneraries, but this herb more particularly so.

An annual with reddish stems up to two feet (61 cm) high with pink flowers. The whole plant has a strong smell.

Where to find it: Common on waste ground, woodland and banks of ditches.

Flowering time: Early to midsummer.

Astrology: It is under the dominion of Venus.

Medicinal virtues: It is commended against the stone and to stay bleeding. It speedily heals wounds and is effectual in old ulcers in the privy parts or elsewhere. A decoction of it has been of service in obstructions of the kidneys and in gravel.

Modern uses: The crushed fresh leaves can be used as a compress for healing wounds. The plant is sedative and astringent. A strong infusion – 1 oz (28 g) to ½ pt (284 ml) of boiling water – is used as a gargle and mouthwash for sore throat and mouth, and also as a lotion for eye irritation. A cloth soaked in the infusion is useful as an application for irritating skin conditions.

The dried herb made into an infusion – using 1 oz (28 g) to 1 pt (568 ml) of boiling water – is taken in doses of 2 fl oz (56 ml) three or four times a day for peptic ulcer, simple diarrhoea and internal haemorrhage. This infusion is also suitable for diabetics as it lowers blood sugar levels.

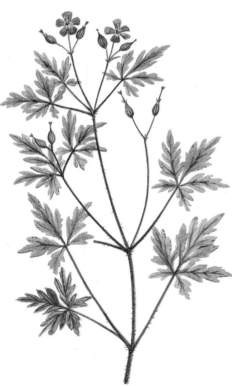

Herb Robert GERANIUM ROBERTIANUM

HERB TRUE-LOVE

The leaves or berries are good as antidotes against all kinds of poison, especially that of Aconites, and pestilential disorders.

True-love, also called One-berry and Herb Paris, has a small creeping root which produces stems with leaves, some bearing berries. At the top are four leaves set like a cross or ribband tied in a true-love's knot and a yellowish-green star-shaped flower, in the centre of which forms the blackish-purple berry, the size of a grape and full of juice.

Where to find it: Woods and copses, borders of fields and waste ground.

Flowering time: Spring to summer.

Astrology: Venus owns it.

Medicinal virtues: The roots in powder, taken in wine, ease the pains of the colic. The leaves are very effectual for healing wounds and filthy old sores and ulcers, and for dispersing tumours and swellings in the privy parts, the groin and to allay all inflammations.

The juice of the leaves applied to felons, or nails of the hands and feet, heals sores or imposthumes at the roots of them.

Modern uses: Although said to be an antidote to poison, True-love is an emetic, narcotic and aphrodisiac. An ointment made from the seeds has been used as an application to tumours. In small doses, the plant is anti-spasmodic, whereas in overdosage delirium and convulsions are produced. The seeds and berries have been used as an aphrodisiac, the action being similar to Opium. A tincture made from the fresh plant is used in homoeopathic medicine for inflammation of the brain.

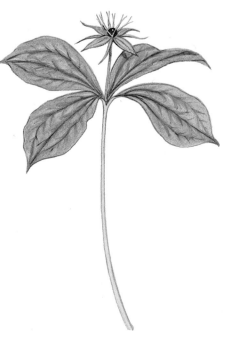

Herb True-love PARIS QUADRIFOLIA

HOLLY

The bark and leaves are excellent, being used in fomentations for broken bones, and such members as are out of joint.

The well-known evergreen bush or tree with glossy green, prickly leaves and red or yellow berries. Also called Holm or Hulver-bush.

Where to find it: Often planted as a hedge, but grows in woodland.

Flowering time: Late spring, early summer. The berries ripen in autumn and stay on the tree through the winter.

Astrology: The tree is saturnine.

Medicinal virtues: The berries are profitable in the colic. If a dozen of them are eaten in the morning when they are ripe and not dried, they purge the body of gross and clammy phlegm; but if the berries are dried and beaten into a powder, they bind the body and stop fluxes and the terms in women.

Modern uses: The leaves contain theobromine which has a weak diuretic effect on the kidneys, dilates coronary and other arteries. An infusion of the leaves produces sweating and is used in fevers and rheumatism. The berries are poisonous, being violently emetic and purgative, but have been used to treat dropsy. The powdered berries are anti-haemorrhagic. For catarrhal complaints, coughs, colds and 'flu an infusion is made of ½ oz (14 g) of chopped Holly leaves to 1 pt (568 ml) of boiling water. The dose is 1 fl oz (28 ml).

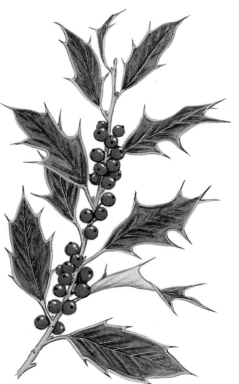

Holly ILEX AQUIFOLIUM

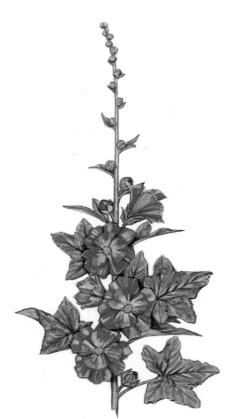

Hollyhocks ALTHAEA ROSEA
(= ALCEA ROSEA)

ALTHAEA ROSEA (= ALCEA ROSEA)

HOLLYHOCKS

It is mostly used in gargles for the swelling of the tonsils, and the relaxation of the uvula.

This is a tall garden plant, six or seven feet (1.8 or 2.1 m) high, with thick round stalks and large round hairy leaves. The flowers are of a pale red colour.

Where to find it: Formerly from China, it grows freely in gardens.

Flowering time: Mid to late summer.

Astrology: It is of the nature of the Common Marsh Mallow (*Althaea officinalis*) but less mollifying. Like all Mallows, it is under Venus.

Medicinal virtues: All parts have a rough, austere taste, especially the root, which has a very binding nature. Use the root to advantage, both inwardly and outwardly, for incontinence of urine, immoderate menses, bleeding wounds, spitting of blood, the bloody flux and other fluxes of the belly.

It is also of efficacy in a spongy state of the gums, attended with looseness of the teeth and soreness in the mouth.

Dried and reduced to a powder, or boiled in wine, and partaken of freely, it prevents miscarriage, helps ruptures, dissolves coagulated blood from falls and blows and kills worms in children.

Modern uses: The Hollyhock can be eaten, but is not very tasty. The flowers are soothing and diuretic and used as a pectoral tonic. They should be picked when in full bloom and dried. The infusion – of ½–1 oz (14–28 g) to 1 pt (568 ml) of boiling water – is taken in doses of 2 fl oz (56 ml), three or four times a day, for coughs and bronchitis. See Mallow.

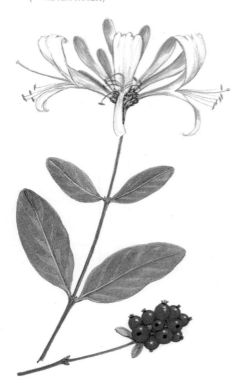

Honeysuckle LONICERA PERICLYMENUM

LONICERA PERICLYMENUM

HONEYSUCKLE

The oil made by infusion of the leaves, is healing and warming, and good for the cramp and convulsions of the nerves.

A climbing shrub, also known as the Woodbine or Perfoliate Honeysuckle, it produces flowers of a pale red colour, made up of several long slender tubes, with broad lips, and small red berries.

Where to find it: Grows in hedgerows and is cultivated in gardens.

Flowering time: All summer.

Astrology: A hot martial plant in the sign of Cancer.

Medicinal virtues: The leaves are the only parts used and are put into gargarisms for sore throats. Some recommend a decoction for a cough and the phthisic and to open obstructions of the liver and spleen.

Modern uses: The Honeysuckle is laxative, expectorant, diuretic, diaphoretic and emetic. It contains natural antibiotics and salicylic acid from which aspirin is produced.

The leaves are used as an infusion, one part to 100 parts of boiling water, as a laxative. The flowers, used in the same proportions, are taken for coughs, catarrh and asthma, or may be made into a syrup by adding honey until the mixture thickens. The dose is one teaspoonful.

Taken in large doses, the plant is emetic and toxic.

HUMULUS LUPULUS

HOPS

A decoction of the tops cleanses the blood, cures the venereal disease, and all kinds of scabs.

A perennial climber with Vine-like leaves. The clusters of scaly-headed flowers of a pale greenish-yellow are female flowers; male flowers are tiny and white.

Where to find it: Cultivated in gardens and also found wild in hedgerows.

Flowering time: Mid to late summer.

Astrology: It is under the dominion of Mars.

Medicinal virtues: It will open obstructions of the liver and spleen, cleanse the blood, loosen the belly, cleanse the reins from gravel and provoke the urine. The decoction of the tops cures the itch and breakings out of the body, tetters, ringworms, spreading sores, morphew and all discolourings of the skin.

The decoction of the flowers and tops helps to expel poison. Half a dram (890 mg) of the seed in powder, taken in drink, kills worms in the body, brings down women's courses and expels urine. A syrup made of the juice and sugar cures yellow jaundice and eases the headache that comes of heat.

Modern uses: A bitter aromatic tonic, with sedative and diuretic properties. The flowers contain a natural antibiotic. Hops will produce sleep when nothing else will. A pillow stuffed with Hops is the country remedy for inducing a good night's sleep.

Poultices made from the flowers are used for boils and painful swellings. An infusion of 1 oz (28 g) of the flowers to 1 pt (568 ml) of water acts as a bitter tonic and will rectify indigestion and improve appetite. The herb stimulates oestrogen production and in men curbs excessive sexual desire and is a remedy for spermatorrhoea. A tincture is available from herbalists. The dose is 5–20 drops.

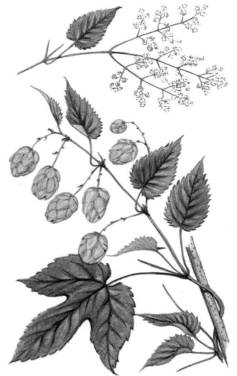

Hops HUMULUS LUPULUS

BALLOTA NIGRA

HOREHOUND (Black)

It is recommended as a remedy against hysteric and hypochondriac affections.

Black Horehound is taller and more branched than the White. The flowers are reddish-purple and labiated like the Nettle family.

Where to find it: Common in waste places, roadsides and hedges.

Flowering time: Midsummer.

Astrology: A herb of Mercury.

Medicinal virtues: This has not as much virtue as the White Horehound. Only the leaves and tops are used. Beaten with salt, the leaves applied to a wound cures the bites of mad dogs, and the juice, mixed with honey, cleanses foul ulcers. An intense bitter, it strengthens weak stomachs.

It is endowed with the properties of a balsam, acting as a powerful alterative and capable of opening obstructions of any kind. It also promotes the menses.

Some praise it very much as a pectoral in coughs and shortness of breath, but it is necessary to observe some caution. It ought only to be administered to gross phlegmatic people and not to thin plethoric persons. The powder is good to kills worms.

Modern uses: Black Horehound is an anti-spasmodic, a stimulant and a vermifuge. It has a relaxing effect on heart tissue and is used by some herbalists as a circulatory tonic to help lower blood pressure. It also acts on the hormonal system and will normalise heavy or scanty menstruation. The whole herb is used, but because of its unpleasant nature it is usually prescribed as a fluid extract in doses of half a teaspoonful.

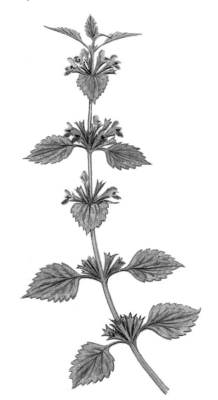

Horehound (Black) BALLOTA NIGRA

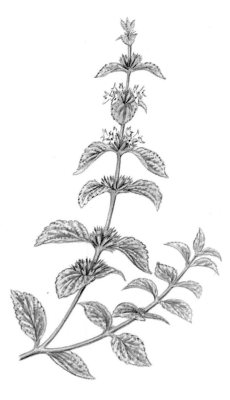

Horehound (White) MARRUBIUM VULGARE

HOREHOUND (White)

The syrup of Horehound is excellent for cold rheums in the lungs of old people, and for those who are asthmatical or short-winded.

Common Horehound has square hairy stalks about two feet (61 cm) high with crumpled leaves and small white flowers.

Where to find it: Roadsides and dry waste places.

Flowering time: Midsummer.

Astrology: A herb of Mercury.

Medicinal virtues: A decoction of the dried herb, with the seed, or the juice of the fresh herb taken with honey, is a good remedy for a cough, or for consumption. Taken with the roots, it helps to expectorate tough phlegm from the chest.

It is given to women to bring down their courses, to expel the afterbirth and also to people who have taken poison.

The leaves used with honey, purge foul ulcers, stay running and creeping sores, and help pains in the sides. The juice, with wine and honey, helps to clear the eyesight and, snuffed up the nostrils, it purges away the yellow jaundice. Combined with Oil of Roses, and dropped into the ears, it eases the pains in them.

It opens obstructions of the liver and spleen and is used outwardly to cleanse the chest and lungs. A decoction is available for those with hard livers or who have the itch or running tetters. The powder, or decoction, kills worms.

Modern uses: A valuable herb in modern practice, Horehound is a pectoral tonic mainly used for its expectorant properties. For coughs it is usually combined with other agents such as Colt's Foot, Marsh Mallow and Ground-ivy, in various proportions. Syrup of Horehound is still widely used for chills, asthma and other lung conditions and is an ingredient of many over-the-counter medicines. The syrup is made by adding honey or sugar to a strong infusion. An ordinary infusion of the whole herb is made by adding 1 oz (28 g) of the dried herb to 1 pt (568 ml) of boiling water and infusing for 20 minutes. The dose is 2 fl oz (56 ml) three or four times a day.

Taken hot, Horehound induces perspiration and helps to reduce temperature in mild fevers. In large doses it acts as a laxative. It is a suitable herb to give to children with coughs.

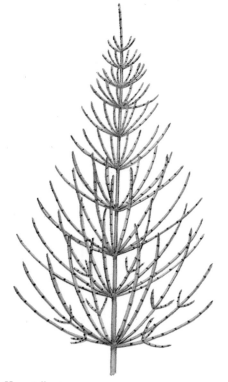

Horsetail EQUISETUM ARVENSE

HORSETAIL

It is very powerful to stop bleeding either inward or outward, the juice of the decoction being drunk, or the juice, decoction, or distilled water applied outwardly.

There are many kinds of this herb, which are but knotted rushes, some with leaves and others without.

Where to find it: Wet, boggy ground.

Flowering time: It produces catkins in midsummer.

Astrology: This herb belongs to Saturn.

Medicinal virtues: It stays laxes or fluxes in man or woman and heals inward ulcers and excoriation of the entrails and bladder. It solders together fresh wounds and cures ruptures in children. The decoction, taken in wine, provokes urine and helps the stone and strangury.

The distilled water taken two or three times a day, a small quantity at a time, also eases the guts and is effectual for coughs. Used as a warm fomentation, the juice or distilled water is of service in inflammations, pustules, or red wheals, and eases the swelling heat and inflammation of the fundament, or privy parts, in men or women.

Modern uses: Equisetum is an astringent diuretic used for acute inflammation of the urinary tract and incontinence. It is given as a decoction, ½ oz (14 g) of the dried herb being added to 1 pt (568 ml) of cold water and allowed to soak for a few hours. It is then brought to the boil, simmered for 20 minutes and cooled. The dose is 2 fl oz (56 ml) three or four times a day.

This preparation is also used as a gargle for oral infections. *Equisetum* is rich in silica, a mineral constituent of skin and nails, and will often help skin complaints such as eczema and acne, if used internally and externally.

CYNOGLOSSUM OFFICINALE

HOUND'S TONGUE

The root baked under the embers, wrapped in paste and a suppository made thereof, and put into or applied to the fundament, does very effectually help the painful piles or haemorrhoids.

A perennial about three feet (91 cm) high with large, woolly leaves and clusters of sullen, red, funnel-shaped flowers.

Where to find it: By hedges and roadsides.

Flowering time: Early to midsummer.

Astrology: The plant is governed by Mercury.

Medicinal virtues: The root is cold, drying and binding and useful for catarrhal defluxions. It is excellent for all kinds of fluxes and haemorrhages as well as for gonorrhoea. It is a vulnerary and helpful in scrofulous tumours, taken inwardly, and applied outwardly as a cataplasm. It cures the bites of mad dogs, if some of the leaves are applied to the wound. The bruised leaves or their juice boiled in hog's lard and applied to the scalp helps the falling away of the hair. It is also applied to any part that is scalded or burnt.

The distilled water of the herb and roots can be used as a wash to heal all manner of wounds and all foul ulcers due to venereal disease.

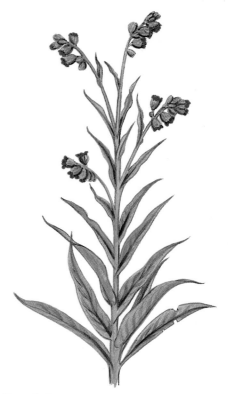

Hound's Tongue CYNOGLOSSUM OFFICINALE

Modern uses: The herb is soothing and helps to reduce pain. It is also astringing. An ointment can be made from the powdered root and used to relieve the irritation and pain of piles. An ointment made from Pilewort is, however, more popular.

SEMPERVIVUM TECTORUM

HOUSELEEK

The leaves gently rubbed on the places stung by nettles or bees, will quickly remove the pain.

Houseleek has a great many thick succulent leaves set together to form a stalk about a foot (30 cm) high. There are thinner and longer leaves on top and spikes of starry red flowers.

Where to find it: Mainly cultivated in gardens; but it prefers rocky, chalky ground, and will grow on old roofs and walls.

Flowering time: Midsummer.

Astrology: A herb of Jupiter.

Medicinal virtues: The juice is good in hot agues. It cools and restrains all violent inflammations, St Anthony's fire, scalds and burns, shingles, fretting ulcers, cankers, tetters, ringworms and eases the pain of the gout.

The juice also takes away warts and corns in the hands or feet. Applied to the temples, it takes away headache. The bruised leaves laid upon the crown of the head stay bleeding at the nose quickly.

Modern uses: The fresh leaves have the medicinal properties, the sap being astringent and cooling. The leaves are crushed and used as a cold poultice to relieve burns and stings and applied to the forehead to ease migraine and feverish headaches. The leaves also give relief if applied directly as a warm poultice to painful haemorrhoids. Alternatively, an ointment can be used by adding the juice to melted wax. The juice applied daily to a corn will soften it.

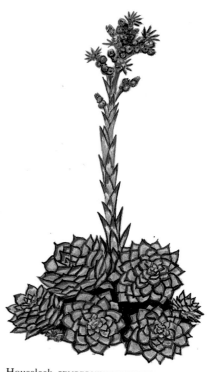

Houseleek SEMPERVIVUM TECTORUM

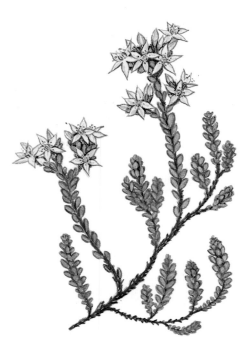

Houseleek (Wall Pepper) SEDUM ACRE

HOUSELEEK (Wall Pepper)

It is good for the scurvy.

A perennial with stalks four or five inches (10 or 13 cm) long, completely covered with thick, fat, triangular, blunt leaves and bearing yellow star-shaped flowers. Also called Biting Stonecrop.

Where to find it: It grows on old walls and the roofs of low houses, on rocks and sandy soil.

Flowering time: Late spring, early summer.

Astrology: A herb of Jupiter.

Medicinal virtues: It has a very hot biting taste and many know it as Pepperwort. Its qualities are directly opposite to the Small Houseleek (*Sedum rupestre*) and other *Sedums* and more apt to raise inflammations than to cure them; it ought not to be put into the *Unguent Populeon* nor into any other medicine for inflammation.

It is good for scurvy taken inwardly as a decoction and used outwardly as a fomentation. It is also commended for the king's-evil.

Modern uses: A decoction of the herb is used in the treatment of high blood pressure, but small doses only can be used as it is emetic and purgative in large doses. It contains an irritating substance which can cause blisters if applied to the skin. It is also contra-indicated in pregnancy as it may cause abortion. A tincture of the fresh plant given in small doses is prescribed by homoeopaths for anal fistulas and haemorrhoids. It is not recommended for domestic use.

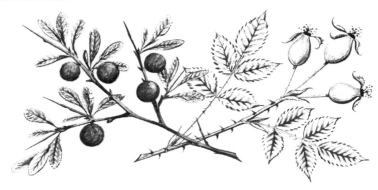

HYACINTH

It will cure the whites.

This is the Bluebell or Wild Hyacinth, a perennial bulb. The graceful stem bears drooping, bell-shaped flowers.

Where to find it: It grows beneath hedges and in gardens and masses itself in woodland.

Flowering time: Spring.

Astrology: Not assigned to any planet.

Medicinal virtues: The root is full of a slimy juice, a decoction of which promotes the urine. Dried and reduced to a powder, it is of a balsamic and styptic nature. Its virtues are little known. The fresh roots are poisonous and may be made into starch.

Modern uses: The bulk is a diuretic and a styptic, but used fresh is poisonous. Its main indication for use has been leucorrhoea, a profuse vaginal discharge. However the effective dose of the dried powdered bulb is only three grains (195 mg) and not to be exceeded and, therefore, this remedy is not recommended for domestic use.

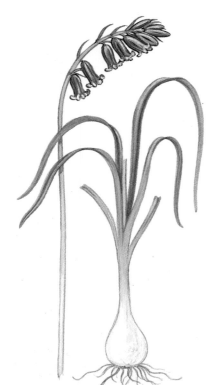

Hyacinth HYACINTHOIDES (= ENDYMION) NON-SCRIPTA

HYSSOPUS OFFICINALIS

HYSSOP

It amends and cherishes the native colour of the body spoiled by the yellow jaundice.

This Hyssop grows to about a foot (30 cm) or more high, with many stalks, square at first, but becoming round as they come to flower. The leaves are long and narrow, and the blue flowers grow in long spikes.

Where to find it: It is cultivated in gardens.

Flowering time: Late summer.

Astrology: The herb is Jupiter's and the sign Cancer.

Medicinal virtues: Hyssop boiled with honey and Rue, and drank, helps those that are troubled with coughs, shortness of breath, wheezing and rheumatic distillations upon the lungs. Taken with Oxymel, it purges gross humours by stool. With honey it kills worms in the belly; and with fresh new figs bruised, helps to loosen the belly – more forcibly if Fleur-de-lys and Cresses be added.

It is an excellent medicine for quinsy, or swelling in the throat if used as a gargle. The head anointed with the oil, kills lice. It is good for falling-sickness, expectorates tough phlegm and is effectual in all cold griefs or diseases of the chest and lungs when taken as a syrup.

Modern uses: It is mainly used as a cough and chest medicine. An infusion of the dried herb – 1 oz (28 g) to 1 pt (568 ml) of boiling water – is taken in doses of 2 fl oz (56 ml) three or four times a day. It can be combined in equal parts with other cough remedies such as Horehound and Colt's Foot. In addition to its pectoral properties, Hyssop is also useful in fevers, if the infusion is drunk frequently so that perspiration is induced. As a stimulant, Hyssop increases blood circulation and reduces blood pressure. Fluid extracts, tinctures and syrups are available from herbalists.

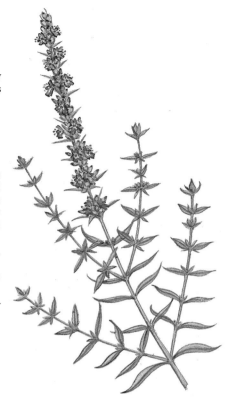

Hyssop HYSSOPUS OFFICINALIS

GRATIOLA OFFICINALIS

HYSSOP (Hedge)

It approaches the nature of the Foxglove in qualities as well as in form; and should be very moderately used, as its powers are very great.

A perennial growing to about a foot (30 cm) high with purplish-pink flowers. It is also called Gratiola.

Where to find it: By watersides and ditches and on boggy land.

Flowering time: Early to midsummer.

Astrology: A herb of Mars.

Medicinal virtues: A most violent purgative. It is not safe to take inwardly unless rectified by the art of the alchymist, and only the purity of it given. Used thus, it is helpful for the dropsy, gout and sciatica. Used in ointments it kills worms, the belly being anointed with it. The powdered root given in small doses is excellent against the worms. It also removes all the mucous matter from the intestines which harbours them.

Modern uses: The herb and root are dried and powdered and used in small doses for jaundice and liver congestion. It promotes urine flow and is laxative. In large doses it is emetic and purgative. Deaths have been recorded due to its use as an abortion agent. It is not recommended for domestic use. As a cardiotonic it relieves cardiac oedema, via the urine.

A tincture of the fresh flowering plant is used in homoeopathic medicine for rheumatic and arthritic conditions, the dose being five drops.

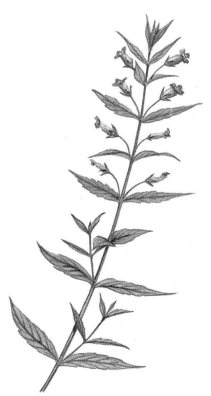

Hyssop (Hedge) GRATIOLA OFFICINALIS

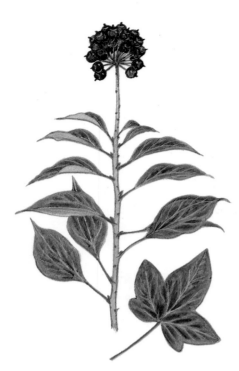

Ivy HEDERA HELIX

HEDERA HELIX
IVY

It is an enemy to the nerves and sinews, being much taken inwardly, but very helpful to them being outwardly applied.

Common Ivy is a well-known evergreen climber with small yellowish flowers and purplish-black berries.

Where to find it: It grows in woods twining itself around the trees, and on stone walls of houses and churches.

Flowering time: Midsummer. The berries are ripe in winter.

Astrology: It is under the dominion of Saturn.

Medicinal virtues: About a dram (1.7 g) of the flowers, powdered and drank twice a day in red wine, helps the lax and bloody flux. The berries powdered and drunk in wine two or three days together prevent and heal the plague. It also provokes the urine and women's courses. The fresh leaves boiled in vinegar and applied warm to the sides give much ease to those troubled with the spleen, ache or stitch. The same applied to the temples with Rose-water and Oil of Roses eases a long-standing headache.

The fresh leaves boiled in wine will cleanse old ulcers if used as a wash. This will also cure all burns and scalds. The juice of the berries or leaves snuffed up the nose purges the head and brain of thin rheum and cures the ulcers and stench therein.

Modern uses: The internal use of Ivy is not recommended as it can cause blood-cell destruction. The berries are toxic and, used externally, can cause skin blisters. However, the leaves can be used in poultices and fomentations for ulcers, enlarged glands, boils and abscesses.

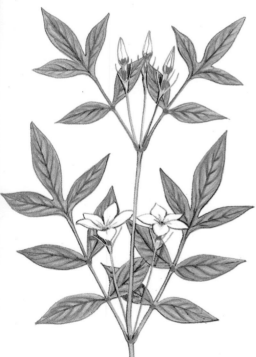

Jessamine JASMINUM OFFICINALE

JASMINUM OFFICINALE
JESSAMINE

It disperses crude humours, and is good for cold and catarrhous constitutions, but not for the hot.

This is the common White Jasmine, a climber which may grow to a height of twenty feet (6 m). The white flowers are like longish tubes with a pleasant agreeable smell. They are followed by berries.

Where to find it: It will grow in gardens, but is a native of the northern parts of India and Persia.

Flowering time: Early to midsummer.

Astrology: It is governed by Jupiter in the sign of Cancer.

Medicinal virtues: Only the flowers are used. It warms the womb and heals schirrhi therein and facilitates the birth. It is useful for coughs and difficulty in breathing. The oil made by infusion of the flowers, is used for perfumes. It is also good for hard and contracted limbs. If used as a liniment, or taken in a drink or clysters, it opens, warms and softens the nerves and tendons.

It removes diseases of the uterus and is of service in pituitous colics. A poultice of the leaves, boiled in wine, dissolves cold swelling and hard tumours.

Modern uses: The berries are considered to be toxic. A syrup made from the flowers is useful for coughs and catarrh. A homoeopathic tincture made from the berries is indicated in the treatment of tetanus and convulsions. The essential oil is used in aromatherapy massage as a treatment for menstrual pain and for respiratory disease. It is also considered to be an aphrodisiac, an anti-depressant and nerve sedative. A few drops of the oil can be used in the bath or two drops can be taken internally on a lump of sugar.

JUNIPER TREE

There is no better remedy for wind in any part of the body, or the colic, than the chymical oil drawn from the berries.

The Juniper is an evergreen bush with thick-set branches, narrow bluish-green leaves, small yellow flowers, and purplish berries each containing three-cornered seeds.

Where to find it: Heathland.

Flowering time: Late spring and early summer.

Astrology: A solar shrub.

Medicinal virtues: The berries are a counter-poison and resist the pestilence. It is a remedy against dropsy, brings down the terms, helps the fits of the mother, expels the wind and strengthens the stomach. It provokes the urine and is available for dysenteries and strangury. The berries are good for coughs, shortness of breath, consumption, pains in the belly, rupture, cramps, convulsions and speedy delivery to pregnant women.

They strengthen the brain, fortify the sight by strengthening the nerves, are good for agues, gout and sciatica, and strengthen the limbs. It is also a speedy remedy for those who have the scurvy, to rub the gums with it. The berries stay all fluxes, help the haemorrhoids and kill worms in children. They also break the stone, procure appetite and are good for palsies and falling-sickness.

Modern uses: The berries are diuretic and antiseptic and may be taken in the form of an infusion – 1 oz (28 g) of the berries to 1 pt (568 ml) of boiling water – for cystitis, the dose being 2 fl oz (56 ml) three or four times a day. The oil is carminative and one or two drops can be taken on a lump of sugar for indigestion and flatulence.

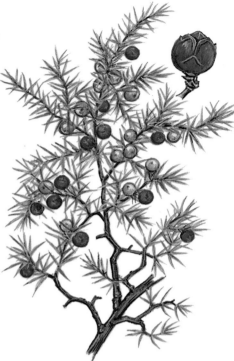

Juniper Tree JUNIPERUS COMMUNIS

KIDNEYWORT

It helps sore kidneys, torn by the stone, or exulcerated within.

Kidneywort, also called Navelwort, Wall Pennyroyal and Pennywort, has long branches bearing flowers, whitish-green in colour, shaped like little bells.

Where to find it: It grows on stone walls, rocks and in stony ground, particularly at the bottom of old trees.

Flowering time: Late spring.

Astrology: Venus challenges this herb under Libra.

Medicinal virtues: The juice or distilled water when drunk is good to cool inflammations and unnatural heats, a hot stomach, a hot liver, or the bowels.

The herb, juice or distilled water applied outwardly, heals pimples, St Anthony's fire and other outward heats. It provokes the urine, is available for dropsy and helps to break the stone.

Being used in the bath or made into an ointment, it cools the painful piles or haemorrhoidal veins. It gives ease to hot gout, the sciatica and inflammations and swellings in the testicles. It helps the kernels or knots in the throat, called the king's-evil.

The juice heals kibes and chilblains, if bathed with it, or annointed with ointment made from it. It is also used to stay the blood of fresh wounds and to heal them quickly.

Modern uses: A cooling diuretic not in popular use since the last century when it had a reputation as a remedy for epilepsy. The leaves can be used to make a poultice to apply to painful haemorrhoids, or made into an ointment by digesting them in hot wax and straining.

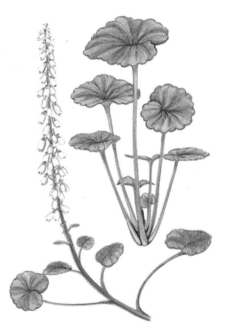

Kidneywort UMBILICUS RUPESTRIS
(= COTYLEDON UMBILICUS)

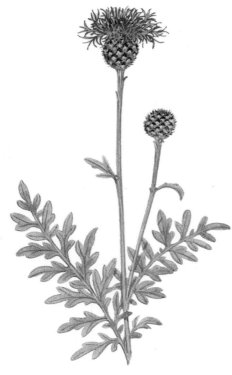

Knapweed (Common)
CENTAUREA SCABIOSA

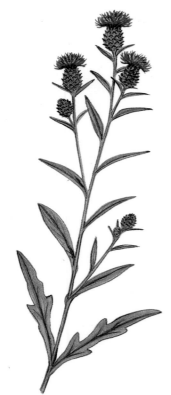

Knapwort (Harshweed) CENTAUREA JACEA

CENTAUREA SCABIOSA

KNAPWEED (Common)

It is of especial use for sore throat, swelling of uvula and jaws, and excellently good to stay bleeding, and heal up all fresh wounds.

A perennial, also known as Greater Knapweed, with broad, dark leaves, dented at the edges, and somewhat hairy. It bears dark purplish-red flowers.

Where to find it: It grows in moist places, borders of fields, hedges and on waste ground.

Flowering time: Early summer.

Astrology: Saturn owns this herb.

Medicinal virtues: It stops bleeding of the mouth and nose and veins that are broken inwardly. It is also good for those bruised by a fall. A decoction of the roots in wine is drunk and applied outwardly. It gently heals up running sores, both cancerous and fistulous, and will do the same for scabs of the head.

Modern uses: The roots and seeds have diuretic, diaphoretic and tonic properties. A decoction of the root made by boiling 1 oz (28 g) of the dried root in 2 pts (1.1 l) of water for 20 minutes is used in tablespoonful doses for catarrh. An ointment made by digesting the powdered root in hot paraffin wax, and straining, is useful for cuts and bruises.

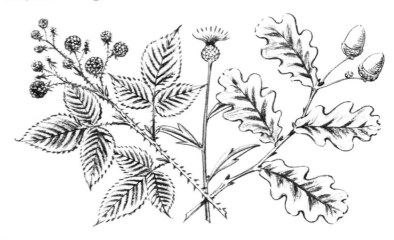

CENTAUREA JACEA

KNAPWORT (Harshweed)

The bruised herb is famous for taking away black and blue marks out of the skin.

This is also known as the Brown Knapweed and resembles the Common Knapweed. The flowers are large and of a lively purple.

Where to find it: Hilly pastures in chalk districts.

Flowering time: Midsummer.

Astrology: This is under Saturn.

Medicinal virtues: An astringent which is best given by decoction. However, the quantity given to have any effect must be large and thus it is seldom used.

It is opening, attenuating and healing. It will cleanse the lungs of tartareous humours and is helpful against coughs, asthma, difficulty of breathing and cold distempers. It is good for diseases of the head and nerves.

Modern uses: A smaller variety, the Black Knapweed (*Centaurea nigra*) is more popular with herbalists. As an astringent it is useful for piles, a decoction of the herb being taken in doses of 1–2 fl oz (28–56 ml) three times a day. This will also be useful for sore throat if used as a gargle. An infusion of the flowering part is helpful in diabetes mellitus.

KNOTGRASS

The juice is effectual to stay bleeding at the mouth, if drank in red wine.

This is also known as Coral Necklace. It has creeping stems with oval leaves and white or pink flowers.

Where to find it: Waysides and near paths into fields.

Flowering time: Late spring to early autumn.

Astrology: Saturn owns this herb.

Medicinal virtues: The juice applied to the forehead or temples stays bleeding at the nose. It reduces the heat of the blood and stomach and stops blood and other humours, including the bloody flux and women's courses.

It provokes urine, and helps the strangury. It expels the stone from the kidneys and bladder. A dram (1.7 g) of the powdered herb boiled in wine and drank is profitable for those bitten or stung by venomous creatures.

The distilled water cleanses foul ulcers, cancers, sores, imposthumes and green and fresh wounds and speedily heals them. Dropped into the ears, the juice will cleanse all runnings in them.

Modern uses: This particular Knotgrass, a member of the Caryophyllaceae family, is now very rare and Knotgrass these days usually refers to *Polygonum aviculare*, a common weed which has very similar properties. Indeed it may be that these two plants have been confused in the past by herbal writers. The leaves of *P. aviculare* are more pointed. As an astringent it is used for haemorrhages, including bleeding piles, and diarrhoea. It also helps to expel urinary tract stones. One teaspoonful of the powdered herb is used to make an infusion, one cupful being taken twice a day.

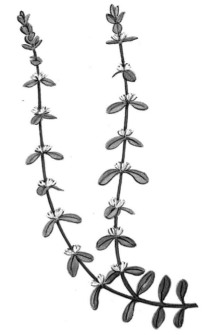

Knotgrass ILLECEBRUM VERTICILLATUM

LADY'S BEDSTRAW

The decoction of the herb or flower is good to bathe the feet of travellers and lacqueys, whose long running causeth weariness and stiffness in their sinews and joints.

It is also called Cheese-rennet, Gallion, Pettinugget and Maid-hair; and by some Wild Rosemary. The plant riseth up a yard (91 cm) high or more with very fine small leaves and many long tufts or branches of yellow flowers. There is also a variety with white flowers, less plentiful, and the leaves a little bigger.

Where to find it: Meadows and pastures, and by hedges.

Flowering time: Late spring. The seed is ripe from mid to late summer.

Astrology: They are both herbs of Venus, and therefore strengthen the parts, both internal and external, which she rules.

Medicinal virtues: The decoction of the yellow-flowered variety is good to fret and break the stone, provoke urine, stayeth inward bleeding and healeth inward wounds. The herb or flower bruised and put into the nostrils, stayeth their bleeding likewise.

The flowers and herb being made into an oil by being set in the sun, and changed after it hath stood ten or twelve days, or into an ointment, being boiled in axungia, or salad oil, with some wax melted therein after it is strained, do help burnings with fire or scaldings with water.

If the decoction be used warm and the joints afterwards anointed with ointment, it helpeth the dry scab and the itch in children. The herb with the white flower is also very good for the sinews, arteries and joints to comfort and strengthen them after travel, cold and pains.

Modern uses: A blood purifier and diuretic used in urinary tract disease, but to a limited degree.

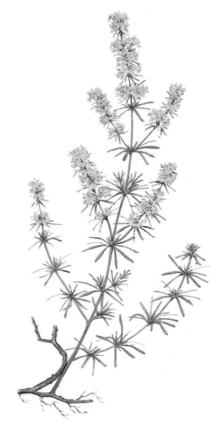

Lady's Bedstraw GALIUM VERUM

LADY'S MANTLE

When drank and outwardly applied, it help women who have over-flagging breasts, causing them to grow less and hard.

This plant branches from near the ground, and bears many hairy star-like leaves and greenish-yellow heads from which white flowers arise.

Where to find it: It grows in pastures and at the sides of woods.

Flowering time: Late spring, early summer.

Astrology: Venus claims this herb.

Medicinal virtues: It is for wounds that are inflamed and is effectual to stay bleeding, vomiting and flux, and to ease bruises and ruptures.

The distilled water drank for twenty days helps conception. To retain the birth, the woman should sit in a bath made from the decoction. It is a good wound-herb both inwardly and outwardly. The decoction can be used as a fomentation, or drank.

Modern uses: An astringent and styptic, it is mainly used as a remedy for excessive menstruation. It can be taken as an infusion, 1 oz (28 g) of the herb to 1 pt (568 ml) of boiling water, being taken in doses of 2 fl oz (56 ml) or as a vaginal injection or douche. To check simple diarrhoea use the powdered root as a decoction, a dose being taken after each evacuation.

Lady's Mantle ALCHEMILLA VULGARIS

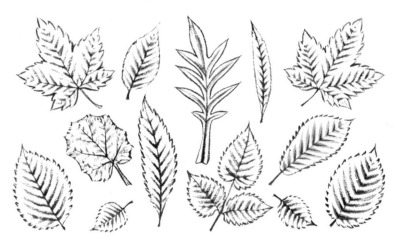

LADY'S SMOCK

This is very little inferior to Watercress in all its operations.

Also commonly known as Cuckoo Flower, it resembles Bittercress. It grows in small bunches of tender stalks with dark green leaves and produces flowers of a blushing white colour.

Where to find it: Wet places and at the sides of brooks.

Flowering time: Late spring, early summer.

Astrology: Under the dominion of the Moon.

Medicinal virtues: Good for the scurvy. It provokes the urine, breaks the stone and effectually warms a cold and weak stomach, restores lost appetite and helps digestion.

Modern uses: The plant contains vitamin C which confirms the observation that it is good for scurvy. It also has tonic and expectorant properties making it useful for coughs. The best way to use Lady's Smock is fresh in salads just like Watercress. The Large Bittercress (*Cardamine amara*) is collected when in flower and used as a tonic for the stomach in much the same way.

Lady's Smock CARDAMINE PRATENSIS

LANG DE BOEUF

Good to purge melancholy.

Also known as Bristly Ox-tongue, this is a close relative of Goat's Beard. It rises from a thick brown root and sends forth rough, hairy leaves, narrow and sharp-pointed. The yellow flowers grow at the top of the branches, each one set in a cup of rough leaves.

Where to find it: In gardens and fields. It likes clay soils.

Flowering time: Mid to late summer.

Astrology: It is under Jupiter.

Medicinal virtues: It is best preserved in a conserve of the flowers. A decoction of the whole plant is deobstruent. The tops are frequently put into wine and cool tankards to purge melancholy. They are also alexipharmic and good in malignant fevers.

Modern uses: Ox-tongue has been mainly used as pot herb. It is not popular with herbalists at the present time, although it is fairly common.

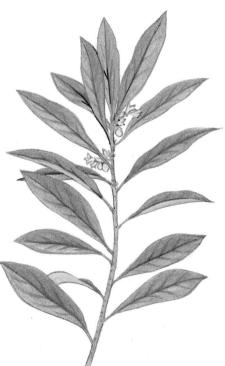

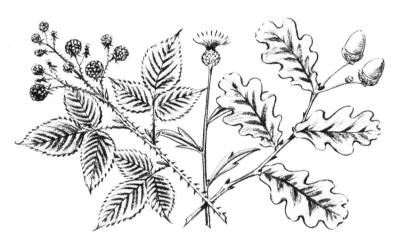

Lang de Boeuf PICRIS
(= HELMINTHIA) ECHIOIDES

DAPHNE LAUREOLA

LAUREL (Spurge)

Very happy effects have been produced by the use of this plant in rheumatic fevers.

This is the Spurge Laurel, a low shrub, seldom growing more than two or three feet (61 or 91 cm) high, with a woody stem and ash-coloured bark. The flowers are a sad, yellowish-green and have an unpleasant smell.

Where to find it: In woods and hedgerows.

Flowering time: Early spring.

Astrology: Not assigned to any planet.

Medicinal virtues: It is a rough purgative and is an efficacious medicine for worms, but it requires caution in its administration. In unskilful hands it might be productive of dangerous consequences.

The whole plant has the same qualities, but the bark is the strongest and a dose of not more than ten grains (650 mg) should be given. An infusion of the leaves is a good emetic and purgative and cures the dropsy. Dried and powdered, the leaves are useful in venereal disease.

Modern uses: It is emetic and laxative, but unpredictable results may occur. It is not recommended for domestic use. Several cases of poisoning have been reported. The leaves and bark will cause abortion. The leaves have been used to improve the menstrual flow, but there are much safer remedies available, such as Yarrow.

Laurel (Spurge) DAPHNE LAUREOLA

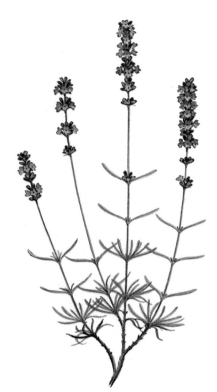

Lavender LAVANDULA ANGUSTIFOLIA
(= L. OFFICINALIS)

LAVENDER

It strengthens the stomach, and frees the liver and spleen from obstructions.

The common Lavender is a shrubby plant having many woody branches and long narrow leaves. The purple-blue flowers are borne on long spikes.

Where to find it: Cultivated in gardens, but found wild in mountainous Mediterranean countries.

Flowering time: Midsummer.

Astrology: Mercury owns this herb.

Medicinal virtues: It is of especial use for pains in the head and brain, following cold, apoplexy, falling-sickness, the dropsy or sluggish malady, cramps, convulsions, palsies and faintings. It provokes women's courses, and expels the dead child and afterbirth.

The flowers steeped in wine help those to produce water that are stopped, or troubled with the wind and colic, if the place be bathed with it. A decoction made of the flowers of Lavender, Horehound, Fennel and Asparagus root with a little Cinnamon, is profitable to help the falling-sickness and giddiness or turning of the brain. The decoction used as a gargle is good against toothache.

Two spoonfuls of the distilled water of the flowers help them that have lost their voice. Applied to the temples or nostrils, it reduces the tremblings and passions of the heart, and faintings and swoonings, but it is not safe to use when the body is replete with blood and humours. The oil used with the Oil of Spike is of a fierce and piercing quality and ought to be carefully used, a very few drops being sufficient for inward or outward maladies.

Modern uses: Lavender is stimulating and carminative. Its aromatic properties make it useful in pharmacy to add to lotions and creams. An infusion is made from the powdered flowers – one teaspoonful to 1 pt (568 ml) of boiling water – and sipped to prevent fainting and to allay nausea. Lavender water made from the essential oil is used in therapeutic baths to reduce nervous excitement and as a perfume. The oil has a sedative action on the heart and will lower blood pressure. A small amount added to bland oils makes a useful application in skin diseases, such as eczema and psoriasis, and a rub for rheumatic conditions.

Caution is needed when using the essential oil as it is extremely potent. The dosage of the oil for internal conditions is no more than one or two drops.

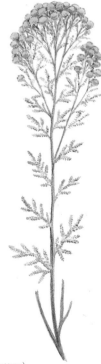

Lavender (Cotton)
SANTOLINA CHAMAECYPARISSUS

LAVENDER (Cotton)

It is an antidote for all sorts of poison.

A shrubby plant with roundish leaves which are retained all winter. The stalks have long white hoary leaves and many yellow flowers.

Where to find it: It is cultivated in gardens as an edging plant, but is a native of the Mediterranean countries.

Flowering time: Mid to late summer.

Astrology: It is under Mercury.

Medicinal virtues: The leaves and sometimes the flowers are used. The leaves and flowers boiled in milk and taken fasting will destroy worms. It is good against obstructions of the liver, the jaundice and to promote the menses. It is an antidote for the bites and stings of venomous creatures.

A dram (1.7 g) of the powdered leaves taken every morning on an empty stomach stops the running of the reins in men, and whites in women. The seed, beaten to a powder and taken as worm-seed, kills worms in children and people of riper years. Bathing in a decoction of the herb helps scabs and the itch.

Modern uses: An infusion of the herb – 1 oz (28 g) to 1 pt (568 ml) of boiling water – is used as a worm remedy in children and to promote menstruation in women whose periods are irregular. The infusion is taken in doses of 2 fl oz (56 ml).

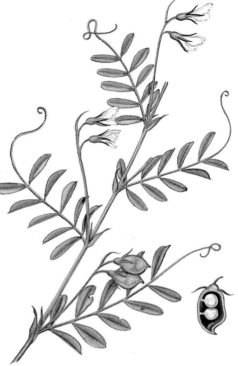

LENS CULINARIS (= ERVUM LENS)

LENTILS

They bind the body and stop looseness.

Lentils are the common name for one of the pulses. This variety has long-winged leaves and small white flowers which are followed by short flattish pods containing two round seeds.

Where to find it: In fields in most temperate regions.

Flowering time: Late spring. The seed is ripe in midsummer.

Astrology: They are under Venus.

Medicinal virtues: The flour or meal made from the seeds, which ripens in midsummer, can be made into an emollient cataplasm and will stop the fluxes.

The seeds, eaten with their skins, bind the body, but the liquid they are boiled in loosens the belly. The flowers are used outwardly in cataplasms for the same purposes as Bean flowers. See Beans.

Modern uses: Lentils have been an important food since ancient times, because of their protein content. Sprouted Lentils now have a reputation as a 'health food'. The seeds sprout quickly if covered in water overnight, are strained, and then rinsed twice a day so that they stay moist. The sprouts turn protein into peptogen and are rich in vitamins. They do not need so much cooking as Beans.

Lentils LENS CULINARIS (= ERVUM LENS)

LACTUCA SATIVA

LETTUCE (Common Garden)

It abates bodily lust.

The Salad Lettuce is so universally known that its description is unnecessary.

Where to find it: An important crop in farms and gardens.

Flowering time: Summer.

Astrology: The Moon owns it.

Medicinal virtues: The juice of the plant is mixed with Oil of Roses and applied to the temples to procure sleep and to cure a headache arising from a hot cause. Eaten boiled, lettuce loosens the belly, helps digestion, quenches thirst, increases milk in nursing mothers, and eases griping pains in the stomach.

It represses venereous dreams if outwardly applied to the testicles with a little Camphire. If applied to the region of the heart or liver, it will reduce heat and inflammation therein. The juice of the distilled water into which some White Sanders or Red Roses are placed, can be used instead to comfort and strengthen the parts and also to temper the heat of the urine.

The seeds or distilled water works the same effects but is forbidden to those who spit blood or are imperfect in their lungs.

Modern uses: Lettuce is rich in iron and vitamins and is cooling to the blood. Homoeopaths use a tincture of the whole plant as a remedy for impotence.

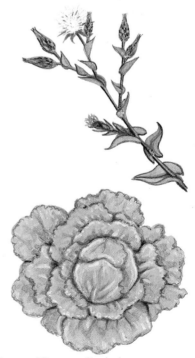

Lettuce (Common Garden)
LACTUCA SATIVA

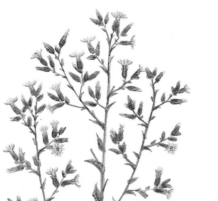

LACTUCA VIROSA

LETTUCE (Great Wild)

It eases the most violent pains of the colic.

Also known as Prickly Lettuce or Lettuce-opium, it grows to five or six feet (1.5 or 1.8 m) high, the lower leaves being a foot (30 cm) long and five (13 cm) inches wide. The flowers are a light yellow. Its milky juice has a smell like Opium.

Where to find it: The sides of ditches and in hedges.

Flowering time: Midsummer to early autumn.

Astrology: It is under the government of Mars.

Medicinal virtues: A syrup made from a strong infusion of the plant makes an excellent anodyne, easing pain and gently disposing the patient to sleep. It has none of the violent effects of other opiates. The best way of giving it is to dry the juice which runs from the roots by incision and add 1 oz (28 g) to a gallon (4.5 l) of wine. It will dissolve therein and make an excellent quieting medicine. A teaspoonful is given in a glass of water. It will ease spasms and convulsions and stop fluxes of all kinds arising from irritation.

Modern uses: The leaves and dried juice, or latex, are used as a sedative and analgesic in place of Opium. The syrup has expectorant properties and will soothe an irritable cough if given in doses of two teaspoonfuls. A tincture is available from herbalists, the dose being 20–30 drops.

Lettuce (Great Wild) LACTUCA VIROSA

PELTIGERA CANINA

LICHEN (Dog)

It is recommended for the bites of mad dogs if used in the following manner: take nine or ten ounces (255 or 284 g) of blood from the body for four mornings successively, and give the patient the following in warm cow's milk: take ash-coloured Liverwort, half an ounce (14 g), Black Pepper, two drams (3.5 g), both finely powdered, mixed, and divided into four equal parts. Having first taken the four doses, let the person, for one month, bathe two or three times a day in the sea, and the longer he stays in the better.

Dog Lichen spreads itself along the ground by outgrowths of its fleshy thallus. The red spore producing structures are borne on the edges of the lobes.

Where to find it: Moist, shady places.

Flowering time: It flowers not.

Astrology: Under the dominion of Jupiter and under the sign of Cancer.

Medicinal virtues: A good herb for all diseases of the liver, to cool and cleanse it and to help inflammation and the yellow jaundice. Bruised and boiled in beer and drank, it cools the liver and kidneys and helps the running of the reins in men and the whites in women. It is a good remedy to stay the spreading of the tetters, ringworm and other fretting or running sores and scabs.

Modern uses: The whole plant is used in the form of an infusion – 1 oz (28 g) to 1 pt (568 ml) of boiling water – and taken in doses of 2 fl oz (56 ml) as a liver tonic. It is laxative. It is best combined with other remedies for the liver such as Dandelion. The American Lichen is also used as an infusion for indigestion and liver disorders.

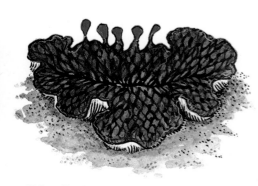

Lichen (Dog) PELTIGERA CANINA

LILY OF THE VALLEY

The spirit of the flowers distilled in wine, restores speech.

   A perennial with a slender creeping root, producing two or three oblong leaves about six inches (15 cm) long and a group of white, bell-shaped flowers.

Where to find it: Heathland and open land, but will also grow in a shady spot in the garden.

Flowering time: It flowers in late spring.

Astrology: It is under the dominion of Mercury and therefore strengthens the brain.

Medicinal virtues: The distilled water dropped into the eyes helps inflammation there. The spirit of the flowers distilled in wine helps the palsy, is good in apoplexy and comforts the heart and vital spirits. It is also of service in disorders of the head and nerves, such as epilepsy, vertigo and convulsions of all kinds and swimming in the head.

Modern uses: An important cardiac tonic resembling the action of Foxglove but without its toxicity. However caution must be exercised in using it, as overdosage causes vomiting and purging. *Convallaria* increases the power of the heart but slows its pace. It also acts as a diuretic and is therefore of use in dropsy. An infusion is made from the whole plant – 1 oz (28 g) to 2 pt (1.1 l) of boiling water – and taken in doses of one tablespoonful. Self-medication is not recommended for heart disease. Herbalists use a tincture made from the plant.

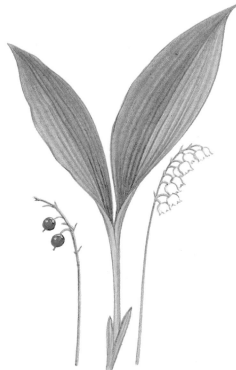

Lily of the Valley CONVALLARIA MAJALIS

NYMPHAEA ALBA (= N. ODORATA)

LILY (Water)

It settles the brain of frantic persons.

   The white Water Lily has large, thick, dark green leaves which float on the water. The flower is snow white and the roots are black.

Where to find it: Pools, standing water and slow running streams and rivers.

Flowering time: Summer.

Astrology: It is under the dominion of the Moon.

Medicinal virtues: The seed or root is effectual to stay fluxes of blood or humours, arising from wounds or from the belly. The roots are stronger and will restrain all fluxes, running of the reins and the passing away of seed when one is asleep. Its frequent use extinguishes venereous actions. The leaves used inwardly or outwardly are good for all agues. The syrup of the flowers procures rest. The distilled water of the flowers takes away freckles, spots, sunburn and morphew from the face and other parts of the body. The oil of the flowers cools hot tumours, eases pains and helps sores.

Modern uses: The root is used as an anaphrodisiac to reduce sexual excitement. It is also a strong astringent and will check diarrhoea. A decoction is made from the root and administered in doses of 2 fl oz (56 ml). Combined with powdered Slippery Elm, it is used in poultices for boils, ulcers and inflammatory diseases of the skin. The decoction is also used as a lotion for sore skin and as a gargle for sore throat. It can also be injected into the vagina to check leucorrhoea.

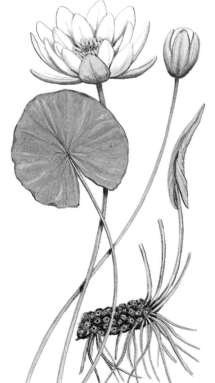

Lily (Water) NYMPHAEA ALBA
(= N. ODORATA)

113

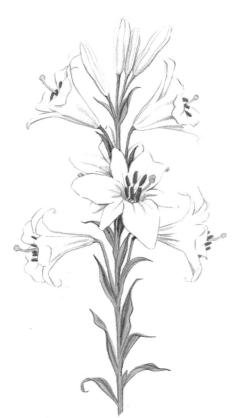

Lily (White Garden) LILIUM CANDIDUM

LILY (White Garden)

The roasted root mixed with hog's grease makes a good poultice to ripen and break plague-sores.

This is the white Meadow Lily, or Madonna Lily, now grown extensively in gardens.

Where to find it: It prefers soil that is sandy and well-drained.

Flowering time: Early summer.

Astrology: Under the dominion of the Moon.

Medicinal virtues: The flowers and roots are used, but mainly for external applications. They are emollient, suppling and anodyne and are good to dissolve and ripen hard tumours and swellings and to break imposthumations.

In pestilential fevers, the roots should be bruised and boiled in wine, and the decoction drank. The juice, baked with Barley-meal and eaten, is good for the dropsy. An ointment made of the roots and hog's grease is excellent for ulcers and to unite sinews that have been cut. It is also used for swellings in the privies and for scalds and burns. The root made into a decoction gives delivery to women in travail and expels the afterbirth.

Modern uses: Astringent and soothing, the decoction taken in doses of 2 fl oz (56 ml) is mainly used for vaginal discharge. A poultice is made from the root to treat external ulcers.

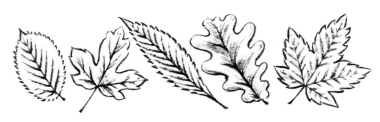

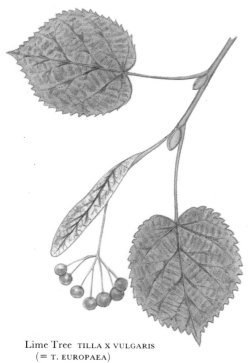

Lime Tree TILLA X VULGARIS (= T. EUROPAEA)

LIME TREE

Excellent for palpitations of the heart.

Also known as the Linden tree, it grows to well over a hundred feet (30 m) high, and has a smooth bark and spreading branches. The yellowish-white flowers are followed by clusters of round fruits.

Where to find it: Woods and open forests. Also cultivated in parkland and gentlemen's gardens.

Flowering time: Midsummer.

Astrology: It is governed by Jupiter.

Medicinal virtues: The flowers are the only parts used, and are a good cephalic and nervine, excellent for apoplexy, epilepsy and vertigo.

Modern uses: A nervine tonic used for tension headaches and hysteria. An infusion is made from one teaspoonful of the powdered flowers or leaves to 1 pt (568 ml) of boiling water and taken in doses of 2 fl oz (56 ml). A decoction of the bark stimulates the body to produce bile and is therefore useful for some cases of indigestion. The infusion is soothing for chronic coughs and catarrh, and will also check simple diarrhoea. The tincture is available from herbalists, who prescribe it for high blood pressure due to nervous tension.

LIQUORICE

The root of this plant is deservedly in great esteem, and can hardly be said to be an improper ingredient in any composition of whatever intention.

The English Liquorice resembles a young Ash tree sprung up from seed. It has narrow long green leaves and flowers like pea blossoms, but of a pale blue colour. The roots run very deep into the ground.

Where to find it: It grows wild in warm climates, originally coming from Spain and Italy. It is cultivated elsewhere.

Flowering time: Late summer.

Astrology: It is under the dominion of Mercury.

Medicinal virtues: The root boiled in water with some Maidenhead and figs makes a good drink for those who have a dry cough or hoarseness, wheezing or shortness of breath, and for pains in the chest and lungs. It is also good for pains of the reins, strangury and heat of the urine. The juice is also effectual in all diseases of the lungs and chest. A strong decoction of the root given to children loosens the bowels and takes off feverish heats which attend costiveness.

The juice or extract is made by boiling the fresh roots in water, straining the decoction and, when the impurities have settled, evaporating it over a gentle heat till it no longer sticks to the fingers. It is better to cut the roots into small pieces before boiling to obtain maximum extraction. A pound (454 g) of Liquorice in 3 pt (1.6 l) of water boiled down to 2 pt (1.1 l) is best for all purposes. The juice can be obtained by squeezing the roots between two rollers. When made carefully, it is sweeter than the root itself.

Modern uses: A widely used remedy for coughs and lung complaints. It is soothing, expectorant and anti-spasmodic. For coughs with sore throat it is often combined with Linseed and made into an infusion. One ounce (28 g) of powdered Liquorice and one teaspoonful of powdered Linseed are simmered in 3 pt (1.6 l) of water for 20 minutes. The same can be taken for stomach ulcers.

People with high blood pressure should not use Liquorice, as it may exacerbate this condition.

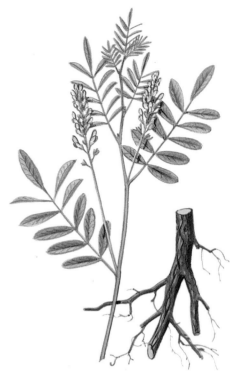

Liquorice GLYCYRRHIZA GLABRA

LOOSESTRIFE

This herb is good for all manner of bleeding at the mouth or nose.

Some know it as the Yellow Willowherb or Yellow Loosestrife. It has several brown hairy stalks two feet (61 cm) high or more with pale green leaves and bright yellow flowers.

Where to find it: By the sides of rivers and other watery places.

Flowering time: Summer.

Astrology: It is a herb of the Moon.

Medicinal virtues: Given either to drink or taken by clyster, this herb is good for wounds that are bleeding, fluxes of the belly and the bloody flux. It stays also the abundance of the women's courses. If the herb be bruised and the juice applied, it will quickly close up the lips of a wound.

It is good as a gargle for sore throats.

Modern uses: This is an astringent which will check haemorrhaging from the nose and also reduce menstrual bleeding. The whole herb is used when dried as an infusion in the proportions of 1 oz (28 g) to 1 pt (568 ml) of boiling water and given in doses of 2 fl oz (56 ml).

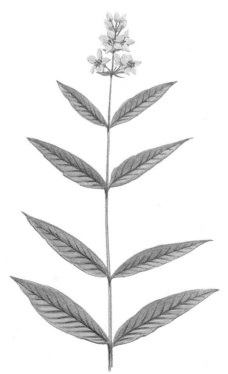

Loosestrife LYSIMACHIA VULGARIS

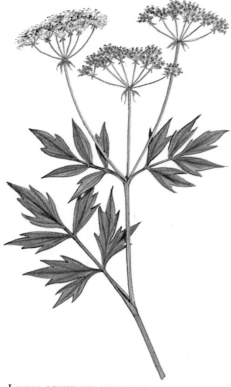

Lovage LEVISTICUM OFFICINALE

LEVISTICUM OFFICINALE

LOVAGE

The leaves bruised and fried in hog's lard and laid hot to any blotch or boil will quickly break it.

A perennial growing five or six feet (1.5 or 1.8 m) high with a thick root. It has large winged leaves and bears large umbels of yellowish flowers. The whole plant has a pleasant aromatic smell.

Where to find it: A native of mountainous districts in the Mediterranean, but cultivated in herb gardens.

Flowering time: Midsummer.

Astrology: It is an herb of the Sun under the sign of Taurus.

Medicinal virtues: It opens, cures, and digests humours and provokes women's courses and urine. Half a dram (890 mg) of the powdered root, taken in wine, warms a cold stomach, helps digestion and consumes all raw and superfluous moisture therein.

It eases all inward gripings and pains, dissolves wind, and resists poison and infection. A decoction of the herb is a remedy for ague, and pains of the body and bowels due to cold. The seed works more powerfully for all the conditions except the last.

The distilled water of the herb used as a gargle helps the quinsy in the throat. If drank three or four times, it helps the pleurisy. It takes away redness and dimness of the eyes if dropped into them and it removes spots and freckles from the face.

Modern uses: The root is used to expel wind from the stomach and to increase excretion through the kidneys in fevers. It also helps to ease painful menstrual periods. The powdered leaves are used as a culinary herb. An infusion of the root is a good way to take it, using 1 oz (28 g) to 1 pt (568 ml) of boiling water.

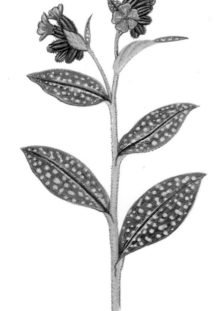

Lungwort PULMONARIA OFFICINALIS

PULMONARIA OFFICINALIS

LUNGWORT

It is of great use in diseases of the lungs.

The plant Lungwort (*Pulmonaria officinalis*) is recognised by its spotted leaves and violet-blue flowers. There is also a kind of moss (*Sticta pulmonaria*) with broad, greyish, rough leaves, which has similar properties.

Where to find it: The moss grows on Oak and Beech trees and is also known as Oak Lungs. The flowering Lungwort is found in woods and shady places.

Flowering time: *Pulmonaria officinalis* flowers in spring. *Sticta pulmonaria* flowers not.

Astrology: Jupiter owns this herb.

Medicinal virtues: For coughs, wheezings and shortness of breath. As an astringent it can be used in lotions to stay the moist humours that flow to ulcers and hinder their healing. It is also used to wash ulcers of the privy parts. It is drying and binding and will stop inward bleeding and too great a flux of the menses.

As a syrup it is good for consumptions and disorders of the chest and as a remedy against the yellow jaundice.

Modern uses: Because the name Lungwort has been applied to both a flowering plant and a moss there has been confusion among even the best herbal writers, who have mixed up the slightly differing attributes of both remedies, and even the common names. It is *Pulmonaria officinalis* that is commonly known as Jerusalem Cowslip, and is the 'Lungwort' mainly used by modern herbalists. This is emollient, expectorant and astringent. It is used as an infusion, the whole plant being collected in late spring and dried. It will be found useful for most respiratory conditions, including coughs, bronchitis, pharyngitis and bronchial catarrh. For coughs use equal parts of Colt's Foot and Lungwort. The infusion of Lungwort is also indicated for those with haemorrhoids and simple diarrhoea.

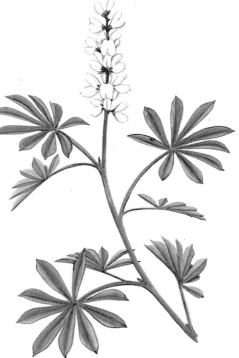

LUPINUS ALBUS

LUPIN

The seeds are somewhat bitter in taste . . . but good to destroy the worms.

The White Lupin has a hairy stalk with digitated leaves and white flowers like pea blossoms.

Where to find it: A cultivated plant, common in gardens.

Flowering time: Early summer.

Astrology: It is governed by Mars in Aries.

Medicinal virtues: The seeds are used internally to bring down the menses, expel the afterbirth and secundines. Outwardly they are used against deformities of the skin, scabby ulcers, scald heads and other cutaneous distempers.

Modern uses: The seeds soaked in water to soften them are applied externally to ulcers. Taken internally, they stimulate the kidneys, bring on the menstrual period and will destroy intestinal worms. Caution is required in self-medication as the seeds of some species of Lupin are poisonous. It is best to purchase herbal remedies from a reliable source.

Lupin LUPINUS ALBUS

RUBIA TINCTORUM

MADDER

The leaves and roots beaten and applied to any part that is discoloured with freckles, morphew, white scurf or any such deformity of the skin, cleanses thoroughly and takes them away.

It has thick roots, weak stems which often lie on the ground, and long spikes of yellow flowers, which are followed by small moist black berries.

Where to find it: A cultivated plant, it produces red and yellow dyes, but is a native of the warmer Mediterranean countries.

Flowering time: Midsummer.

Astrology: It is a herb of Mars.

Medicinal virtues: The roots have a weak, bitterish astringent taste. A strong decoction is diuretic and good for obstructions of the visceral organs, dispersing congealed blood and the dropsy and curing the jaundice. It cleanses the kidneys and urinary organs of stone and gravel and eases the sciatica. It is effectual for bruises both inward and outward. A decoction of the leaves makes a good fomentation to bring down the courses.

Modern uses: Not much used medicinally, although the roots, leaves and seeds have a reputation for improving the menstrual flow and for liver complaints. The powdered herb is taken in doses of 10–30 grains (0.65–1.9 g).

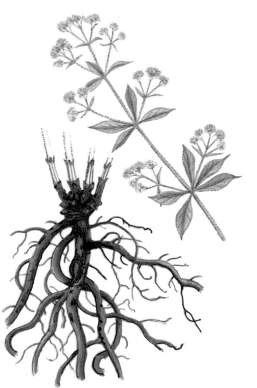

Madder RUBIA TINCTORUM

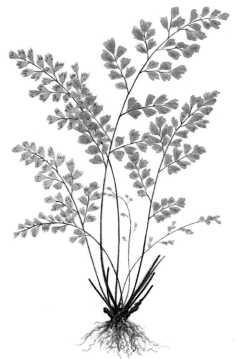

Maidenhair (Common)
ADIANTUM CAPILLUS VENERIS

ADIANTUM CAPILLUS VENERIS

MAIDENHAIR (Common)

Maidenhair should be used green, and in conjunction with other ingredients, because their virtues are weak.

This is a perennial evergreen fern, with small rounded green leaves and with spores spotted on the backs of them.

Where to find it: Stone walls, rocks and in moist caves.

Flowering time: There is no flower. The seed appears in late summer.

Astrology: This and all other Maidenhairs are under Mercury.

Medicinal virtues: A good remedy for coughs, asthma and pleurisy. It is also a gentle diuretic and useful in jaundice, gravel and other impurities of the kidneys.

Modern uses: An infusion of the leaves is used for catarrh. One ounce (28 g) of the leaves is infused in 1 pt (568 ml) of boiling water. For coughs, honey is added to make a syrup. The plant is also known as Maidenhair Fern or True Maidenhair. Another fern, *Asplenium trichomanes*, is also referred to as Common Maidenhair. Golden Maidenhair (*Adiantum aureum*) is recommended as a scalp treatment. It is boiled in water and used to wash the hair to prevent thinning. The White Maidenhair (*Asplenium ruta muraria*) has similar properties, the leaves being used for coughs, shortness of breath, and scalp problems, such as excess scurf.

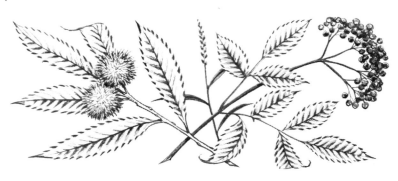

MALVA SYLVESTRIS

MALLOW (Common)

When boiled in water, the strong decoction is good to take off the strangury.

The Common Mallow grows three or four feet (0.9 or 1.2 m) high, with a thick round stem, roundish indented leaves and large reddish-mauve flowers.

Where to find it: Hedgerows, edges of fields and waste ground.

Flowering time: Late spring, early summer.

Astrology: All Mallows are under Venus.

Medicinal virtues: The whole plant is used, but the root has most virtue. The leaves, dried or fresh, are put into decoctions for clysters. The root may be dried, but it is best fresh, if chosen when there are only leaves growing from it, not a stalk.

Boiled in water, the strong decoction when drank provokes the urine, sharp humours of the bowel and gravel.

Sweetened with a syrup of Violets, it cures painful urination. A conserve of Mallow flowers, a syrup of the juice, a decoction of Turnips, or Willow, or a Syrup of Ground-ivy is also good for this.

Modern uses: The leaves and flowers are soothing to the urinary tract, intestines, and respiratory organs. An infusion of 1 oz (28 g) of the leaves or flowers in 1 pt (568 ml) of boiling water is taken in doses of 2 fl oz (56 ml) for cystitis, coughs and colds and for intestinal inflammation.

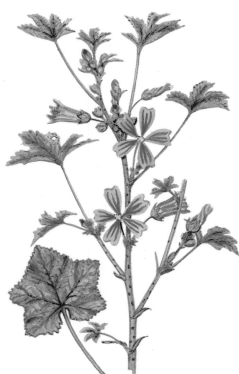

Mallow (Common) MALVA SYLVESTRIS

MANDRAKE

The root was formerly supposed to have the human form, but it really resembles a Carrot or a Parsnip.

Also known as Satan's Apple, it has a large brown root, sometimes single, sometimes divided into three parts. The plant produces several large dark green leaves about a foot (30 cm) long and four or five inches (10 or 13 cm) broad with pointed ends and a foetid smell. The flowers are bell-shaped and about the height and size of a Primrose, and are followed by a fruit about the size of a small apple.

Where to find it: A cultivated plant originally from the warmer parts of southern Europe.

Flowering time: Mid to late summer.

Astrology: It is governed by Mercury.

Medicinal virtues: The fruit has been accounted poisonous, but without cause. The leaves are cooling and are used for ointments and other external applications.

The fresh root operates very powerfully as an emetic and purgative, so that few constitutions can bear it. The bark of the dried root acts a rough emetic.

Modern uses: The root is strongly purgative and emetic and not recommended for domestic use. The dried powdered leaves can be used as an ointment for irritating skin conditions by digesting in hot wax and straining. A tincture made from the fresh plant is used by homoeopaths. It should not be confused with English Mandrake (*Bryonia dioica*) or American Mandrake (*Podophyllum peltatum*).

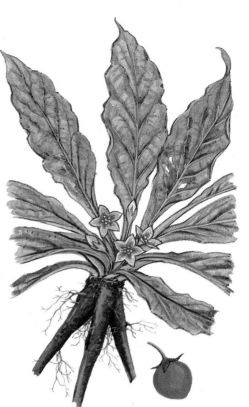

Mandrake MANDRAGORA OFFICINARUM
(= ATROPA MANDRAGORA)

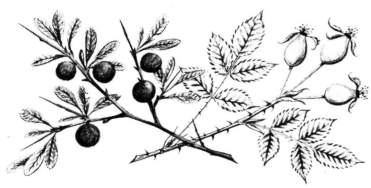

MAPLE TREE

The decoction of the leaves or bark strengthens the liver.

There are many varieties of this tree, including the American Sugar Maple which provides an excellent syrup.

Where to find it: It grows in hedgerows and in gentlemen's gardens.

Flowering time: It blossoms from early to late spring.

Astrology: It is under the dominion of Jupiter.

Medicinal virtues: A decoction of the leaves or bark opens obstructions of the liver and spleen and eases pains from them. The larger Maple, if tapped, yields a considerable quantity of liquor, of a sweet and pleasant taste, which may be made into wine. The wood boiled as sugar-cane leaves a powder hardly to be distinguished from sugar.

Modern uses: The bark of the Red Maple is astringent and a decoction of it is used as a lotion for sore eyes. Maple syrup is regarded as a 'health' food and is available from health stores. It can be used as a substitute for sugar.

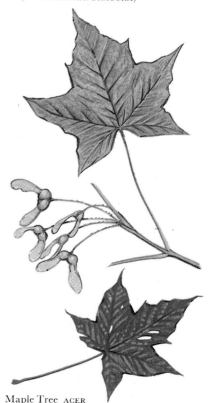

Maple Tree ACER

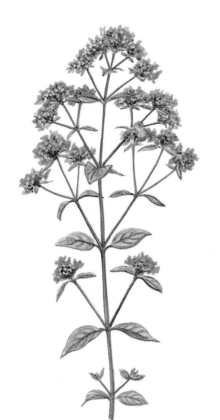

Marjoram (Common Wild)
ORIGANUM VULGARE

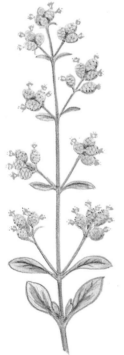

Marjoram (Sweet) ORIGANUM MAJORANA

ORIGANUM VULGARE

MARJORAM (Common Wild)

There is scarcely a better herb growing for relieving a sour stomach.

The Wild or Field Marjoram has a creeping underground root, which throws up hard brownish square stalks with small dark green leaves and tufts of purplish-red flowers.

Where to find it: Borders of cornfields and well-drained stony soil.

Flowering time: Late summer.

Astrology: It is under the dominion of Mercury.

Medicinal virtues: It strengthens the stomach and head, relieving loss of appetite, coughs and consumption of the lungs. It provokes urine and the terms in women, helps the dropsy, scurvy, scabs, itch and yellow jaundice. The juice dropped into the ears helps deafness, pain and noise in them.

The whole plant is a warm aromatic and an infusion of the dried leaves is extremely grateful to nervous cases. The essential oil poured on to lint and put into the hollow of an aching tooth removes the pain. The powdered leaves or tops are given for headaches. For flatulence and indigestion use a conserve of the tops.

Modern uses: A valuable herb with diaphoretic, expectorant and carminative properties. It is used for coughs, flatulence and at the start of fevers. It stimulates the menstrual flow. The herb is used as an infusion – 1 oz (28 g) to 1 pt (568 ml) of boiling water – the dose being 2 fl oz (56 ml) three or four times a day. The fresh plant simmered in seed oil or wax can be applied with massage for rheumatic complaints.

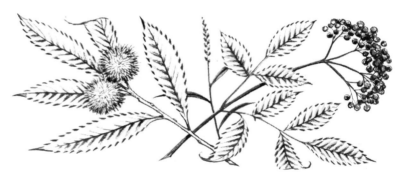

ORIGANUM MAJORANA

MARJORAM (Sweet)

The powder snuffed up into the nose provokes sneezing and thereby purges the brain.

A culinary herb growing to about ten inches (25 cm) high, with small white or pink flowers.

Where to find it: Mainly in gardens, but also in pastures and the cornfields.

Flowering time: Late summer.

Astrology: A herb of Mercury under Aries.

Medicinal virtues: An excellent remedy for the brain. It is warming and comforting in cold diseases of the head, stomach, sinews and other parts taken inwardly or outwardly applied. Drinking the decoction helps diseases of the chest, obstructions of the liver and spleen, old griefs of the womb and windiness and loss of speech by resolution of the tongue.

The decoction made with some Pellitory of Spain, and Long Pepper, if drunk, is good for dropsy, for those who cannot make water and against pains in the belly. Used as a pessary it provokes women's courses. Made into a powder and mixed with honey it takes away the marks of blows and bruises.

The oil is warm and comforting to the joints that are stiff.

Modern uses: The attributes of Sweet Marjoram are similar to the Wild, but the latter is more commonly used nowadays in medicine. Oil of Marjoram is excellent as an application to bruises and sprains. It also stimulates the menstrual flow. As a tonic combine with an equal part of Chamomile and take as an infusion.

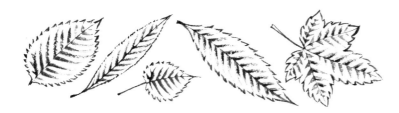

ALTHAEA OFFICINALIS

MARSH MALLOW

The decoction opens the strait passages and makes them slippery, whereby the stone may descend the more easily, and without pain, out of the reins, kidneys and bladder, and eases the pains thereof.

A perennial growing three or four feet (0.9 or 1.2 m) high with hairy white stalks, spreading branches, soft and hairy leaves and palish-pink flowers.

Where to find it: Salt marshes, damp low-lying land, river banks and coastal regions.

Flowering time: Late spring, early summer.

Astrology: Venus.

Medicinal virtues: The leaves and roots boiled in water, with Parsley or Fennel roots and applied warm to the belly, helps to open the body and cool hot agues. It gives abundance of milk to nursing mothers. The decoction of the seed in milk or wine helps pleurisy and other diseases of the chest and lungs.

The juice drank in wine helps women to a speedy and easy delivery. The leaves bruised and laid to the eyes with a little honey, takes away the imposthumations of them. For stings of bees or wasps, the leaves bruised and rubbed into the place will take away the pain, inflammation and swelling.

A poultice made of the leaves with some Bean or Barley-flour, and Oil of Roses, is an especial remedy against all hard tumours and inflammations, imposthumes, or swellings of the testicles. The juice boiled in oil takes away roughness of the skin, scurf or dry scabs in the head. An excellent gargle to heal sore throat or mouth is made by boiling the flowers in oil or water and adding a little honey and Alum. The roots boiled in wine or honeyed water and drank is of special use for coughs, hoarseness, shortness of breath and wheezing.

The roots and seeds boiled in wine or water are profitable against ruptures, cramps or convulsions of the sinews, and boiled in white wine for kernels that rise behind the ears, and inflammations or swellings in women's breasts. The mucilage of the roots, with Linseed and Fenugreek, is much used in poultices, ointments and plasters to mollify and digest hard swellings and to ease pains in any part of the body.

Modern uses: An emollient and soothing agent which has a relaxing effect on the body's internal passages. It is mainly used for inflammation and irritation of the alimentary canal, urinary and respiratory organs. It is available from herbalists as a fluid extract, tincture, concentrated decoction or syrup. The powdered root can be combined with Slippery Elm powder for use in poultices. For domestic use an infusion of the leaves is excellent for most purposes where a soothing agent is required. Use 1 oz (28 g) of the leaves to 1 pt (568 ml) of boiling water and take three or four times a day in doses of 2 fl oz (56 ml). The syrup is helpful in pericarditis.

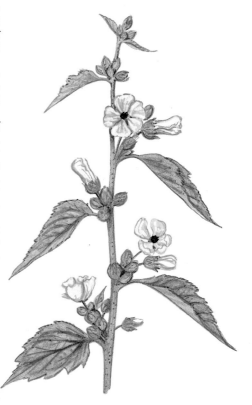

Marsh Mallow ALTHAEA OFFICINALIS

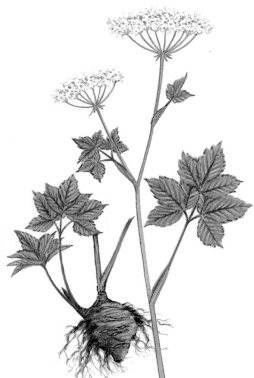

PEUCEDANUM (= IMPERATORIA) OSTRUTHIUM

MASTERWORT

The root . . . stands high as a remedy of great efficacy in malignant and pestilential fevers.

Common Masterwort grows to about three feet (91 cm) high and bears umbels of white flowers. The dark green leaves are winged and resemble those of Angelica.

Where to find it: Originally from Australia and alpine regions, it is now cultivated in gardens.

Flowering time: Late summer.

Astrology: It is a herb of Mars.

Medicinal virtues: The root is hot and available for colds and diseases of the head, stomach and body, dissolving very powerfully upwards and downwards. It is most efficacious if given in a light infusion. It is also used in a decoction with wine against all cold rheums, distillation upon the lungs, or shortness of breath.

It provokes urine and helps to break the stone and expel gravel from the kidneys. It also provokes women's courses and expels the dead-birth. It is singularly good for feminine disorders. Also use it for the dropsy, cramps and falling-sickness. The decoction in wine used as a gargle draws down phlegm from the brain. If the taste be too offensive, use the water distilled from the herb and root.

Modern uses: A decoction of the root – 1 oz (28 g) to 1 pt (568 ml) of boiling water – is taken in doses of 2 fl oz (56 ml) for asthma, flatulence and delayed menstruation.

Masterwort PEUCEDANUM
(= IMPERATORIA) OSTRUTHIUM

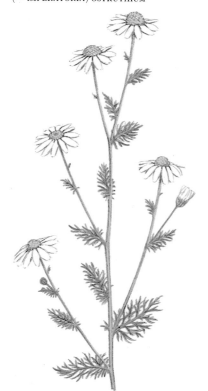

ANTHEMIS COTULA

MAYWEED (Stinking)

It has some of the virtues of Chamomile, but has a far more disagreeable taste.

It grows to a foot (30 cm) high and is also known as Stinking Chamomile as it resembles Chamomile, but the leaves have an unpleasant smell. The flower is white with a high yellow disc.

Where to find it: Cornfields and waste ground.

Flowering time: Late spring, early summer.

Astrology: It is governed by Venus.

Medicinal virtues: It is used for the same purposes as Chamomile, that is to dissolve tumours, expel wind and to ease pains and aches in the joints and other parts. It is also good for women whose matrix has fallen. They should bathe their feet in a decoction of it. Internally the leaves operate by the urine and in some constitutions by the stool. But by both ways roughly, so it should be very cautiously tampered with.

Modern uses: The flowers are preferred to the leaves. They are used to make a poultice to apply to piles and are administered as an infusion to stimulate menstruation. If given internally too strong it can cause vomiting. The dose of the infusion varies from 1–4 fl oz (28–114 ml).

Mayweed (Stinking) ANTHEMIS COTULA

FILIPENDULA (= SPIRAEA) ULMARIA

MEADOWSWEET

An excellent medicine in fevers attended with purgings.

A fragrant meadow herb with small white flowers that appear like umbels at the tops of the stalks.

Where to find it: By river-sides and in moist meadows.

Flowering time: Early summer.

Astrology: Jupiter is regent of this herb.

Medicinal virtues: The flowers are alexipharmic and sudorific and good in fevers and all malignant distempers. They are astringent, binding and useful in all fluxes.

An infusion of the freshly gathered tops of this plant promotes sweating. It is a good wound-herb taken inwardly or externally applied. A water distilled from the flowers is good for inflammations of the eyes.

Modern uses: Since the discovery that Meadowsweet contains methyl salicylate, it has been used as an anti-rheumatic agent with successful results. Its astringency makes it a specific for simple diarrhoea. It has also earned the tag of the 'herbal bicarbonate of soda', and is useful for dyspepsia. Its diuretic property makes it of use in dropsy and oedema of the limbs.

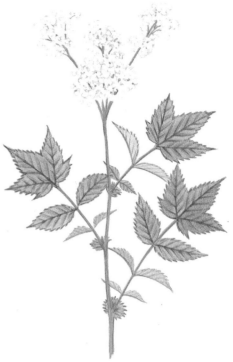

Meadowsweet
FILIPENDULA (= SPIRAEA) ULMARIA

MELILOTUS OFFICINALIS

MELILOT

The juice dropped into the eyes, is a singular good medicine to take away the film that dims the sight.

A common biennial, also known as King's Clover and Ribbed Melilot, growing two or three feet (61 ot 91 cm) high. The flowers are yellow and grow on long spikes. They are followed by a rough, round pod.

Where to find it: It grows amid the corn and in hedges.

Flowering time: Early to midsummer.

Astrology: Not assigned.

Medicinal virtues: Boiled in wine and applied as a compress, Melilot softens all hard tumours and inflammations in the eyes, or the fundament and privy parts of men or women. Sometimes the yolk of a roasted egg, fine flour, Poppy seed, or Endive is added to it.

It helps spreading ulcers in the head if washed with a lye made of it. To ease pains of the stomach, it is carefully applied fresh or boiled with any of the aforementioned things. If dropped into the ears, it will ease the pains in them. Steeped in vinegar or Rose-water, it will mitigate a headache.

Combined with Chamomile flowers, Melilot flowers are used in clysters to expel wind and ease pains, or put into poultices to assuage swelling tumours in the spleen and other parts and to help inflammations in any part of the body.

The head washed with the distilled water of the herb and flowers strengthens the memory and preserves the head and brain from pain and apoplexy.

Modern uses: The plant contains coumarin, which is anticoagulant. It is mainly used as a remedy for flatulence and to improve the taste of nauseous medicines. The whole plant is collected when in flower and used as an infusion – 1 oz (28 g) to 1 pt (568 ml) of boiling water. The dose is 2 fl oz (56 ml) three or four times a day. The infusion makes a useful eye lotion for inflammation of the eyelids, mainly because of its astringency. The infusion is anti-thrombotic and is taken as a tonic for the venous system and as a sedative for neuralgia and insomnia.

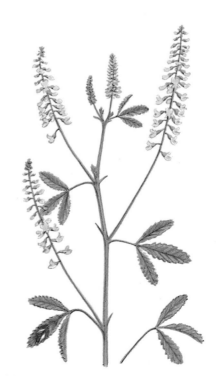

Melilot MELILOTUS OFFICINALIS

MERCURY (French)

The juice takes away warts.

An annual growing about a foot (30 cm) high with angular stalks and narrow leaves with yellowy-green flowers, either male or female. Also known as Annual Mercury.

Where to find it: Waste ground.

Flowering time: Early summer.

Astrology: It is under the dominion of the Moon.

Medicinal virtues: The leaves and stalks are aperitive and mollifying. The decoction purges choleric and serous humours. It is also used in clysters. A decoction of the seeds with Wormwood is commended for the yellow jaundice.

Modern uses: Mucilaginous, diuretic and purgative. The properties are similar to Dog's Mercury, but milder. The leaves are boiled and eaten as a pot herb in some parts of Europe, but the herb is not now recommended for collection and use in domestic medicine. Boiling the leaves reduces their acrid nature.

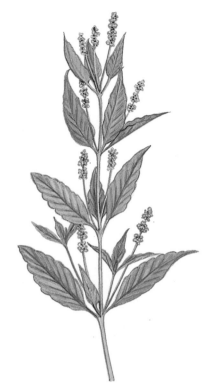

Mercury (French) MERCURIALIS ANNUA

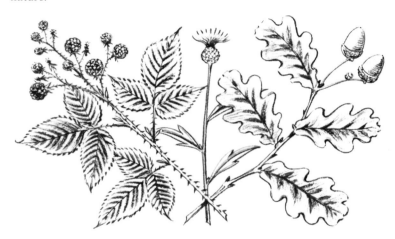

MEZEREON SPURGE

The whole plant has an exceeding acrid, biting taste and is very corrosive.

A hardy deciduous shrub growing to about four feet (1.2 m) with purplish-red flowers almost the whole length of the branches. A red berry appears in midsummer.

Where to find it: A garden shrub, but also found wild in scrubland and woodland.

Flowering time: Late winter, early spring.

Astrology: It is saturnine.

Medicinal virtues: An ointment prepared from the bark or the berries is applied to foul ill-conditioned ulcers. A decoction is made of one dram (1.7 g) of the powdered bark of the root to three pints (1.6 l) of water, boiled down to two pints (1.1 l). This taken during the course of a day for a considerable time has been found efficacious in resolving and dispersing venereal swellings and excrescences. Caution is required in administration and the medicine must only be given to people of robust constitutions and very sparingly even to those. If given in too large a dose, or to a weakly person, it will cause bloody stools and vomiting.

A light infusion is the best mode of giving it. It is good in dropsy and other stubborn disorders.

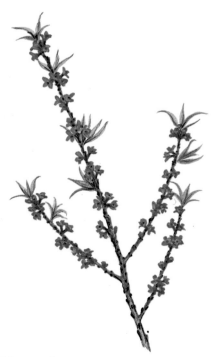

Mezereon Spurge DAPHNE MEZEREUM

Modern uses: It is mainly used in homoeopathic form for mental depression. Specially prepared tablets are available only from homoeopathic chemists. It has been used domestically for rheumatism, syphilis and obstinate skin diseases, but severe poisoning has been caused. Only very small doses should be taken, no more than 10 grains (650 mg) of the powdered bark or two or three drops of the fluid extract. A small amount is sometimes incorporated in compound decoction of Sarsaparilla, which is used as a blood purifier.

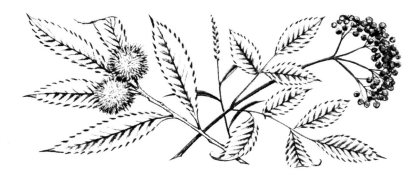

MENTHA SPICATA (= M. VIRIDIS)

MINT (Garden or Spear)

The juice of Garden Mint taken in vinegar, stays bleeding and stirs up venery, or bodily lust.

Spearmint is one of the most popular herbs grown in gardens. In good ground it will grow two or three feet (0.9 or 1.2 m) high. The purplish flowers grow in long spikes.

Where to find it: Commonly cultivated in herb gardens, but is found wild in scattered places. It was originally from the Mediterranean countries.

Flowering time: Midsummer.

Astrology: It is an herb of Venus.

Medicinal virtues: Two or three branches in the juice of four pomegranates stays the hiccough and vomiting. It is good to repress the milk in women's breasts. If the leaves be steeped or boiled in milk before being drunk, it is profitable to the stomach and restrains the milk from curdling.

Use of it often will stay women's courses and the whites. Applied to the forehead or temples, it eases pains in the head. The heads of young children can be washed with it to help against sores and scabs.

The dried powder taken after meat helps digestion and those that are splenetic. Taken in wine, it helps women in childbearing. It is good against gravel and stone in the kidneys and the strangury. The decoction gargled in the mouth amends an ill-favoured breath and cures the sore mouth and gums.

Mint is a herb that is useful in all disorders of the stomach, including weakness, loss of appetite, pain and vomiting. It also stops gonorrhoea, fluor albus and immoderate flow of the menses.

A cataplasm of the green leaves applied to the stomach, stays vomiting, and to women's breasts prevents hardness and curdling of milk.

Modern uses: Mainly used for culinary purposes, but is added to medicines because of its pleasant taste. It is anti-flatulent, anti-spasmodic and stimulating, and often used in paediatric medicines. The plant is gathered in late summer just as it begins to flower. It yields an oil similar to Peppermint oil and with similar properties. Two or three drops of oil can be taken on a lump of sugar for flatulence. Adding eight drops of the oil to 1 pt (568 ml) of water makes *Aqua menthae*, or Mint Water, which can be given to babies with colic. The infusion of 1 oz (28 g) of dried herb to 1 pt (568 ml) of boiling water is also excellent for nausea and wind.

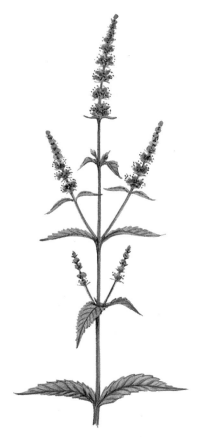

Mint (Garden or Spear) MENTHA SPICATA (= M. VIRIDIS)

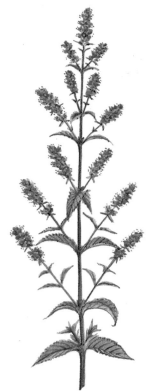

Mint (Pepper) MENTHA PIPERITA

MINT (Pepper)

It is useful for complaints of the stomach, such as wind and vomiting, for which there are few remedies of greater efficacy.

The leaves of Peppermint are broader and shorter than Spearmint, but the flowers are larger growing in loose oblong spikes of purple.

Where to find it: In gardens and in moist places, such as the banks of rivers.

Flowering time: Mid to late summer.

Astrology: A plant of Venus.

Medicinal virtues: It is good in poultices and fomentations to disperse curdled milk in the breasts and to be used with milk diets. All Mints are astringent and great strengtheners of the stomach. Their fragrance betokens them cephalics. They take off nauseousness, retchings and looseness. The simple water given to children removes the gripes.

Modern uses: The plant yields Peppermint Oil, which contains menthol. It is anti-spasmodic, relieving pains in the alimentary canal. The dosage is one to three drops on sugar.

Mint removes nausea and flatulence and allays vomiting. Peppermint Water, used for griping pains in the tummy, is made by adding a few drops of the oil to a pint of distilled water (Aqua Mentha Pip. Dest.) and administering in doses of ½–1 fl oz (14–28 ml). Peppermint Tea, made by infusing 1 oz (28 g) of the herb in 1 pt (568 ml) of boiling water, is good used early in colds or fevers. It is often combined with Elderflowers and Yarrow and given hot to cut a cold overnight. The tea is also helpful in treating insomnia, anxiety and dizziness.

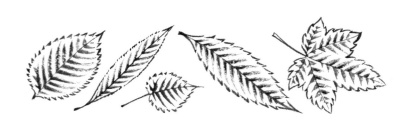

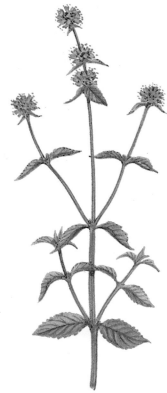

Mint (Water) MENTHA AQUATICA

MINT (Water)

It expels wind out of the stomach and opens obstructions of the womb.

The commonest of the wild Mints. It has hairy stalks, large leaves and purple flowers growing in round spikes. It is a smaller plant than Garden Mint.

Where to find it: River banks, marshes and other wet places.

Flowering time: Midsummer to mid autumn.

Astrology: A herb of Venus.

Medicinal virtues: The distilled water of the herb is carminative and anti-spasmodic, relieving colic and other disorders of the bowels, instantaneously. It is good to remove gravel, and hysteric depressions.

Modern uses: Astringent and emetic, it is mainly used for looseness of the bowels being given by infusion. It also stimulates the menstrual flow. Made too strong, the infusion becomes emetic. Taken hot, the infusion induces perspiration and is valuable in fevers and inflammatory conditions.

MISTLETOE

A cephalic and nervine medicine, useful for convulsive fits, palsy and vertigo.

The well-known parasitic plant that grows on the branches of trees, including the Oak, which is considered to be the best. It produces green-yellow flowers and white berries.

Where to find it: Most commonly found growing on Apple trees. But also grows on Ash, Hazel, Crab Apple, Maple, Willow, Lime and Hawthorn trees.

Flowering time: Spring.

Astrology: Under the dominion of the Sun, with a little of the nature of Jupiter.

Medicinal virtues: The berries produce a sticky substance known as bird-lime. This is a powerful attractive and is good to ripen hard tumours and swellings. The juice from the fresh wood dropped into the ears is effectual in curing imposthumes in them. The powdered leaves made into a drink are food for the falling-sickness.

Modern uses: Mistletoe is an important article in both herbal and homoeopathic medicine. It is anti-tumour, diuretic, cardiotonic and hypotensive. A specially prepared homoeopathic tincture is used in the treatment of cancer. It is used externally and given by injection. Herbalists use Mistletoe to strengthen the heart and to reduce blood pressure. Combined with Valerian root and Vervain in equal parts, it makes an excellent nervine tonic. The powdered leaves are used in the treatment of epilepsy, but dosage is critical. Large doses cause convulsions and affect heart function. The powder is given in doses of 10–60 grains (0.65–3.9 g).

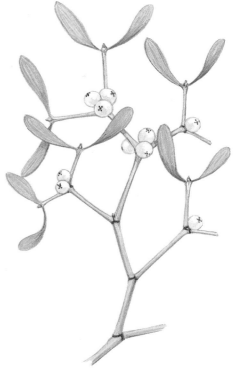

Mistletoe VISCUM ALBUM

MONEYWORT

It is good to stay all fluxes in man or woman.

A perennial creeping plant with yellow flowers. It is known by some as Creeping Jenny and by others as Herb Twopence. The slender branches run along the ground two or three feet (61 or 91 cm).

Where to find it: It grows in moist ground, in grass and by the sides of hedges.

Flowering time: Summer.

Astrology: Venus owns it.

Medicinal virtues: It stays laxes, bloody fluxes, the flowing of women's courses, bleeding inwardly and outwardly and quells stomachs that are given to casting.

It is also good for ulcers or excoriations of the lungs, or other inward parts. It will quickly heal wounds and spreading ulcers. The juice is effectual for overflowings of the menses and the dried powdered roots are good in purgings.

Modern uses: The whole herb is used for its astringency. An ointment is made by digesting the powdered herb in wax and oil and applied to wounds. A decoction of the herb is used as a lotion for wounds and sore places. The powdered leaves have been used internally in doses of 10 grains (650 mg) for haemorrhages. The properties of Moneywort, which is not much used, are similar to Loosestrife (*Lysimachia vulgaris*).

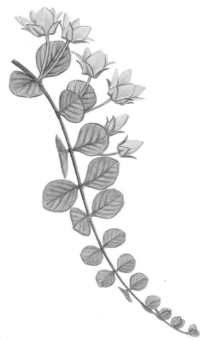

Moneywort LYSIMACHIA NUMMULARIA

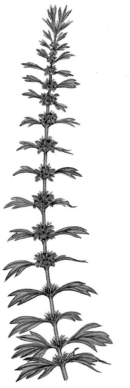

Motherwort LEONURUS CARDIACA

LEONURUS CARDIACA

MOTHERWORT

There is no better herb to take melancholy vapours from the heart and to strengthen it.

A perennial plant growing to three or four feet (0.91 to 1.2 m) high, with spreading branches, deeply indented leaves and hooded, red or pinkish flowers. It is a member of the Dead-nettle family.

Where to find it: Roadside verges and waste ground, where it has escaped from herb gardens.

Flowering time: Late summer.

Astrology: Venus owns this herb and it is under Leo.

Medicinal virtues: It makes mothers joyful and settles the womb; that is why it is called Motherwort. It is of use for trembling of the heart, and fainting and swooning. It may be kept in syrup or as a conserve. A spoonful of the powder, drank in wine, helps women in sore travail. It provokes the urine and women's courses, cleanses the chest of cold phlegm and kills worms in the belly. It helps cramps and convulsions.

Modern uses: A heart tonic for angina pectoris, it also helps to lower blood pressure. It regulates circulatory disturbances during the menopause, such as palpitations. It is a sedative, inducing tranquillity in simple anxiety or when there is restlessness during fevers. In this it resembles the action of Valerian root. It regulates menstruation, encouraging the monthly flow when it is scanty, and eases painful periods.

The herb is collected in late summer and dried. The powdered herb is given as an infusion in doses of 2 fl oz (56 ml). Tinctures and liquid extracts are available from herbalists.

ARTEMESIA VULGARIS

MUGWORT (Common)

The tops, leaves and flowers . . . are aromatic and most safe and excellent in female disorders.

An aromatic perennial plant growing to three or four feet (0.9 or 1.2 m) with angular reddish-brown stems and leaves that are smooth and green on top and white and hairy underneath. The button-like flowers are a yellowish-brown.

Where to find it: Waste ground, watersides, and near footpaths and hedges.

Flowering time: Midsummer.

Astrology: A herb of Venus.

Medicinal virtues: An excellent tea for female disorders. The flowers and buds should be put into a teapot and boiling water poured over them. When cool, add a little sugar and milk. Drink this twice a day or oftener. Sitting over the infusion helps bring down the courses, hastens delivery of the baby and helps to expel the afterbirth. It is also good for obstructions and inflammations of the mother. It breaks the stone and provokes the water. Made into an ointment with hog's grease, it takes away wens, hard knots and kernels that grow about the neck. This is more effective if some Daisies be put with it. The fresh herb or juice is a remedy for the taking of too much Opium. Three drams (5.3 g) of the dried, powdered leaves taken in wine is a speedy and certain help for the sciatica.

Modern uses: The leaves and roots are used. It is a remedy for scanty menstruation and is taken by infusion in teaspoonful doses. It can be mixed with Marigold flowers, Cramp Bark and Black Haw in equal parts. Use one teaspoonful of the mixture to a cup of boiling water.

As a nervine it is useful for convulsions, a teaspoonful of the powdered leaves being taken in water three times a day.

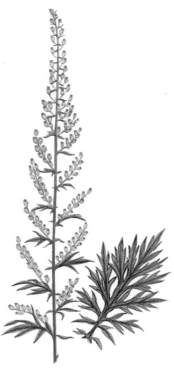

Mugwort (Common) ARTEMESIA VULGARIS

MULBERRY TREE

The juice of the leaves is a remedy against the bites of serpents, and for those that have taken Aconite.

There are two kinds of Mulberries, the Common Black (*M. nigra*) and the White (*M. alba*). It is a large tree growing to 30 foot (9 m) high with a brown rugged bark. The flowers grow in clusters and the deep purple fruit is oblong and about an inch (25 mm) long.

Where to find it: A cultivated tree originally from Asia Minor and Persia, where it grows wild.

Flowering time: The fruit ripens in late summer, early autumn.

Astrology: Mercury rules the tree.

Medicinal virtues: The ripe berries open the body, but the unripe bind it, especially when they are dried. They then stay fluxes, laxes and women's courses. The bark of the root kills broad worms in the belly. The juice from the berries made into a syrup helps inflammations or sores in the mouth or throat.

A decoction made of the bark and leaves is good to wash the teeth with when they ache. The leaves bound into place stay bleeding at the mouth or nose, or the bleeding of the piles.

Modern uses: The bark is laxative and removes intestinal worms. The fruits are also laxative. They are administered as a convalescent syrup to help patients overcome the effects of fever. They are rich in grape sugar, which provides easily assimilated energy. The syrup is made by adding just under twice as much sugar to the expressed juice of the berries. The dose is half to one teaspoonful.

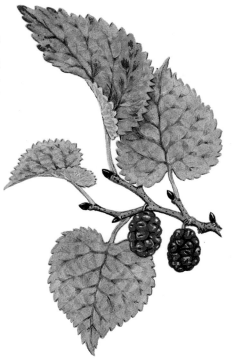

Mulberry Tree MORUS NIGRA

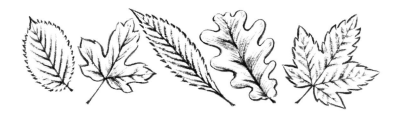

MULLEIN (Black)

A specific against the pain and swelling of the haemorrhoids or piles.

Black or Dark Mullein resembles White Mullein, but is smaller and lacks the white downy covering.

Where to find it: Grassy banks, hedgerows and roadsides, but is not so commonly found as White Mullein.

Flowering time: Midsummer.

Astrology: A saturnine plant.

Medicinal virtues: The leaves are used and are accounted a good pectoral agent, particularly for coughs and the spitting of blood. They are likewise good for colicky pains and griping in the abdomen. Fomentations are used outwardly for the piles.

Modern uses: This and the White are considered to have very similar properties and that which is most easily obtainable is used. It may be mixed with other remedies for lung disorders, such as Colt's Foot, Lungwort and Horehound, according to the specific condition being treated.

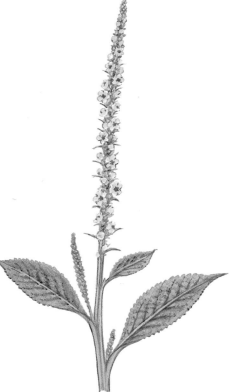

Mullein (Black) VERBASCUM NIGRUM

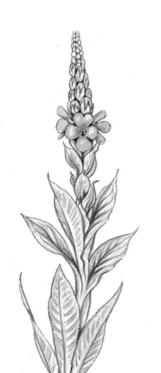

Mullein (Great) VERBASCUM THAPSUS

MULLEIN (Great)

The seed bruised and boiled in wine and laid on any member that has been out of joint, and newly set again, takes away all swelling and pain.

The Great Mullein, more usually known as Aaron's Rod, has large woolly white leaves on a stalk rising four or five feet (1.2 or 1.5 m) high and yellow flowers in a long spike.

Where to find it: Sunny banks and waste places, waysides and lanes.

Flowering time: Midsummer.

Astrology: Under the dominion of Saturn.

Medicinal virtues: A small quantity of the root is commended against laxes and fluxes of the body. The decoction is profitable for cramps, convulsions and chronic coughs, and used as a gargle it eases toothache.

The oil made by infusing the flowers is good for the piles. A decoction of the leaves together with Sage, Marjoram and Chamomile flowers is used to bathe in for colds, stiff sinews and cramps.

Three fluid ounces (85 ml) of the distilled water of the flowers drank morning and evening is a remedy for the gout. The juice expressed from the leaves or flowers or the powder of the dried roots applied to warts will take them away.

The dried flowers powdered are taken for bowel complaints or colicky pains. To dissolve swellings, tumours and inflammations of the throat, take the decoction of the root and leaves.

Modern uses: The leaves and flowers are used. A tea, made by using one teaspoonful of powdered leaves to a cup of boiling water, is excellent for most lung complaints, including asthma, bronchitis and croup.

A tea made from the powdered flowers is pain-relieving and sedative. The infused oil, which is a good application for piles, is made by pouring olive oil onto fresh Mullein flowers in a jar and allowing them to macerate in a warm place, preferably in the sun for three weeks. The more flowers that are used the stronger the oil will be. The oil is strained before use. It is anti-inflammatory and has been used successfully for ear troubles, two or three drops being introduced into the ear two or three times a day.

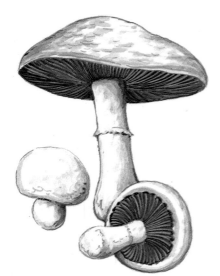

Mushroom (Garden) AGARICUS CAMPESTRIS

MUSHROOM (Garden)

Inwardly, they are unwholesome, and unfit for the strongest constitutions.

This is an edible Mushroom with a soft white head and a grey or flesh colour underneath. The head is expanded almost flat, forming a large flap. It has an agreeable smell.

Where to find it: It grows on dung or putrefied earth, but is also cultivated in gardens.

Flowering time: The mushroom has no flowers or leaves, but it can be grown all year round.

Astrology: Mushrooms are under Mercury in Aries.

Medicinal virtues: The Mushroom is roasted and made into a poultice or boiled with White Lily roots and Linseed in milk. It is used as an application to boils and abscesses and ripens them better than any preparation that can be made. The poultices are also of service against quinsies and inflammatory swellings.

Modern uses: Mushrooms and Toadstools are not used by modern medical herbalists but some varieties are used by homoeopaths, including the Poison Mushroom (*Agaricus emeticus*), Fly Agaric (*Amanita muscaria*) and Death Cap (*Amanita phalloides*), all of which are poisonous if eaten.

BRASSICA NIGRA

MUSTARD (Black)

An excellent sauce for clarifying the blood.

An annual growing three or four feet (0.91 or 1.2 m) high with small yellow flowers. The seed pod is long and pointed and contains about a dozen dark brown seeds which have a hot, biting taste.

Where to find it: Waste places, roadsides, beside streams and on sea cliffs.

Flowering time: Early summer.

Astrology: A herb of Mars.

Medicinal virtues: Excellent for weak stomachs, but unfit for choleric people. It strengthens the heart and resists poisons. Those with weak stomachs should take one dram (1.7 g) each of Mustard seed and Cinnamon beaten to a powder with half a dram (890 mg) of powdered Mastic and Gum Arabic dissolved in Rose-water and made into troches of half a dram (890 mg) each. One troche is to be taken an hour or two before meals. Old people may take much of this medicine with advantage. Mustard seed has the virtue of heat, discussing, ratifying and drawing out splinters of bones from the flesh.

It is good for falling-sickness or lethargy and to bring down the courses. A decoction of the seed in wine resists poison, the malignity of Mushrooms and the bites of venomous creatures, if taken in time. Taken in an electuary the seed stirs up lust, helps the spleen and pain in the sides and gnawings of the bowels.

An outward application eases the pain of sciatica and the gout and aching joints.

Modern uses: Mustard seeds are used mainly in poultices for acute local pain and congestive lung conditions, such as bronchitis.

The poultices are made by mixing the powdered seeds into a paste with warm water and spread onto brown paper. The poultices should be removed when they make the skin red. Mustard oil, a powerful irritant, is incorporated into liniments for rheumatic pain.

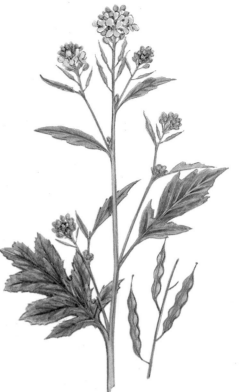

Mustard (Black) BRASSICA NIGRA

SISYMBRIUM OFFICINALE

MUSTARD (Hedge)

By the use of the decoction a lost voice has been recovered.

An annual plant growing to one or two feet (30 or 61 cm) with a blackish-green stalk with rugged leaves and small yellow flowers in long spikes. These flower by degrees so that the plant is in flower over a longish period. The yellow seed is sharp and strong to the taste.

Where to find it: By hedge-sides and on waste ground and at the roadside.

Flowering time: Midsummer.

Astrology: Mars owns this herb.

Medicinal virtues: It is used for hoarseness and diseases of the chest and lungs. A decoction of the plant is taken or the juice made into a syrup with honey and sugar. It is profitable for coughs, wheezing and shortness of breath and, if used in clysters, for jaundice, pleurisy, pains in the back and loins, and colic.

The seed is a remedy against poison and venom, and worms in children. It is good for sciatica, aching joints, ulcers and cankers in the mouth, throat, or behind the ears and for hardness and swelling of the testicles or of women's breasts.

Modern uses: The whole plant is used as an expectorant for coughs and to relieve hoarseness. It has an affinity for the vocal chords. An infusion of 1 oz (28 g) of the dried leaves to 1 pt (568 ml) of boiling water can be taken in doses of 2 fl oz (56 ml), three or four times a day.

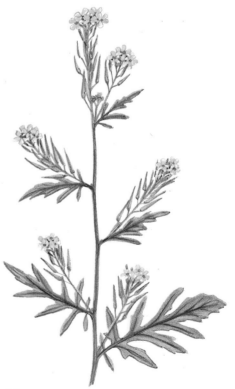

Mustard (Hedge) SISYMBRIUM OFFICINALE

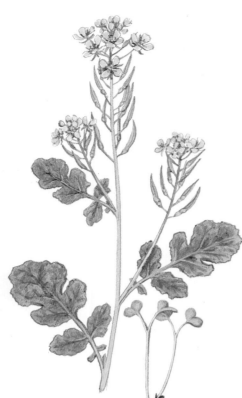

Mustard (White) SINAPIS ALBA

SINAPIS ALBA

MUSTARD (White)

Whenever a strong stimulating medicine is wanted to act on the nerves, and not excite heat, there is none preferable to Mustard seed.

An annual growing to about 18 inches (46 cm) with rough, hairy leaves, and deep yellow flowers, larger than other mustards. The seeds are white and contained in hairy pods. Although larger than other Mustard seeds, they are not quite as hot.

Where to find it: Not so common as other varieties, but found on cultivated land and areas rich in lime.

Flowering time: Late spring to late summer.

Astrology: A herb of Mars.

Medicinal virtues: The young shoots can be used in salads and are very wholesome. The seed, bruised and infused in wine or ale, is of service against the scurvy and dropsy, provoking urine and the menses. Outwardly applied, Mustard is drawing and ripening: and laid on paralytic members it recalls the natural heat.

Poultices made with Mustard flowers, breadcrumbs and vinegar, are frequently applied to the soles of the feet in fevers and may be used to advantage in old rheumatic and sciatic pains.

Modern uses: The seed is used in much the same way as Black Mustard seed. Taken internally the seeds are laxative, mainly because of the mucilage they produce, but small doses only are advised, as they may inflame the stomach. In making poultices, the white seeds can be mixed with the black. Such applications are very stimulating and redden the skin, but they are useful in treating bronchitis and rheumatic pains.

MYRTUS COMMUNIS

MYRTLE TREE

Good for the falling down of the womb.

The Myrtle is a little tree or bush with evergreen leaves which are pleasantly aromatic. The flowers are white, and are followed by a small round black berry.

Where to find it: It grows wild in southern Europe, but elsewhere is an ornamental garden plant.

Flowering time: Late summer.

Astrology: A tree of Mercury.

Medicinal virtues: The leaves and berries are drying and binding and therefore good for diarrhoea and dysentery. They are used also for spitting of blood, catarrhal defluxions on the chest, fluor albus and dropped womb or fundament. They are used inwardly in infusions, and outwardly in injections.

Modern uses: The leaves are made into an infusion and used as a vaginal douche for leucorrhoea and prolapse of the womb.

URTICA DIOICA

NETTLE (Common)

It consumes the phlegmatic superfluities in the body of man, that the coldness and moisture of winter has left behind.

The well-known Stinging Nettle is a perennial growing to about four feet (1.2 m). It has a creeping root, sharp-pointed leaves and greenish flowers. The irritant substance which causes the sting when the prickly hairs are touched is a mixture of histamine and formic acid.

Where to find it: It is very common growing near hedges and on waste ground.

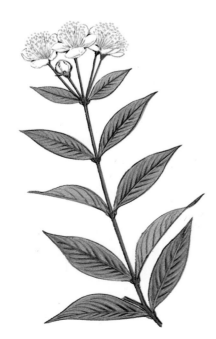

Myrtle Tree MYRTUS COMMUNIS

Flowering time: Early summer to early autumn.

Astrology: A herb of Mars.

Medicinal virtues: The roots or leaves, or the juice of them, boiled and made into an electuary with honey and sugar, is a safe and sure medicine to open the passages of the lungs, which is the cause of wheezing and shortness of the breath. It helps to expectorate phlegm and to raise the imposthumed pleurisy. As a gargle it helps the swelling of the mouth and throat.

A decoction of the leaves provokes the courses and urine and expels gravel and stone. It kills worms in children, eases pain in the sides and dissolves wind in the spleen.

The seed taken as a drink is remedy against the bites of dogs and the poisonous qualities of Hemlock, Henbane, Nightshade and Mandrake. The bruised seed or leaves put into the nostrils takes away the polypus. The juice of the leaves or a decoction of the root is used as a wash for fistulas and gangrenes and for corroding scabs or itch.

Modern uses: Nettles are rich in vitamins and minerals. They should be collected just before they flower and dried. The leaves are used mainly for their diuretic properties and an infusion relieves high blood pressure and cystitis. The mineral-rich leaves are used in the treatment of anaemia and as a blood tonic and purifier.

A decoction of the root is astringent and indicated for diarrhoea and dysentery.

Homoeopaths use a fresh plant tincture for eczema.

As an infusion, Nettle leaves are taken in doses of 2 fl oz (56 ml). The dose of the powdered herb is 5–10 grains (325–650 mg). Tinctures and fluid extracts are available from herbalists.

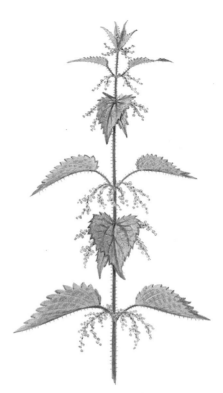

Nettle (Common) URTICA DIOICA

SOLANUM NIGRUM

NIGHTSHADE (Common)
Be sure you do not mistake the Deadly Nightshade for this plant.

This is an annual plant growing only about a foot (30 cm) high with broad, pointed leaves that are soft and full of juice. The flowers are white with yellow anthers and are followed by greenish berries which go black as they ripen. Also called Black Nightshade.

Where to find it: Under walls, by paths and at the sides of hedges and fields. It is often found growing on rubbish heaps.

Flowering time: Midsummer to mid autumn.

Astrology: A cool saturnine plant.

Medicinal virtues: It is used to cool hot inflammations, either inwardly or outwardly. It is in no way dangerous, as most of the Nightshades are, but must be used moderately.

The safest way to take it internally is as the distilled water of the whole herb. The juice with vinegar is good for an inflamed mouth and throat. The juice of the herb or berries with Oil of Roses and a little vinegar and ceruse beaten together in a lead mortar is used to anoint all hot inflammations in the eyes.

It does good for the shingles and ringworm and all running, fretting and corroding ulcers. A pessary dipped into the juice and dropped into the matrix, stays the immoderate flow of the courses. A cloth moistened in the juice and applied to the testicles, and any swelling therein, gives ease.

Modern uses: There is controversy regarding the poisonous nature of this plant and this is probably due to the amount of toxic substance, solanine, varying in strength from season to season. It is definitely not recommended for domestic use. The berries are poisonous to children. Homoeopaths make a tincture as a remedy for epilepsy. Used externally, the bruised fresh leaves are analgesic and anti-inflammatory.

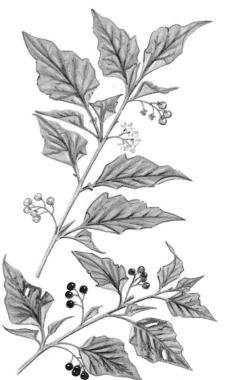

Nightshade (Common) SOLANUM NIGRUM

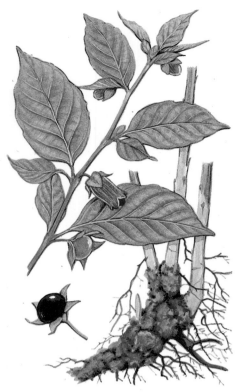

Nightshade (Deadly) ATROPA BELLADONA

NIGHTSHADE (Deadly)

This Nightshade bears a very bad character as being of a poisonous nature.

The largest of the Nightshades, growing to five feet (1.5 m) with spreading roots and leaves like the Common Nightshade only larger. The flowers are a dismal purple and hang down like bells. The berries are like black cherries, full of juice.

Where to find it: Woodland clearings in the shade of the trees.

Flowering time: Midsummer.

Astrology: Not assigned to any planet.

Medicinal virtues: It is not good at all for inward uses, but leaves and root may with good success be applied outwardly by way of poultice to inflammatory swellings.

An ointment made of the juice does wonders in old ulcers, even of a cancerous nature. The leaves applied to the breasts will dissipate hard swellings. A poultice made of the roots boiled in milk has been found serviceable for ill-conditioned tumours and foul ulcers. Sometimes even the outward application is dangerous, the poisonous nature of the plant affecting the skin. It can affect the pupil of the eye so that it will not contract even in the brightest light.

Modern uses: The medical profession makes most use of *A. belladonna*, employing it in liniments, plasters, tinctures, suppositories and ointments. Ophthalmologists use atropine from the plant as a mydriatic to dilate the pupil before eye examinations.

Extracts of the root are mainly used in lotions and other external applications – as an anodyne in neuralgia, gout, rheumatic pain and sciatica.

Taken internally, it is narcotic, diuretic and sedative. It suppresses glandular secretions and reduces inflammation.

It is not to be used as a domestic remedy.

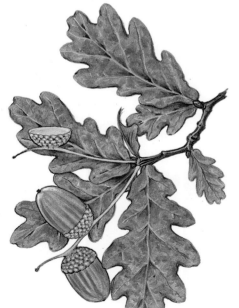

Oak Tree QUERCUS ROBUR

OAK TREE

The distilled water of the buds, before they break out into leaves, is good . . . to assuage inflammations and to stop all manner of fluxes.

The Oak is familiar to most. It is a large tree with spreading head and a thick trunk producing flowers in catkins and seeds as acorns.

Where to find it: Very common in many countries where it forms large forests.

Flowering time: Mid to late spring. The acorns are ready in autumn.

Astrology: A tree of Jupiter.

Medicinal virtues: The inner bark of the tree and the skin covering the acorn are used to stay the spitting of blood and the flux. The decoction of the bark and the powdered acorns stay vomiting, spitting of blood, bleeding at the mouth, or other flux of blood. It will also stay the involuntary flux of natural seed. The powdered acorn taken in wine provokes urine and resists poison from venomous creatures.

The distilled water of the leaf buds cools the heat of the liver, breaks the stone and stays women's courses. The distilled water of the leaves is one of the best remedies for the whites.

Modern uses: A powerful astringent used to check diarrhoea – 1 oz (28 g) of the powdered bark is boiled in 2 pt (1.1 l) of water until it measures 1 pt (568 ml). It is then strained and taken in doses of 2 fl oz (56 ml). The decoction is also antiseptic and used as a vaginal injection for leucorrhoea and as a gargle for a sore throat. It can also be applied as a lotion to bleeding piles.

AVENA SATIVA

OATS

The meal of Oats boiled with vinegar and applied, takes away freckles and spots in the face, and other parts of the body.

A cereal plant with a fibrous root, a hollow stalk growing to about three feet (91 cm), with long narrow green leaves and flowers in a loose inflorescence.

Where to find it: A cultivated cereal.

Flowering time: Mid to late summer.

Astrology: Not assigned to any planet.

Medicinal uses: Oats fried with Bay salt and applied to the sides take away the pains of stitches and wind in the sides of the belly.

A poultice made of the meal of Oats, and some Oil of Bay added, helps the itch and leprosy and also fistula of the fundament.

Modern uses: Considered by modern herbalists to be a useful nervine tonic, which also exerts a beneficial effect on the musculature of the heart. The tincture available from herbalists is also used as a uterine tonic and antispasmodic. The dose is 10–30 drops in hot water.

Taken as a gruel, Oatmeal is nutritious and easily digested by fever patients and those with gastro-intestinal inflammation. Homoeopaths prepare a tincture from the flowering plant as a remedy for arthritic conditions.

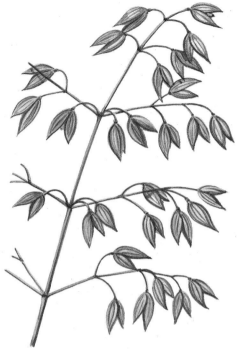

Oats AVENA SATIVA

ALLIUM CEPA

ONION

They are flatulent, or windy, but provoke the appetite, increase thirst, ease the bowels and provoke the courses.

Where to find it: Cultivated in gardens, but a native plant of the Middle East.

Flowering time: Early summer.

Astrology: Owned by Mars.

Medicinal virtues: Onions increase sperm. They kill worms in children if they drink the water in which the Onions have been steeped all night. Roasted Onions, eaten with honey or sugar and oil, help an inveterate cough and expectorate tough phlegm.

Snuffed up the head, the juice purges the head and helps lethargy, but eaten often is said to procure pains in the head.

The juice is good for scalds and burns, and used with vinegar it takes away blemishes, spots and marks in the skin. Onions are injurious to people of bilious habit, affecting the head, eyes and stomach.

Modern uses: The properties of Onion are similar to Garlic. It is antiseptic, diuretic and expectorant. The juice is made into a syrup with honey and used as a medicine for coughs, asthma and bronchitis. Homoeopaths prescribe pills made from the Onion for hay fever and rhinitis. A tincture of Onion made by steeping an Onion in alcohol is diuretic and used to expel sediment from the bladder and to treat dropsy.

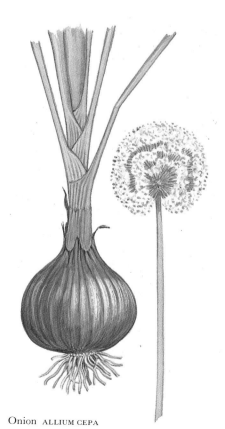

Onion ALLIUM CEPA

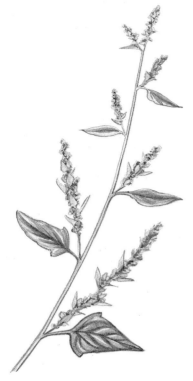

ATRIPLEX PATULA

ORACH

It cures headaches, wandering pains, and the first attacks of rheumatism.

A fairly common annual growing three or four feet (0.9 or 1.2 m) high with whitish stalks, faint green leaves and greenish-white flowers. It is also known as Arrach, of which there are several varieties – Orache or Iron Root.

Where to find it: Waste places, roadsides, cultivated ground. It prefers clay or heavy soils.

Flowering time: Midsummer to early autumn.

Astrology: It is under Venus.

Medicinal virtues: The seeds are gathered when just ripe and a pound (454 g) of them, bruised, is placed in three quarts (3.4 l) of moderate strength spirit. The whole is left to stand for six weeks, affording a light and not unpleasant tincture.

A tablespoonful of the tincture, taken in a cup of water-gruel, has the same effect as a dose of Ipecacuanha, except that its operation is milder and it does not bind the bowels afterwards.

After taking the dose, the patient should go to bed. A gentle sweat will follow, carrying off whatever offending matter the motions have dislodged, thus preventing long disease.

As some stomachs are harder to move than others, a second tablespoonful may be taken if the first does not perform its office.

Modern uses: The herb can be eaten boiled like greens or used in salads. The seeds are not used in herbal practice. Ipecacunanha is used as an emetic and added to medicines to prevent an overdose being taken. In smallish doses it induces sweating and expectoration of mucus.

Orach ATRIPLEX PATULA

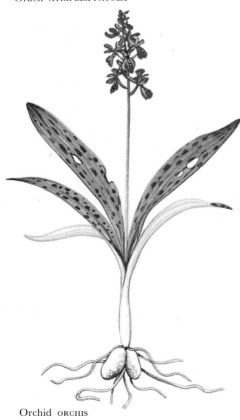

ORCHIS

ORCHID

They provoke venery, strengthen the genital parts and help conception.

There are many varieties of orchids, but it is the tuberous roots only that are used and a description of them will be sufficient.

Where to find it: Meadows.

Flowering time: Mid spring to late summer.

Astrology: They are hot and moist and under the dominion of Venus.

Medicinal virtues: The roots, bruised and applied to the place, heal the king's-evil. They also kill worms in children.

Applied outwardly as a cataplasm, they dissolve hard tumours and swellings.

A preparation is made from the roots and known as salep. The new root is separated from its brown skin by dipping it in hot water and rubbing it with a coarse linen cloth. They are placed in a moderate oven on a tin plate for five or six minutes, in which time they will lose their milky whiteness and acquire a transparency like horn. They are then dried and hardened in the air for several days. Such a salep contains a great deal of nourishment and will support the system during famine, or those who travel long distances without food.

Modern uses: Because Orchids are protected species, they are now rarely available for medicinal purposes. Salep has been produced in Turkey for centuries. The dried root is powdered and made into a nourishing drink and was very popular before coffee was in vogue. Potions made from the fresh tubers were administered by witches for their aphrodisiac properties.

Orchid ORCHIS

SEDUM TELEPHIUM

ORPINE

It cools any inflammation upon any hurt or wound, and eases the pain.

The common Orpine has large, broad, flattened leaves, dented on the edges. The flowers are pinkish-white and grow in tufts and produce seed like dust.

Where to find it: Shadowy fields and woods. It also grows in gardens.

Flowering time: Midsummer.

Astrology: The Moon owns this herb.

Medicinal virtues: This plant is seldom used for internal medicines. The distilled water is profitable for gnawings and excoriations in the stomach and bowels and for ulcers in the lungs, liver or other inward parts. It stays the bloody flux, and other fluxes.

The juice mixed with salad oil is applied for burns and scalds. The bruised leaves are applied to wounds to heal them and to the throat to ease the quinsy. The roots may also be bruised and applied to wounds and bruises.

Modern uses: The plant is astringent and has been used for checking diarrhoea, a decoction of the leaves being made by boiling them in milk and taking 2 fl oz (56 ml) three or four times a day. It is not a remedy in current use. Others, like Blackberry root, are more popular.

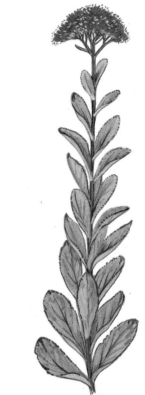

Orpine SEDUM TELEPHIUM

PAEONIA OFFICINALIS

PAEONY

The root, fresh gathered, cures the falling-sickness.

The well-known garden perennial. The stems are brown and the flowers a beautiful purplish-red. The roots run deep into the ground.

Where to find it: A garden plant that thrives in most soils.

Flowering time: Late spring.

Astrology: A herb of the Sun and under the Lion.

Medicinal virtues: The roots have more virtues than the seed, next the flowers, and then the leaves.

The root is washed, crushed and infused for at least 24 hours. It is then strained and a good draught taken morning and evening for several days. This will cure the falling-sickness in old as well as young, if the disease be not of too long standing and past cure. The body can be prepared by taking a drink-posset made of Betony.

The root or the seed beaten to a powder, and given in wine, is effectual for cleansing the womb after childbirth and easing the mother. Taken morning and night, the black seed is effectual for nightmare and melancholy dreams.

The distilled water or syrup made of the flowers works the same, but more weakly.

Modern uses: An infusion of the powdered root – 1 oz (28 g) to 1 pt (568 ml) of boiling water – is taken in doses of 2 fl oz (56 ml) three or four times as an anti-spasmodic remedy for spasms, convulsions and epilepsy. It is an effective liver tonic.

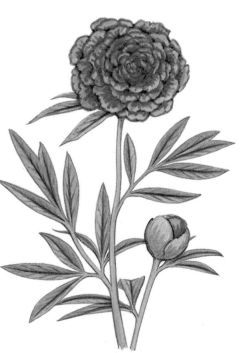

Paeony PAEONIA OFFICINALIS

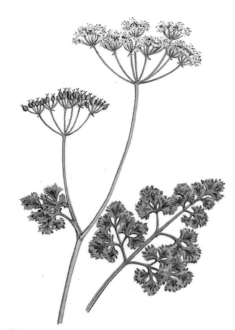

Parsley (Common) PETROSELINUM CRISPUM
(= P. SATIVUM)

PARSLEY (Common)

The distilled water is a familiar medicine with nurses to give children when troubled with wind in the stomach or belly, and it is also of service to upgrown persons.

The well-known culinary herb has long, thick, white roots and dissected leaves and produces small umbels of white flowers. It grows to about two feet (61 cm).

Where to find it: Originally from the Mediterranean, Parsley is now widely cultivated. It is found wild growing on old walls and rocks.

Flowering time: Summer.

Astrology: It is under the dominion of Mercury.

Medicinal virtues: It is comforting to the stomach and helps to provoke urine and the courses, to break wind, both in the stomach and bowels, and opens the body. The root is stronger, and may be boiled and eaten like Parsnips. The seeds have similar uses, but are also good to break the stone and ease the pain thereof.

The leaves laid to the eyes inflamed with heat, or swollen, helps them. If used with bread or meal, or fried with butter, and applied to women's breasts that are hard through the curdling of their milk, it abates the hardness and takes away the black and blue marks coming of bruises or falls.

Take of Parsley seed, Fennel, Anise and Caraway, of each one ounce (28 g), of the roots of Parsley, Burnet, Saxifrage and Caraway, of each an ounce and a half (42 g). Let the seeds be bruised and the roots washed and cut small. Let them lie all night and steep in a bottle of white wine and in the morning be boiled in a close earthen vessel to a third of the quantity. Strain and clear it and take four ounces (113 g) night and morning fasting. This opens obstructions of the liver and spleen and expels the dropsy and jaundice by urine.

Modern uses: Parsley tea is made from the dried leaves, 1 oz (28 g) being added to 1 pt (568 ml) of boiling water, and taken in doses of 1–2 fl oz (28–56 ml).

The seeds contain an oil which is used in doses of 3–10 drops to promote the menstrual flow and to ease menstrual pain. A fluid extract is prepared from the roots by herbalists; but for domestic use a decoction can be made by boiling them in water and administering in doses of 2 fl oz (56 ml) for jaundice, dropsy and urinary tract stone.

PARSLEY PIERT

If a dram of the powder be taken in white wine it will bring away gravel from the kidneys, without much pain.

A small herb with green flowers so small they can hardly be seen. It rarely grows more than four inches (10 cm) high.

Where to find it: Fields, waste ground, sandy soil.

Flowering time: Summer.

Astrology: Not assigned to any planet.

Medicinal virtues: It provokes urine and breaks stone. A strong infusion of the whole plant is good against gravel, jaundice and other complaints arising from obstructions of the viscera. It also helps the strangury.

Modern uses: A popular herb in modern practice. It increases the urinary flow but is soothing and, therefore, of importance as a remedy for cystitis and urinary tract stones. An infusion of the fresh plant is the best way to use it. It can also be combined in equal parts with other similarly acting herbs, such as Buchu leaves, or with diuretics and demulcents, such as Juniper berries and Marsh Mallow.

Parsley Piert
APHANES (= ALCHEMILLA) ARVENSIS

PARSLEY (Rock or Milk)

The powder promotes the menstrual discharge.

This plant has a long striated stalk with small grassy leaves divided into narrow and pointed segments. It grows from one to three feet (30 to 91 cm) high with small white flowers in large umbels.

Where to find it: Hills by the sea and exposed areas.

Flowering time: Late summer.

Astrology: Not assigned to any planet.

Medicinal virtues: The seeds are mild and gentle and given in powder to increase the secretion of the kidneys. It is good in colic and gravel, and for the dropsy and jaundice.

Modern uses: A rare plant and therefore hardly used. Its properties are similar to another variety, *Peucedanum officinale*, described under Fennel (Sow or Hog's). Dill or Fennel can be used as a substitute.

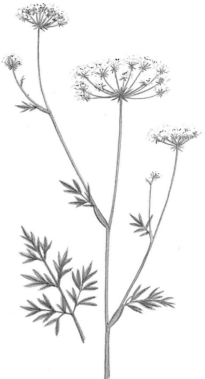

Parsley (Rock or Milk)
PEUCEDANUM PALUSTRE

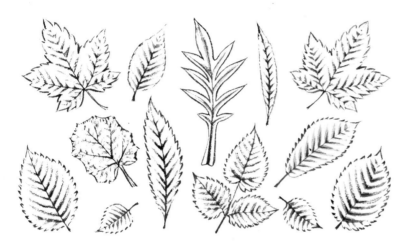

BERULA ERECTA (= SIUM ANGUSTIFOLIUM)

PARSNIP (Upright Water)

Useful for obstructions of the liver, spleen and the womb.

An aquatic plant with large, deep green leaves and large umbels of white flowers on top of the tall, hollow and channelled stalks. Also known as Lesser Water Parsnip.

Where to find it: Slow-flowing rivers and lakes.

Flowering time: Late spring, early summer.

Astrology: Not assigned to any planet.

Medicinal virtues: The seeds are reduced to a powder and applied outwardly to cancerous tumours in the breasts. A scruple taken internally stops purging and haemorrhages, particularly excessive menstrual discharges and spitting of blood. In larger doses it cures intermittent fevers and agues. A strong decoction is good for sore mouths.

The roots boiled in vinegar, and applied as a poultice, cleans and disposes of old putrid sores. The juice is good to bathe sore and inflamed eyes.

Modern uses: There are other varieties, for example the Great Water Parsnip, (*Sium latifolium*) and the Creeping Water Parsnip (*Sium nodiflorum*). The roots of these are considered to be poisonous. They are not recommended for domestic use. None of the varieties are considered to have medicinal properties and are not used professionally.

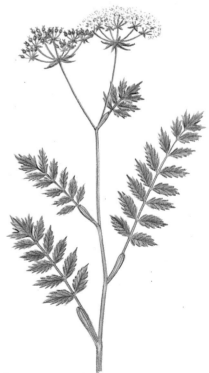

Parsnip (Upright Water) BERULA ERECTA
(= SIUM ANGUSTIFOLIUM)

139

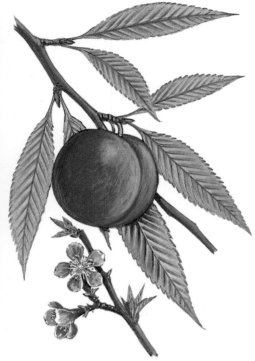

Peach Tree
PRUNUS (= AMYGDALUS) PERSICA

PRUNUS (= AMYGDALUS) PERSICA

PEACH TREE

If the kernels be bruised and boiled in vinegar, until they become thick, and applied to the head, it marvellously makes the hair to grow upon bald places or where it is too thin.

It spreads branches well, from which spring reddish twigs, whereon are set long, narrow green leaves. The blossoms are large, and light pink in colour.

Where to find it: Cultivated in warm countries, but thought to be originally from China. It is not found growing wild.

Flowering time: Spring. The fruit ripens in autumn.

Astrology: Venus owns this tree.

Medicinal virtues: Nothing is better than the leaves or flowers of this tree to purge choler and the jaundice from children and young people. They are given as a syrup or as a conserve. The fruit provokes lust. The leaves bruised and laid on the belly kill worms; and boiled in ale and drank, they open the belly.

The liquor that drops from the wounded tree is given with a decoction of Colt's Foot to those troubled with a cough or shortness of breath, adding thereto some sweet wine and Saffron. It is good for hoarseness, loss of voice and helps defects of the lungs, vomiting and spitting of blood.

Modern uses: The leaves are laxative, sedative and expectorant. An infusion is often used with success against whooping cough. The leaves or powdered bark are excellent for inflammatory bowel disease and gastritis. Use 1 oz (28 g) of the leaves of ½ oz (14 g) of the bark to 1 pt (568 ml) of boiling water and take in doses of up to 2 fl oz (56 ml).

The same is also good for cystitis and tenderness of the bladder, because it stimulates the urine flow but is soothing.

An oil expressed from the kernels is similar to Almond oil.

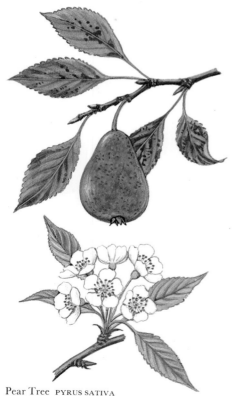

Pear Tree PYRUS SATIVA

PYRUS SATIVA

PEAR TREE

All the sweet and luscious sorts, whether cultivated or wild, help to move the belly downwards, more or less.

The well-known fruit tree. *Pyrus pyraster* is the common Wild Pear.

Where to find it: The Pear is a native fruit of Great Britain and grows wild throughout eastern Europe and west to the Himalayas. The Wild Pear from which the garden varieties have been cultivated grows in woods and coppices.

Flowering time: It blossoms in mid to late spring.

Astrology: This tree is under Venus.

Medicinal virtues: Hard and sour Pears and the leaves bind the belly. The Wild Pear is very good in repelling medicines and if they be boiled with mushrooms it makes them less dangerous. Boiled with a little honey, they help the oppressed stomach. Wild Pears sooner close the lips of fresh wounds than others.

Modern uses: The juice of the Pear is recommended by naturopaths for catarrh and colitis, hypertension, constipation and skin eruptions. It is rich in minerals and vitamins A, B and C. The leaves are not now used in herbal medicine, as they are not considered to be therapeutically active.

PELLITORY OF SPAIN

One of the best purgers of the brain that grows.

A perennial plant resembling Chamomile. At the top it has but one large flower at a place, with a border of many leaves.

Where to find it: Fields, near hedges and paths.

Flowering time: Early to midsummer.

Astrology: It is under Mercury.

Medicinal virtues: An ounce (28 g) of the juice taken in Muscadel an hour before the fit of the ague comes, will effectually drive it away, and at the second or third dose at the furthest.

The herb or dried root chewed in the mouth purges the brain of phlegmatic humours, easing pains in the head and teeth and preventing coughs, phthisics and consumption, the apoplexy and falling-sickness.

The powdered herb or root snuffed up the nostrils produces sneezing and eases headache. Made into an ointment with hog's grease, it helps both the gout and sciatica.

The roots when chewed stimulate the salivary glands, promoting a flow of viscid humours and relieving toothache, headache, lethargy and palsy of the tongue. It is taken internally for paralysis and rheumatism.

Modern uses: Its ability to promote salivation has made it of use for dry mouth and throat, and an excellent remedy for toothache. The root is powdered and made into lozenges or a tincture is applied to the aching tooth with cotton wool.

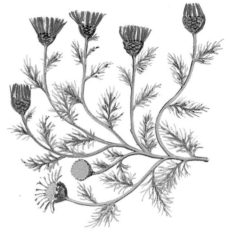

Pellitory of Spain
ANACYCLUS (= ANTHEMIS) PYRETHRUM

PELLITORY OF THE WALL

The juice clarified and boiled in a syrup with honey, and a spoonful drank every morning is good for the dropsy; by taking the dose once a week, that disease will be cured.

A perennial growing one or two feet (30 or 61 cm) high with brownish-red, tender, almost transparent stalks, with broad leaves which taper at the end. The small pale, purplish flowers are followed by black seeds which stick to any garment they touch.

Where to find it: Borders of fields, old walls and rocks, and among rubbish heaps.

Flowering time: Early to midsummer.

Astrology: It is under Mercury.

Medicinal virtues: A remedy for an old and dry cough, shortness of breath and wheezing in the throat. The dried herb is made up into an electuary with honey, or the juice of the herb, or a decoction is made with honey and sugar. Three ounces (85 g) of the juice relieves stoppage of the urine, and expels stone or gravel in the kidneys or bladder.

The bruised herb, sprinkled with some Muscadel, and warmed upon a few quick coals in a chafing-dish and applied to the belly, mitigates pains in the back, sides or bowels, proceeding from wind. The decoction eases the pains of the mother and brings down the courses.

With a little honey added the decoction can be used as a gargle for a sore throat.

The juice made into a liniment with ceruse and Oil of Roses cleanses foul, rotten ulcers and prevents their spreading. Applied to the fundament, it eases the pains of the piles. The juice is effective to cleanse fistulas and heal them.

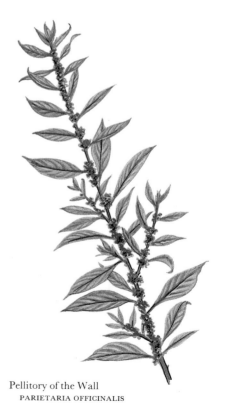

Pellitory of the Wall
PARIETARIA OFFICINALIS

Modern uses: An effective remedy for urinary tract stone, perhaps the most effective single agent available. Herbalists use a prepared tincture, but domestically an infusion is made from the dried herb – 1 oz (28 g) to 1 pt (568 ml) of boiling water – and taken in doses of 2 fl oz (56 ml). This increases urine production and is also indicated for dropsy and suppression of urine. The herb can be combined with Parsley Piert in equal parts.

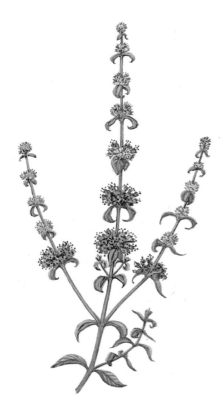

Pennyroyal MENTHA PULEGIUM

MENTHA PULEGIUM

PENNYROYAL

It warms any part to which it is applied and digests corrupt matter.

A perennial belonging to the Mint family. It grows about a foot (30 cm) high with smooth, roundish stalks which have two small, round, pointed leaves at each joint. The pale purple flowers are set in whorls.

Where to find it: Moist commons and near ponds and pools or on the banks of streams.

Flowering time: Late summer.

Astrology: This herb is under Venus.

Medicinal virtues: The herb, boiled and drank, provokes women's courses and expels the dead child and afterbirth. If taken in water and vinegar mingled together, it stays the disposition to vomit. Mingled with honey and salt, it voids phlegm out of the lungs and purges by stool. Applied to the nostrils with vinegar, it revives those who faint and swoon.

The fresh herb bruised and put into vinegar, cleanses foul ulcers and takes away the marks of bruises and blows about the eyes and burns in the face, and the leprosy if drank, and also applied outwardly.

It eases headache, pains in the chest and belly, and gnawing of the stomach. The decoction helps the jaundice and dropsy and clears the eyesight. One spoonful of the juice sweetened with sugar-candy is a cure for whooping cough.

Modern uses: Like other members of the Mint family, Pennyroyal is an excellent remedy for flatulence and colicky pains in the abdomen. But its main use is for promoting menstruation. It is stimulating and warming and is given to children with stomach and bowel upsets and also to ease feverish symptoms in measles and whooping cough. The herb is taken by infusion. Due to the presence of a rich volatile oil, the herb should never be boiled.

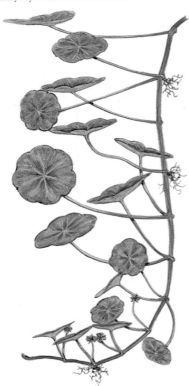

Pennywort (Common Marsh)
HYDROCOTYLE VULGARIS

HYDROCOTYLE VULGARIS

PENNYWORT (Common Marsh)

It is good to break the stone and void it.

A perennial with bluish-green leaves, notched round the edges, and numerous small pinkish flowers in long spikes. Also known as White-rot.

Where to find it: Bogs, fens and marshes, damp walls. It prefers acid soil.

Flowering time: Midsummer.

Astrology: It is under Venus.

Medicinal virtues: A remedy for suppression of urine and the strangury and to remove gravel in the reins and bladder.

Modern uses: Although Pennywort does not appear to be of harm to humans, it does have a reputation for causing foot-rot in sheep. It is very little used, being emetic and purgative, as well as diuretic. The Indian Pennywort (*Hydrocotyle asiatica*), which has similar properties, is a traditional Indian remedy for fevers and bowel complaints. Large doses, however, cause headaches and may induce coma. It is not recommended for domestic use. Its use as a remedy for leprosy is being re-examined by medical researchers. The plant contains a natural antibiotic.

PEPPER

It comforts and warms a cold stomach.

There are three sorts – Black, White and Long. They are climbing, twining tropical plants with white flowers, borne in catkins, and red berries.

Where to find it: It is a native of Java, Sumatra and Malabar.

Flowering time: Summer.

Astrology: Under the dominion of Mars.

Medicinal virtues: It dissolves wind in the stomach or bowels, provokes urine, helps the cough and other chest diseases and stirs up the appetite. The White Pepper, made from the ripe fruits after the rind has been removed, is sharper and more aromatic than the Black, which is made from the unripe berries. The White is used for agues, to warm the stomach, before the coming of the fit. All can be used against quinsy, being mixed with honey and taken inwardly or applied outwardly to disperse the kernels in the throat.

Modern uses: Pepper is a digestive stimulant and anti-flatulent remedy. It is also anti-bacterial and insecticidal. It is incorporated into pills or the powder is taken in doses of 5–15 grains (325–975 mg).

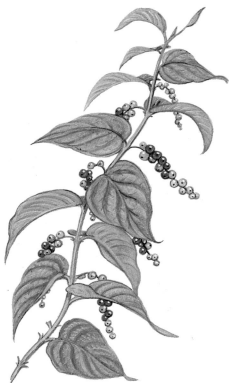

Pepper PIPER NIGRUM

PEPPER (Guinea)

It is a stimulant in phlegmatic disorders, paralytic complaints, and relaxations of the stomach.

There are several kinds of this Pepper, which is also known as Capsicum, Cayenne, Chillies and Paprika. It is a shrub growing up to six feet (1.8 m) high with white flowers, like stars, and yellow centres.

Where to find it: A native of India, but will grow in the garden in hot beds.

Flowering time: Summer.

Astrology: Under Mars.

Medicinal virtues: They are so hot they will raise a blister in the mouth and throat if the seeds or husks be used alone.

The vapour from them causes sneezing, coughing and even vomiting. If the hands touch the nose or eyes after handling them, inflammation will follow. Though dangerous, they have great medicinal properties. The husks are powdered, and to every ounce (28 g), a pound (454 g) of flour is added. This is used to make cakes with yeast. When cooked, the cakes are beaten to a powder and sifted. This powder is then used to season meat, soups and stews. It drives away wind and helps flatuency. It takes away the dimness of the sight if used in meats.

Mixed with honey, the powder helps quinsy and made up with turpentine, and laid on hard knots or kernels in any part of the body, it will dissolve them.

A decoction of the husks makes a good gargle for toothache and preserves the teeth.

Modern uses: A digestive stimulant which eases flatulence. Pills made from the powder stimulate the circulation, helping to ward off disease due to cold and damp.

Because of the intense nature it must be used with caution. Herbalists incorporate it into many prescriptions when they wish to increase circulation. This often serves to make other remedies more potent. It influences heart action first, then arterial circulation and then capillaries and nerves. It is useful in pains in the stomach and bowels and cramps. It acts as a good stimulating liniment for arthritis and rheumatism. Equal parts of tincture of Capsicum, obtainable from herbalists, and glycerine, are shaken together and applied to painful joints.

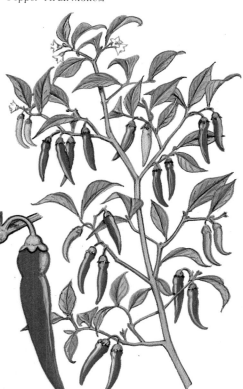

Pepper (Guinea) CAPSICUM FRUTESCENS

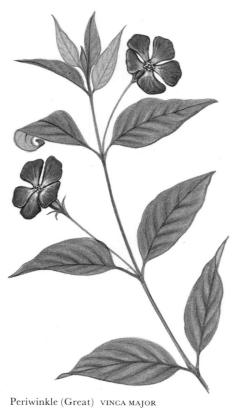

PERIWINKLE (Great)

It is a great binder, and stays bleeding at the mouth and nose, if it be chewed.

A perennial creeping plant with dark, green, shining leaves and pretty pale blue flowers.

Where to find it: Woods and orchards, by the sides of hedges. It is also grown in gardens.

Flowering time: Early spring.

Astrology: Venus owns this herb.

Medicinal virtues: It is a good female medicine and may be used with advantage in hysteric and other fits. An infusion is good to stay the menses. The young tops made into a conserve is good to prevent nightmares. The Small Periwinkle (*Vinca minor*) possesses similar virtues and may be used in its place.

Modern uses: *Vinca major* is an astringent used to check heavy menstrual periods and haemorrhage. The infusion of 1 oz (28 g) of the herb to 1 pt (568 ml) of boiling water is given for diarrhoea, and bleeding piles. The Madagascar Periwinkle is the source of vincristine and vinblastine, which are used as cancer drugs.

Periwinkle (Great) VINCA MAJOR

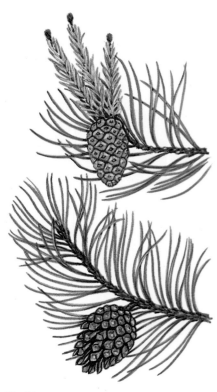

PINE TREE

The kernels are excellent restoratives.

This is the Scots Pine or Norway Pine. It has reddish bark, greyish leaves like needles and sharp-pointed cones. Male flowers are orange-yellow, female flowers pinkish-green.

Where to find it: It grows throughout Europe, but is planted in parks and large gardens as an ornamental tree.

Flowering time: Late spring to early summer.

Astrology: It is a tree of Mars.

Medicinal virtues: From it comes common turpentine, which is thick, whitish and opaque. And from this, the distilled oil sometimes called spirit of turpentine is extracted. The substance left at the bottom of the still is the common rosin, which if taken out before it is drawn too high and then washed in water, is called white or yellow rosin. The black rosin is more evaporated and not washed, but both are of the same nature and are used in ointments and plasters.

In consumptions and after a long illness, the kernels are used as a restorative. They are given in an emulsion beaten up with Barley-water. This is also good for the heat of the urine and other disorders of the urinary passages.

Modern uses: The Pine tree yields several important medicinal compounds. Stockholm tar is the thick, dark, oily substance obtained by distillation of the resin. The turpentine is also called terebenthine from which Ol. Terebenthine is extracted. The tar is antiseptic and expectorant and given for chronic bronchial coughs and consumption. The oil is used in liniments or ointments for sciatica and skin diseases, such as eczema and psoriasis. Syrup of tar is tar water – made by shaking one part of tar with ten of water and decanting – with sugar added. It is taken in doses of one or two teaspoonfuls as an expectorant.

See also Fir.

Pine Tree PINUS SYLVESTRIS

PLANTAIN

It is good to stay spitting of blood and bleedings at the mouth, or the making of foul and bloody water, by reason of any ulcer in the reins or bladder.

A common perennial weed with large, broad leaves and pale greenish-yellow and brown flowers in long greenish spikes.

Where to find it: Waste ground and roadsides.

Flowering time: Early spring to early autumn.

Astrology: This is under Venus. It cures the head by its antipathy to Mars and the privities by its sympathy to Venus. There is not a martial disease that it does not cure.

Medicinal virtues: The clarified juice drank for a few days helps excoriations or pains in the bowels, and distillations of rheum from the head. It stays all manner of fluxes, even women's courses, when too abundant, and staunches the too free bleeding of wounds.

The seed is profitable against dropsy, falling-sickness, yellow jaundice and stoppings of the liver and reins. The juice, or distilled water, dropped into the eyes cools inflammation in them.

The juice mixed with Oil of Roses and the temples and forehead anointed with it, eases pains in the head proceeding from heat. It can also be profitably applied to all hot gouts in the hands and feet. It is also good to apply to bones out of joint, to hinder inflammations, swellings and pains that presently rise thereupon.

The dried and powdered leaves taken in drink kills worms of the belly; boiled in wine, it kills worms which breed in old and foul ulcers. One part of the herb water and two parts of the brine of powdered beef, boiled together and clarified, is a remedy for all scabs and itch in the head and body, tetters, ringworms, shingles and running and fretting sores. All Plantains are good wound-herbs, for wounds and sores, internal and external.

Modern uses: An infusion of the leaves – 1 oz (28 g) to 1 pt (568 pt) of boiling water – is taken in doses of 2 fl oz (56 ml) as a remedy for piles and diarrhoea.

A decoction of the seeds is given to children in tablespoonful doses for thrush. One ounce (28 g) of the seeds is boiled in 1½ pt (852 ml) of water until it measures 1 pt (568 ml). The seeds are mucilaginous and laxative and can be used as a substitute for Linseed.

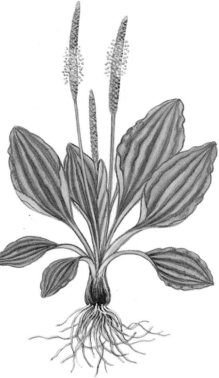

Plantain PLANTAGO MAJOR

PLANTAIN (Buck's Horn)

Commended against venomous bites, especially those of a mad dog.

It looks like a star lying on the ground, with numerous leaves spreading in every direction. They are narrow and jagged like the horn of a buck. The yellow-brown flowers grow on hairy stalks three or four inches (8 or 10 cm) long.

Where to find it: Near the sea on sandy or rocky soil and on heathland.

Flowering time: Early summer.

Astrology: Under Venus.

Medicinal virtues: A moderately drying and binding herb, it is good for wounds, both inward and outward. It is similar in nature to other Plantains.

Modern uses: This can be used as a substitute for *Plantago major*. A decoction of the whole plant or the dried leaves is used as a diuretic to tone the urinary tract and to help expel sediment and stones.

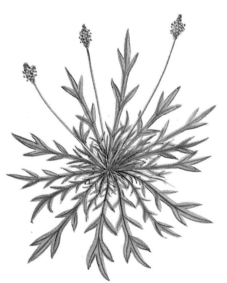

Plantain (Buck's Horn)
PLANTAGO CORONOPUS

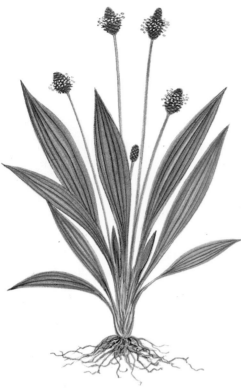

PLANTAGO LANCEOLATA

PLANTAIN (Ribwort)

The juice is commended for the ague to lessen its effects.

A common perennial related to *Plantago major*, but with slender dark green leaves and small brown flowers in a short spike.

Where to find it: Roadside verges, meadows, hedgerows and on dry soils.

Flowering time: Late spring, early summer.

Astrology: A herb of Venus.

Medicinal virtues: The leaves are astringent and vulnerary, and are used in the same manner as the Broad-leaved Plantain.

Modern uses: This is also used as a substitute for *Plantago major*. The whole plant is used. The fresh leaves are used in poultices for wounds, sores and burns and to check bleeding. An infusion made from the leaves can be used as a rectal injection for piles. It is also taken internally, sweetened with honey, for asthma and bronchitis, in doses of 2 fl oz (56 ml).

Plantain (Ribwort) PLANTAGO LANCEOLATA

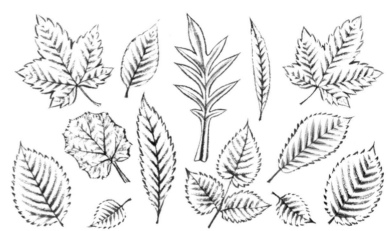

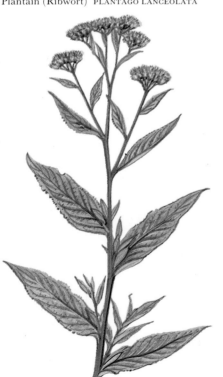

INULA CONYZA

PLOUGHMAN'S SPIKENARD

It is good to promote the menses.

A biennial, about two and a half feet (76 cm) high with broad lanced leaves, rugged on the surface, and dull yellow flowers in a tuft.

Where to find it: By roadsides, rocky slopes, cliffs and copses.

Flowering time: Late summer.

Astrology: It is under the government of Venus.

Medicinal virtues: When bruised the leaves emit an aromatic smell, but they are bitter to the taste. A weak tea is made of the herb to promote the menses and is preferable to any mineral.

Modern uses: The juice can be applied externally to ease itching skin. The infusion of the leaves promotes the menstrual flow and is helpful for wheeziness and internal injury. One ounce (28 g) of the dried leaves is infused in 2 pt (1.1 l) of boiling water and taken in doses of 1–2 fl oz (28–56 ml).

Ploughman's Spikenard INULA CONYZA

PRUNUS DOMESTICA

PLUMS

Plum tree leaves boiled in wine are good to wash and gargle the mouth and throat.

Where to find it: This is the well-known Plum tree which has been cultivated in gardens and orchards for centuries. It is found wild and prefers to grow on sloping ground or at the ridge of a hill.

Flowering time: Early spring.

Astrology: Under Venus.

Medicinal virtues: Their virtues differ with the great diversity of kinds. Sweet Plums moisten the stomach and make the belly soluble, whereas those that are sour quench the thirst more but bind the belly. The dried fruit, under the name of Damask Prunes, loosens the belly, and stewed they procure the appetite, open the body and allay choler.

    The gum that exudes from the tree is good to break the stone. Boiled in vinegar with the leaves and applied to the skin it kills tetter and ringworm. As a gargle or wash the leaves dry the flux of rheum coming to the palate, gums, or almonds of the ears.

Modern uses: The dried leaves are laxative and diuretic and of help in lowering temperature in fevers. They are made into a decoction – ½ oz (14 g) being boiled in 1 pt (568 ml) of water – and taken in doses of 2 fl oz (56 ml). Dried plums, or prunes, are laxative, and are best eaten first thing in the morning. The ripe fruit is delicious and nourishing. The juice alone is laxative and a digestive tonic and is indicated for dyspepsia, piles, obesity and skin eruptions. A wineglassful is taken twice a day.

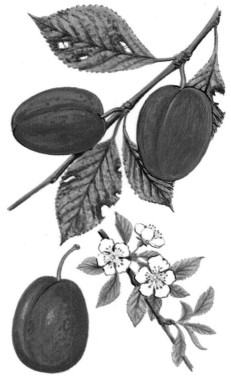

Plum PRUNUS DOMESTICA

POLYPODIUM VULGARE

POLYPODY

It gently carries off the contents of the bowels without irritation.

    This is a perennial herb of the Fern family, distinguishable by the seeds being in roundish spots, distributed on the under surface of the leaf. The root, the thickness of a finger, is covered with brown scales. It tastes sweetish.

Where to find it: Among mossy stones, tree stumps, at the foot of old walls and shady rocky places.

Flowering time: No flower is produced. The fern is ready for use in autumn.

Astrology: It is under Jupiter in Leo.

Medicinal virtues: A mild and useful purge, usually mixed in broths with Beets, Parsley, Mallow, Cummin, Ginger, Fennel and Anise.

    For intestinal complaints, take one ounce (28 g) of the fresh bruised root, add an ounce and a half (42 g) of fresh White Beet roots, a handful of Wild Mallow, and pour on a pint and a quarter (600 ml) of boiling water. Let it stand till next day and then strain. A quarter of a pint (142 ml) of this liquor contains the infusion of two drams (3.5 g) of Polypody root. Sweeten with sugar-candy or honey before taking.

Modern uses: The root is laxative, and can be used fresh or dried. A decoction is made by boiling ½ oz (14 g) of the root in 1 pt (568 ml) of boiling water, and sweetened with honey. Dose 2 fl oz (56 ml), three or four times a day. This remedy also acts as a digestive tonic, stimulating the appetite. It is also helpful in relieving coughs and respiratory infections.

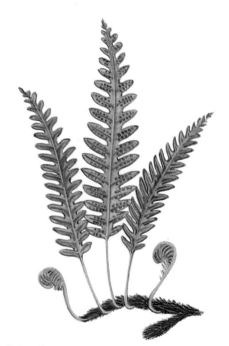

Polypody POLYPODIUM VULGARE

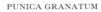

PUNICA GRANATUM
POMEGRANATE TREE
A strong infusion cures ulcers in the mouth and throat and fastens teeth.

A small tree growing to about 15 feet (4.6 m) with brownish bark, long, narrow, willow-like leaves and bright scarlet flowers. The fruit is the size of an orange, with a harder peel, containing sweet juice and numerous seeds embedded in pulp.

Where to find it: Originally from Western Asia, it grows widely in tropical and sub-tropical countries.

Flowering time: Early summer.

Astrology: It is under Mercury.

Medicinal virtues: Both the flowers and the rind of the fruit are strongly astringent. A decoction of them stops bleedings and purgings, and is good for the whites.

Modern uses: A decoction of the bark is used for expelling tapeworm – 2 oz (56 g) of the bark is steeped in 2 pt (1.1 l) of water for 24 hours, then brought to the boil and simmered until 1 pt (568 ml) is left. The bark of the root has similar properties. The dosage is 2 fl oz (56 ml), but it may cause nausea. The dose may need to be repeated and followed by an enema.

A decoction of the rind of the fruit checks diarrhoea and dysentery and, injected into the vagina, it checks leucorrhoea. It is also used as a gargle for sore throats.

The juice of the fruit may also be used to expel worms from the bowel. It should be diluted in equal parts with water or with twice as much Carrot juice. It is also indicated in high blood pressure and arthritis.

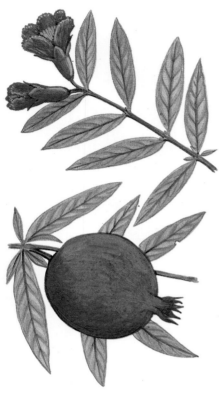

Pomegranate Tree PUNICA GRANATUM

POPULUS NIGRA
POPLAR (Black)
The water that drops from the hollows of this tree takes away warts, wheals and breakings out of the body.

A deciduous tree with broad green leaves somewhat like Ivy and small yellowish-green flowers in catkins. The predominant colour of the flowers comes from the red stamens, however.

Where to find it: Woodland, particularly in damp situations, and by watersides.

Flowering time: Spring.

Astrology: Saturn has dominion over it.

Medicinal virtues: The leaves bruised and applied with vinegar help the gout. The seed drank in vinegar is good against falling-sickness.

Modern uses: An ointment made from the flower buds is used to ease haemorrhoids, applied to the joints in arthritis and rheumatism, and rubbed into the chest when there is bronchitis.

POPULUS ALBA
POPLAR (White)
One ounce of the powdered bark drunk is a remedy for the sciatica, or strangury.

The White Poplar is a decorative tree, the bark, young shoots and underside of the leaves being covered by a dense silvery felt. It grows 80 to 90 feet (24 to 27 m) high.

Where to find it: It likes sand dunes where its suckers help to bind the sand, but it grows throughout Europe, and in Asia north of the Himalayas.

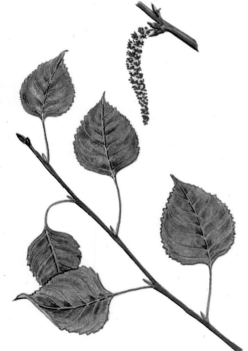

Poplar (Black) POPULUS NIGRA

Flowering time: Spring.

Astrology: Under Saturn.

Medicinal virtues: The White Poplar is of a cleansing property. The juice of the leaves dropped into the ears, eases the pains in them. The young clammy buds or eyes, before they break out into leaves, bruised, and a little honey put to them, is a good medicine for dull sight.

Modern uses: The uses of *Populus alba* are similar to *Populus nigra*. In present day practice, however, White Poplar usually refers to *Populus tremuloides*, also known as the Quaking Aspen. This is the North American counterpart of *Populus tremula*, the Common Aspen which grows wild in Northern Europe and north-east Asia, extending into very cold regions. The buds of these contain much the same constituents as the Black Poplar and can be used for similar purposes. The bark and leaves of *P. tremuloides* used as an infusion restores the digestive system, relaxing the intestinal tract and relieving headache due to liver congestion. It has diuretic properties of value in suppression of urine and can be combined with the leaves of *Arctostaphylos uva-ursi*. It is also indicated for cases of chronic diarrhoea, and dysentery.

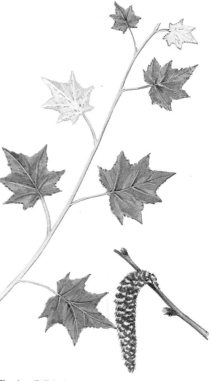

Poplar (White) POPULUS ALBA

PAPAVER SOMNIFERUM

POPPY (White or Opium)

An overdose (of Opium) causes immoderate mirth or stupidity, redness of the face, swelling of the lips, relaxation of the joints, giddiness of the head, deep sleep, accompanied with turbulent dreams and convulsive starting, cold sweats, and frequently death.

The Opium Poppy is an annual with large, whitish-green leaves and a round, smooth stalk growing five or six feet (1.5 or 1.8 m) high. The flowers are large and vary from white to purple. The seed vessel is as large as an orange.

Where to find it: It is mainly cultivated in the Far East for the production of Opium. It does grow wild on waste ground in Europe, but the yield of Opium from such plants is negligible.

Flowering time: Summer.

Astrology: It is under the dominion of the Moon.

Medicinal virtues: Syrup of diacodium is a strong decoction of the seed vessels. It is a gentle narcotic, easing pain and causing sleep. Half an ounce (14 g) is a full dose for an upgrown person, for younger it must be diminished accordingly.

The seeds, beaten into an emulsion, with Barley-water, are good for the strangury, and heat of the urine, but have none of the sleepy virtues of the syrup.

Opium is the milky juice of the plant concreted into a solid form. It has a faint disagreeable smell and a bitterish, hot, biting taste. Taken in proper doses, it procures sleep and a short respite from pain, but great caution is required in administering it for it is very powerful and, consequently, a very dangerous medicine in unskilful hands.

It relaxes the nerves, abates cramps and spasmodic complaints, but increases paralytic disorders. It proves a speedy cure for catarrhs and tickling coughs, but it exasperates all inflammatory symptoms, whether internal or external, by dangerously checking perspiration.

It is good for stopping purgings and vomitings and this is effected by small doses judiciously given. Half a grain (32 mg), or at most, a grain (65 mg), is sufficient in all common cases. It is more advisable to repeat a dose frequently rather than give a larger quantity.

Modern uses: The Poppy yields Opium from which is extracted morphine and codeine. These are used in allopathic medicine. Herbalists use the Wild or Red Poppy (see overleaf), which is non-poisonous.

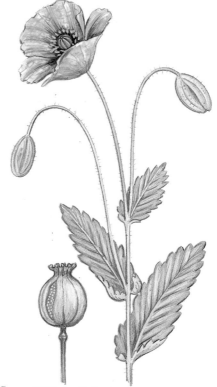

Poppy (White or Opium)
PAPAVER SOMNIFERUM

POPPY (Wild)

A syrup is made of the seed and flowers, which is useful to give sleep and rest to invalids.

The Red Poppy is an annual growing to about one foot (30 cm) with long narrow leaves, a blackish, hairy stalk and scarlet flowers with a black centre.

Where to find it: Fields, waste ground, hedge-sides and gardens.

Flowering time: Late spring to midsummer.

Astrology: The herb is Lunar.

Medicinal virtues: A syrup is made of the seed and flowers to stay catarrhs and defluxions of rheums from the head into the stomach and lungs, which causes a continual cough, the forerunner of consumption. It helps hoarseness of the throat, and loss of voice, which the oil of the seed does likewise.

Boiled in wine and drank, the black seed stays the flux of the belly and women's courses. The Poppy-heads, boiled in water, are given to procure rest and sleep. The leaves act in the same manner.

Modern uses: The flowers are made into a syrup and used to soothe coughs and to induce sleep. An infusion of the petals is helpful in treating asthma, bronchitis, catarrh, whooping cough and angina: ½ oz (14 g) of the dried petals are infused in 2 pt (1.1 l) of boiling water. This can be taken a cupful at a time three or four times a day.

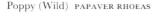

Poppy (Wild) PAPAVER RHOEAS

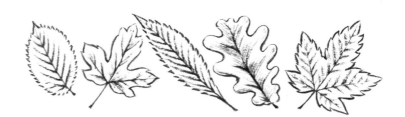

PRIMROSE

The juice of the roots snuffed up the nose, occasions violent sneezing, and brings away a great deal of water, but without being productive of any bad effects.

A woodland perennial with a tuft of leaves and white or pale yellow flowers on long slender hairy stalks.

Where to find it: It is common in woods, thickets and hedges. It particularly likes clay soil.

Flowering time: Early to mid spring.

Astrology: It is under the dominion of Venus.

Medicinal virtues: The dried and powdered roots are good for nervous disorders, but the dose must be small. A dram and a half (2.6 g) of the dried roots, taken in autumn, is a strong, but safe emetic.

Modern uses: The Primrose is similar in action to the Cowslip. It has always been used for gout and rheumatism, preferably in the form of an infusion. One teaspoonful of the dried herb with one of Motherwort is simmered in 1 pt (568 ml) of boiling water until it measures ½ pt (284 ml). This is then administered in three doses of 3 fl oz (85 ml) before meals.

A tincture of the whole plant is sedative and will induce rest and sleep by reducing tension. The dosage varies between 1 and 10 drops. An infusion of the flowers has similar attributes and may be used when the tincture is not available – 1 oz (28 g) of the petals is infused in 1 pt (568 ml) of water and drunk like tea. An infusion of the root taken in tablespoonful doses is effective for nervous headaches.

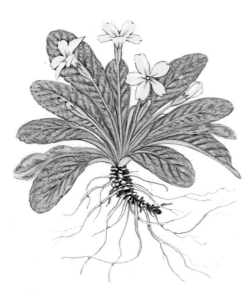

Primrose PRIMULA VULGARIS

CUCURBITA PEPO

PUMPKIN

The seed is cooling and of the nature of the Melon.

An annual creeper with stems up to 30 feet (9 m) long, furnished with large claspers. The leaves are large and rough like Melons. The flowers are large like yellow Lilies in colour. The fruit is very large and contains white, flattish seeds.

Where to find it: Dunghills.

Flowering time: Midsummer. The fruit is ripe in autumn.

Astrology: Under the dominion of the Moon.

Medicinal virtues: It is rarely used in medicine except in the making of emulsions.

Modern uses: The seeds, bruised and liquidised in water, form an emulsion which is used to expel tapeworms. An infusion of the seeds is useful against catarrh and as a demulcent for the bowels and urinary tract when there is irritation. The seed contains anti-tumour properties, and is particularly suitable for the treatment of enlarged prostate. Pumpkin seeds are incorporated in many patent remedies available from health stores.

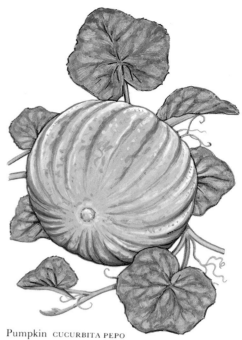

Pumpkin CUCURBITA PEPO

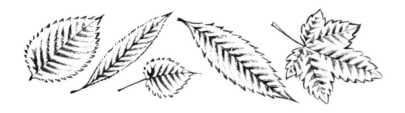

CYDONIA OBLONGA (= PYRUS CYDONIA)

QUINCE TREE

The expressed juice, taken in small quantities, is a mild, astringent stomachic medicine, of efficacy in sickness, vomiting, eructations, and purgings.

The Quince can grow to the height of a good-sized apple tree, with a rough bark and spreading branches. The leaves resemble those of the Apple tree, the flowers are large and pink or sometimes white and the fruit is yellow.

Where to find it: Originally from Persia, it is cultivated in gardens, but is found wild near ponds and lakes.

Flowering time: Spring. The fruits ripen in late autumn.

Astrology: Saturn owns this tree.

Medicinal virtues: A grateful cordial is made by digesting in three pints (1.6 l) of the clarified juice, a dram (1.7 g) of Cinnamon and half a dram (890 mg) each of Ginger and Cloves, by keeping it warm for six hours and then adding a pint (568 ml) of red port, dissolving in it nine pounds (4 kg) of sugar and straining it. A quince jelly is made by boiling the juice with a sufficient quantity of sugar until it attains a due consistency.

The seeds abound with a soft mucilaginous substance which they readily impart to boiling water, making it like white of egg. This is excellent for sore mouths and to soften and moisten the mouth and throat in fevers and other diseases. The green fruit helps fluxes in man or woman, and choleric laxes. Boiled in water, the mucilage heals the sore breasts of women.

Modern uses: The mucilage from the seeds is astringent and soothing to the intestinal tract and used in dysentery and diarrhoea. It is obtained by boiling two teaspoonfuls of the seeds in 1 pt (568 ml) of water for 10 minutes and straining the mixture. It can be taken as desired.

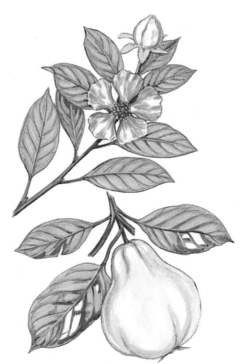

Quince Tree CYDONIA OBLONGA
(= PYRUS CYDONIA)

151

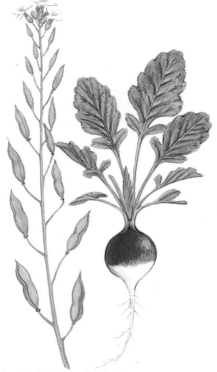

RAPHANUS SATIVUS

RADISH (Common Garden)

It does not give much nourishment, and is very windy.

The well-known salad vegetable. The flowers are white, with violet veins.

Where to find it: Originally from China, it is found wild where it has escaped from cultivation. It also grows in gardens.

Flowering time: Several times a year depending on seeding time, but in its natural habitat it flowers in late spring.

Astrology: It is under Mars.

Medicinal virtues: It is opening, attenuating and anti-scorbutic. It provokes urine and is good for the stone and gravel. The expressed juice of the root, with the addition of a little wine, is an admirable remedy for gravel. The roots eaten plentifully sweeten the blood and juices and are good against scurvy.

Modern uses: The juice stimulates the production of bile and has been used in the treatment of gallstones, and as a liver tonic. It is rich in potassium, sodium, iron and magnesium. The juice is strong and is best combined with six times as much Celery juice or twice as much Carrot juice. It is not suitable for inflammatory conditions of the stomach or where there is kidney disease. A wineglassful of mixed juice is taken every day, starting with a small amount and increasing gradually.

Radish (Common Garden)
RAPHANUS SATIVUS

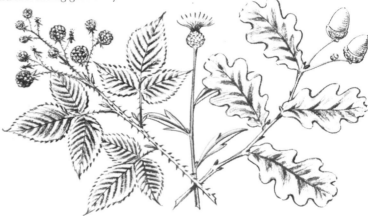

ARMORACIA RUSTICANA (= COCHLEARIA ARMORACIA)

RADISH (Wild or Horse)

The bruised root laid to the part affected with sciatica, joint-ache or the hard swellings of the liver and spleen, helps them all.

The leaves appear before winter and grow to about eighteen inches (46 cm). A second crop of leaves follow, which are rougher, broader and taller. The root is large and white with a taste like mustard.

Where to find it: A cultivated plant, but is found wild in moist and shady places.

Flowering time: Midsummer.

Astrology: It is under Mars.

Medicinal virtues: The juice of the root, when drank, is effectual for the scurvy. Given to children to drink, it kills worms. The distilled water of the herb and root is taken with a little sugar for sciatica.

Modern uses: A digestive stimulant, it is added to food as a vinegar or sauce. An infusion of the root – ½ oz (14 g) to 1 pt (568 ml) of boiling water – is given in doses of 2 fl oz (56 ml) for its strong diuretic properties, which are of value in dropsy. This is also suitable for rheumatism and gout.

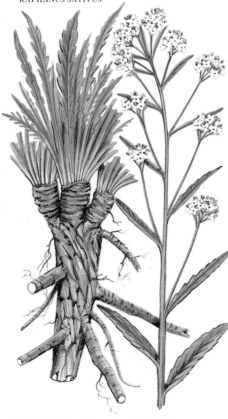

Radish (Wild or Horse) ARMORACIA
RUSTICANA (= COCHLEARIA ARMORACIA)

SENECIO JACOBAEA

RAGWORT

The decoction of the herb is good to wash the mouth or throat that has ulcers or sores therein.

It grows to three or four feet (0.9 to 1.2 m), and is much branched, bearing many flowers, each consisting of a border of green leaves, with a dark yellow thrum in the middle. A very common annual weed, also known as St James's-wort.

Where to find it: In pastures and untilled ground.

Flowering time: Summer.

Astrology: Under the command of Dame Venus.

Medicinal virtues: It cleanses, digests and discusses. The decoction of the herb is used for swellings, hardness or imposthumations, for it thoroughly cleans and heals them. Use it also for the quinsy and king's-evil. It helps to stay catarrh, thin rheums and defluxions from the head into the eyes, nose or lungs.

The juice heals wounds and cleanses old filthy ulcers in the privities, and inward ulcers. It stays the malignant, fretting and running cankers and hollow fistulas.

It is also much commended to help aches and pains either in the fleshy parts or in nerves and sinews. In sciatica, bathe with the decoction or anoint the place with an ointment made from the herb. Mastic and olibanum in powder may be added to the ointment after it is strained.

Modern uses: Ragwort may irritate the liver if taken internally and is, therefore, not recommended for domestic use. An infusion of the herb is purgative and emetic. Herbalists employ Ragwort only for external conditions. The infusion is used as a lotion for ulcers and wounds, and the ointment for inflammation of the eyes. The homoeopathic tincture is used for cystitis.

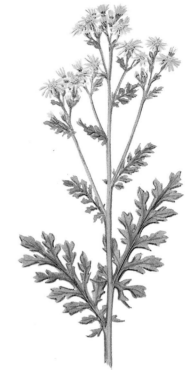

Ragwort SENECIO JACOBAEA

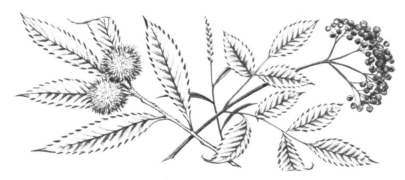

JASIONE MONTANA

RAMPION (Sheep's)

The juice applied externally heals foulness and discolourings of the skin.

A perennial, also known as Sheep's Bit Scabious, which resembles Devil's Bit Scabious. It grows to about three feet (91 cm) with faint-green leaves and fine blue flowers.

Where to find it: Grassland, particularly high pastures, and heathland. It likes a lime-free soil.

Flowering time: Late summer.

Astrology: It is under the dominion of Mercury.

Medicinal virtues: An infusion of the flowers is excellent for disorders of the chest, such as asthma and difficulty of breathing; also for fevers.

Modern uses: The plant resembles Devil's Bit, which is indicated for similar purposes. Sheep's Rampion is not in current use due to its rarity. See Devil's Bit.

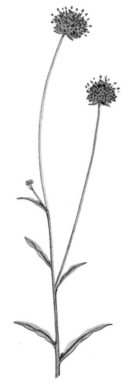

Rampion (Sheep's) JASIONE MONTANA

153

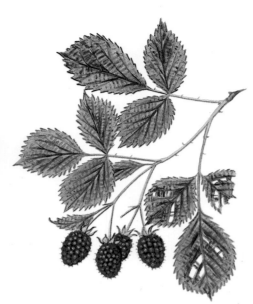

Raspberry RUBUS IDAEUS

RUBUS IDAEUS
RASPBERRY

The fruit . . . is somewhat astringent and good to prevent miscarriage.

The common Garden Raspberry is a hardy deciduous shrub of the Rose family.

Where to find it: It is mainly cultivated, but also grows wild in woodland, where it likes the loamy soil.

Flowering time: Late spring to midsummer.

Astrology: Venus owns this shrub.

Medicinal virtues: The fruit has a pleasant grateful smell and taste, is cordial, strengthens the stomach and stays vomiting. It dissolves the tartarous concretions on the teeth, but is inferior to Strawberries for that purpose.

The juice of the ripe fruit boiled into a syrup is agreeable to the stomach, and prevents sickness and retchings.

Modern uses: The syrup made from the fruits is used to flavour medicines. The leaves are astringent and an infusion of them – 1 oz (28 g) to 1 pt (568 ml) of boiling water – will check simple diarrhoea. The infusion can also be used where there is a fever to encourage sweating. A strong infusion made in the same proportions, but boiled for a few minutes, makes a good gargle for sore throats.

The powdered leaves made into tablets are taken in pregnancy to help childbirth. The infusion can be taken for the same purpose, and for painful menstruation. It has a marked hormonal effect on the musculature of the uterus, stimulating normal contractions and inducing relaxation between them.

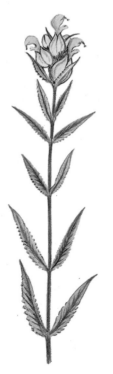

Rattle Grass RHINANTHUS

RHINANTHUS
RATTLE GRASS

The whole seed (of the Yellow Rattle) being put into the eyes, draws forth any skin, dimness of film, from the sight, without pain or trouble.

The common Red Rattle (also called Housewort) has reddish, hollow stalks, with reddish-green leaves and purplish-red flowers. Black seed is produced in small husks which rattle when shaken. The Yellow Rattle usually has just one stalk about two feet (61 cm) high and flowers of fair yellow colour. The seed also rattles in the husks.

Where to find it: Meadows and woods.

Flowering time: Mid to late summer.

Astrology: Both under the dominion of the Moon.

Medicinal virtues: The Red Rattle is profitable to heal fistulas and hollow ulcers, and to stay the flux of humours in them, the abundance of women's courses, or other fluxes, if boiled in wine and drank.

The Yellow Rattle is good for cough, or dimness of the sight, if the herb be boiled with beans, and some honey put thereto, be drunk or dropped into the eyes.

Modern uses: Red Rattle Grass (*Pedicularis sylvatica*) and Yellow Rattle Grass (*Rhinanthus minor*) have fallen from popularity as herbal remedies, mainly because their medicinal properties closely resemble those of the Eyebright (*Euphrasia officinalis*), which is widely used for its ophthalmic and astringent qualities.

REST-HARROW

The decoction with some vinegar used to wash out the mouth, eases toothache.

A perennial shrub with reddish-pink flowers. The stems have thorns making the plant difficult to collect. Also called Spiny Rest-harrow.

Where to find it: Roadsides, waste ground and fields.

Flowering time: Midsummer.

Astrology: It is under the dominion of Mars.

Medicinal virtues: It provokes urine, breaks and expels the stone, if the bark of the root is taken in wine. The decoction powerfully opens obstructions of the liver and spleen. The powdered root, made into an electuary, or lozenges, with sugar, or the bark of the fresh roots boiled until tender and beaten to a conserve with sugar, works to the like effect. The powdered roots strewed upon the brims of external ulcers consumes their hardness and causes them to heal the better.

Modern uses: The flowers and roots are popular with French herbalists for the treatment of urinary tract infection and inflammation. The powdered roots are diuretic and given by decoction. This is indicated in cases of dropsy, kidney stone, cystitis and water retention. The flowers are dried and the infusion used as a gargle or mouthwash for sore throat and gums.

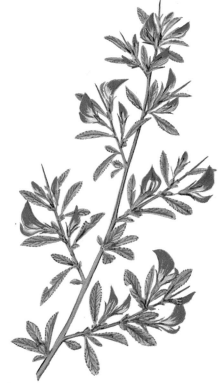

Rest-harrow ONONIS SPINOSA

RHUBARB

In bloody flux, and those loosenesses occasioned by acrid matter remaining in the intestines, this root is very useful.

This has a long thick root, brownish on the outside and full of reddish veins inside. It is similar to Garden Rhubarb.

Where to find it: This is the Rhubarb grown in China and other parts of central and eastern Asia.

Flowering time: Early to midsummer.

Astrology: Under the dominion of Mars.

Medicinal virtues: It is a mild purgative and a mild astringent. It is given more as a strengthener of the intestines than as a purgative. It generally leaves the belly costive and is therefore preferable to other purgatives in obstinate purgings and bloody flux.

Roots which are light in texture, moist, fragrant and sound are chosen being milder in action and more grateful to the stomach. They are more likely to answer the purpose of an astringent, a diuretic or an alterative. In acute fevers where it is dangerous to take purgatives, Rhubarb may be safely given.

Two or three teaspoonfuls of the tincture strengthens the intestines, whereas two or three ounces (56 or 85 g) is frequently necessary as a purgative.

Modern uses: Rhubarb is widely used in pharmaceutical preparations obtainable over the counter in chemists and health food shops. In small doses the powdered root is astringent and checks diarrhoea, but in large doses it irritates the colon causing the bowels to evacuate. The dosage of the powdered root is 3–30 grains (0.2–2 g). Tinctures and fluid extracts are available from herbalists.

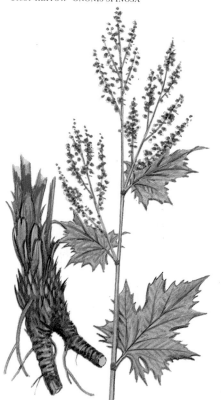

Rhubarb RHEUM PALMATUM

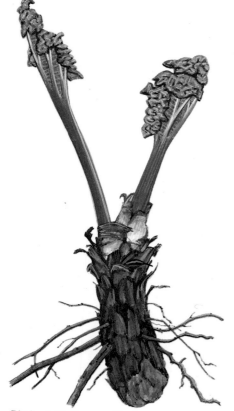

Rhubarb (Culinary or Tart)
RHEUM RHAPONTICUM

RHEUM RHAPONTICUM

RHUBARB (Culinary or Tart)

Good in fluxes and weakness of the stomach.

This is the Garden Rhubarb widely cultivated for its food value.

Where to find it: Although commonly grown in gardens, it was originally from Asia where it grows wild.

Flowering time: Midsummer.

Astrology: Under Mars.

Medicinal virtues: As a purgative it is much weaker than *Rheum palmatum*, but it is more astringent. It stays fluxes and strengthens the stomach and is good where there is spitting of blood or the making of bloody urine. It is also good against venomous bites.

Modern uses: The stems are used for food. A large amount, however, will act as a laxative. Because of its mildness, it is used as a remedy for children's tummy troubles. The powdered root is given in doses varying between 5 and 60 grains (0.32 and 3.9 g) as a gastro-intestinal tonic. It checks diarrhoea, improves the appetite and regulates bowel activity. Rhubarb contains oxalic acid, which may exacerbate people of a gouty rheumatic tendency. The leaves are poisonous and many deaths have been due to their being mistaken for Spinach.

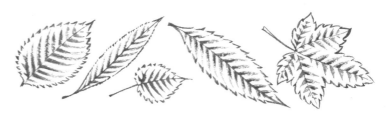

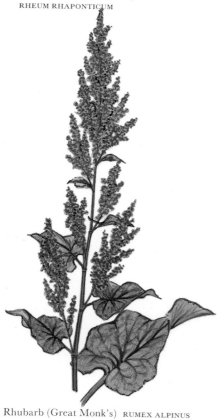

Rhubarb (Great Monk's) RUMEX ALPINUS

RUMEX ALPINUS

RHUBARB (Great Monk's)

The juice of the leaves or roots, or the decoction of them in vinegar, is used as a most effectual remedy to heal running sores.

This is not a Rhubarb, but is a kind of Dock. It has acquired the name of Monk's Rhubarb because it is similar in action to Rhubarb. It is also known as Great Garden Patience or Patience Dock.

Where to find it: It is found near the roadside in high outlying districts. Much more common in mountainous areas, particularly where animals graze.

Flowering time: Midsummer.

Astrology: A herb of Mars.

Medicinal virtues: A dram (1.7 g) of the dried root, with a scruple of Ginger, taken fasting in warm broth, purges the choler and phlegm downwards gently and safely. The seed binds the belly and helps to stay bloody flux. The distilled water heals foul ulcerous sores and allays inflammation. The decoction gargled takes away toothache; and if drank, heals the jaundice. The seed also eases griping pains in the stomach.

The root expels stone, provokes urine and helps the dimness of sight. Boiled in wine and taken it helps the swelling of the throat, called the king's-evil, as well as swellings of the kernels of the ears.

Modern uses: As it is fairly rare outside of the mountainous regions of Europe, it is not widely used by medical herbalists. However, where it is available it is used as a safe laxative. The leaves were used as a vegetable. The root is collected in spring or autumn, dried and powdered. The dose varies with the individual. See also Dock (Common).

RICE

It stays laxes and fluxes of the stomach and belly.

This is the well-known food, obtained from an annual plant which grows in water and produces stems up to ten feet (3 m) long.

Where to find it: It grows wild by ditches and rivers in India and China, but it is mainly cultivated as a staple food.

Flowering time: Summer. The seeds are ready by mid autumn.

Astrology: It is a Solar grain.

Medicinal virtues: A flour of the Rice is put into cataplasms to repel bad humours and applied to women's breasts to stay inflammations. Boiled in milk and hot steel quenched therein does give it a somewhat drying and binding quality.

Modern uses: Used mainly as a food. The Whole Brown Rice is preferred as it is rich in vitamins B and E. White Rice is refined and its over-use should be considered as a health hazard. As a convalescent food Rice is suitable for those with a tendency to diarrhoea.

Rice water, which is a decoction of the seeds, is made by boiling about ½ oz (14 g) of Rice in 1 pt (568 ml) boiling water for half and hour, straining and adding honey to taste. It is a good remedy for diarrhoea due to irritation of the bowels. It is soothing and cooling and also suitable for fevers and painful urination. It can be drunk freely. A poultice made by powdering the Rice and adding to water is excellent for skin inflammation. Brown Rice is obtainable from health food stores.

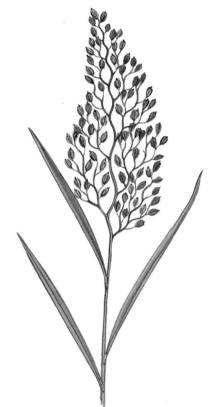

Rice ORYZA SATIVA

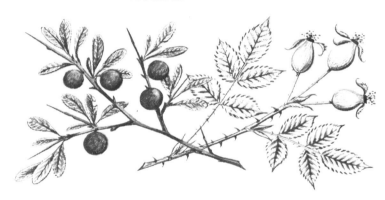

ROCKET CRESS

The juice is excellent in asthmas, and all diseases of the lungs.

There are several plants bearing the name of Rocket. This one is annual or biennial growing to about three feet (91 cm) high with pointed leaves and pale yellow flowers streaked with purple. It is also known as Garden Rocket.

Where to find it: It is grown in gardens, but is also found in hedgerows and meadows.

Flowering time: Late spring to midsummer.

Astrology: Under Venus.

Medicinal virtues: The best way of using this is as a syrup. It will cure inveterate coughs and relieve oppression and obstruction of the chest.

Modern uses: The leaves have been used like cress in salads, but they are very bitter to the taste. As a medicine, it is not in popular use as it is very nauseous. Indeed, it could be used as an emetic in place of Ipecacuanha. Horehound, Lungwort and Colt's Foot are recommended for coughs nowadays.

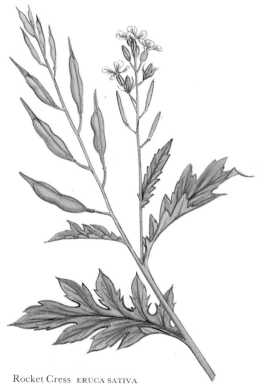

Rocket Cress ERUCA SATIVA

ROOT OF SCARCITY

Its nourishing qualities are so many that it ought to be cultivated every where.

This is a variety of Beetroot and is cultivated in just the same way. It is also known as the Mangel Wurzel.

Where to find it: It is derived from the Sea Beet, which grows wild at the coast and in marshland. It is mainly grown as a winter food for cattle.

Flowering time: Early summer to early autumn.

Astrology: The root is under Saturn.

Medicinal virtues: Insects and vermin, which destroy other roots and plants, will not touch or injure it. It is not affected by mildew, or blasted by drought. It draws the virtues from the soil and prepares it for the reception of corn or other seed.

Cattle sheep and horses readily eat the leaves and poultry may be fed upon the roots if they be cut small and mixed with bran.

When crops fail, this plant will be found one of the cheapest, most valuable and wholesome roots ever introduced, and is preferable to Turnips, Carrots or Beetroot.

Modern uses: The Mangel Wurzel is generally considered to be too tough to be used as a vegetable, although ideal for animals for whom it is a nutritious article. It can be used to produce wine or ale. It is not used medicinally. See Beets.

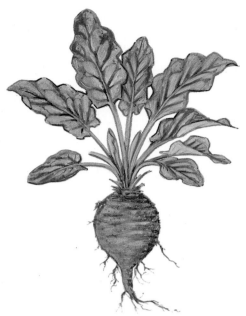

Root of Scarcity BETA ALTISSIMA

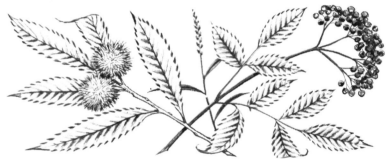

ROSE (Damask)

An excellent purge for children and grown people of a costive habit.

The Damask Rose is an old garden Rose of obscure origin. It does not grow as tall as the White Rose, but is taller and has more prickles than the Red. The flowers are of a pale red colour and have a pleasant scent.

Where to find it: A common garden Rose, but it grows wild in France.

Flowering time: Early to midsummer.

Astrology: Under the dominion of Venus.

Medicinal virtues: A syrup is made from the flowers by infusing them for 24 hours in boiling water, straining and adding twice the weight of refined sugar. A small quantity will keep the bowels regular. A conserve made of the unripe flowers has similar properties.

A conserve made of the fruit of the Wild or Dog Rose (*Rosa canina*) is very pleasant and of considerable efficacy for common colds and coughs. The flowers of the common Red Rose (*Rosa rubra*) are dried and given in infusions and sometimes in powder against overflowing of the menses, spitting of blood and other haemorrhages. An excellent tincture is made from them by pouring a pint (568 ml) of boiling water on an ounce (28 g) of the dried petals and adding 15 drops of oil of vitriol and three or four drams (5.3 or 7 g) of sugar, stirring together and leaving to cool. This tincture, when strained, is of a beautiful red colour. It may be taken for strengthening the stomach and

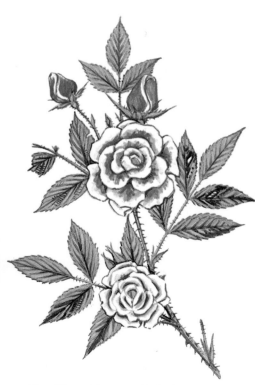

Rose (Damask) ROSA DAMASCENA

preventing vomiting to the amount of three or four spoonfuls twice or three times a day. It is a powerful and pleasant remedy in immoderate discharges of the menses and all other fluxes and haemorrhages.

The Damask Rose, on account of its fragrance, belongs to the cephalics, but it is also valuable for its cathartic quality. An infusion made of half a dram to two drams (0.89 to 3.5 g) of the dried leaves makes a good purge.

Modern uses: This Rose is valued for its perfume and it is from the Damask Rose and similar varieties that Attar of Rose perfume is produced. The official Oil of Rose also comes from the Damask Rose. This is used to make Rose-water, which herbalists incorporate into eye lotions. An infusion of the petals – 1 oz (28 g) to 1 pt (568 ml) of boiling water – can be used domestically as an eye lotion.

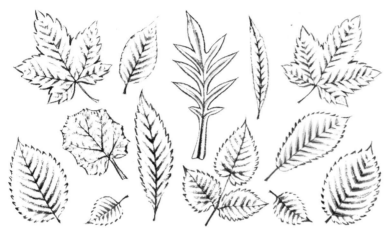

ROSEMARY

It helps a weak memory, and quickens the senses.

A shrub growing to three feet (91 cm) or more high with grey-green sharp-pointed leaves and pale blue flowers, variegated with white.

Where to find it: It will grow in gardens, but prefers to be near the sea.

Flowering time: Mid to late spring, and sometimes again in late summer.

Astrology: The Sun claims dominion over it.

Medicinal virtues: A decoction of Rosemary in wine helps cold diseases of the head and brain such as giddiness and swimmings, drowsiness or dullness, the dumb palsy, loss of speech, lethargy and falling-sickness. It is both drunk and the temples bathed with it.

It eases pains in the teeth and gums and is comfortable to the stomach. It is a remedy for windiness in the stomach, bowels and spleen, and powerfully expels it. Both flowers and leaves are profitable for the whites if taken daily. The leaves used in ointments, or infused in oil, help cold benumbed joints, sinews, or members.

The Oil of Rosemary is a sovereign help for all the diseases mentioned. Touch the temples and nostrils with two or three drops or take one to three drops for inward diseases. But use discretion, for it is quick and piercing, and only a little must be taken at a time.

Modern uses: The dried herb is used by infusion – one teaspoonful to a cup of boiling water – as a remedy for headache due to gastric disturbance. It stimulates bile production by the liver. The oil is anti-flatulent and is taken on sugar, one or two drops only at a time. It is tonic to the scalp and is one of the ingredients in Eau-de-Cologne and many over-the-counter shampoos and hair preparations. For home use the infusion of the dried herb can be used as a hair wash.

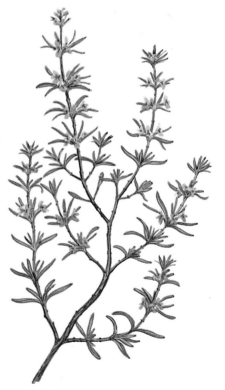

Rosemary ROSMARINUS OFFICINALIS

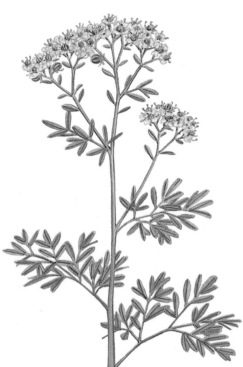

RUE (Garden)

The seed taken in wine, is an antidote against all dangerous medicines or deadly poisons.

Rue is a shrubby plant with tough, woody branches. The leaves are evergreen and have a bitter taste. The flowers are yellow and appear at the ends of the younger shoots.

Where to find it: A cultivated garden shrub. It likes dry, sheltered spots.

Flowering time: Late summer.

Astrology: A herb of the Sun, and under Leo.

Medicinal virtues: It provokes urine and women's courses. A decoction made with dried Dill leaves and flowers eases all inward pains and torments, both drunk and outwardly applied warm. It also helps the pains of the chest and sides, coughs and hardness of breathing, inflammation of the lungs, if drunk, and sciatic and joint pains if anointed.

A draught taken prevents the shaking fits of agues coming on. Boiled in oil it is good to help colicky wind, hardness and windiness of the mother if applied outwardly.

Bruised and put into the nostrils, it stays the bleeding. The decoction with Bay leaves added is used to bathe swellings of the testicles.

An ointment made from the juice with Oil of Roses, ceruse, and a little vinegar, and anointed, cures St Anthony's fire, and all running sores in the head.

Modern uses: An infusion of 1 oz (28 g) of the dried herb in 1 pt (568 ml) of boiling water is taken in doses of 2 fl oz (56 ml) to promote menstruation. Oil of Rue is given in doses of one to three drops for the same purpose. The herb is combined with nervine tonics such as Scullcap and Valerian as a remedy for many nervous conditions including headache, dizziness and palpitations.

Rue (Garden) RUTA GRAVEOLENS

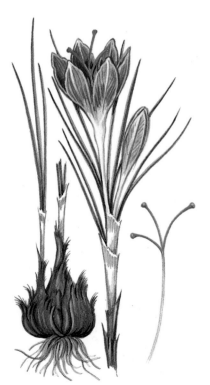

SAFFRON

The use of it ought to be moderate and reasonable; for when the dose is too large, it produces a heaviness of the head and sleepiness. Some have fallen into an immoderate convulsive laughter which ended in death.

It has a tuberous root, about the size of a Nutmeg, and purplish flowers with yellow-red centres. It resembles the Garden Crocus.

Where to find it: A cultivated plant. Most supplies come from Spain.

Flowering time: Early autumn.

Astrology: It is a herb of the Sun and under the Lion.

Medicinal virtues: Not above ten grains (650 mg) must be given at one time. A cordial if taken in immoderate quantity, hurts the heart instead of helping it. It quickens the brain, helps consumptions of the lungs, and difficulty of breathing, is excellent in epidemical diseases, such as pestilence, smallpox and measles. A notably expulsive medicine, it is a good remedy in yellow jaundice. It is a useful aromatic, of a strong penetrating smell and a warm pungent bitterish taste. It is particularly serviceable in disorders of the chest, in female obstructions and hysteric depressions. Saffron is endowed with great virtues. It refreshes the spirits and is good against fainting fits and palpitations of the heart. It strengthens the stomach, helps digestion, cleanses the lungs and is good in coughs.

Modern uses: An infusion of one teaspoonful of the powdered flower pistils to 1 pt (568 ml) of boiling water is administered in doses of 2 fl oz (56 ml) to stimulate menstruation and ease painful periods. It is also anti-flatulent and diaphoretic. Dosage is critical, as Saffron is toxic taken to excess.

Saffron CROCUS SATIVUS

SAFFRON (Meadow)

Indiscreetly used, this root is poisonous.

Also known as Naked Ladies, this is a bulbous perennial, producing numerous leaves and flowers of a pale but elegant purple. It resembles a Crocus.

Where to find it: Damp meadows.

Flowering time: Early autumn.

Astrology: It is under Saturn.

Medicinal virtues: A single grain swallowed by a healthy person as an experiment, produced heat in the stomach, flushes of heat and shiverings, colicky pains and irritation in the loins and urinary passages. Other symptoms included tremor, head pain, rapid pulse, continual production of urine and great thirst.

However, when properly prepared, it is a safe and powerful medicine. The best way is to make it into a syrup by digesting an ounce (28 g) of the roots sliced thin in a pint (568 ml) of white-wine vinegar, over a gentle fire, for 48 hours. It is then strained and two pounds (908 g) of honey mixed into it and gently boiled till it comes to a proper consistency.

This syrup is agreeably acid, gently bites the tongue and is excellent for cleansing it from mucus. Too much causes vomiting and purging, so the dose at first should be no more than half a teaspoonful twice or three times a day. The quantity may be gradually increased, as the stomach will bear it, or as the case may require.

It operates by way of the urine, for which it is a remarkably powerful medicine. It has been given with astonishing success in dropsies and tertian agues and it frequently succeeds as an expectorant when all other means fail.

Modern uses: *Colchicum* is highly regarded as a remedy for gout and arthritis. It has to be used with utmost caution as it is a potent cell poison. Alkaloids contained in the plant have proved to be anti-cancerous and drugs derived from *Colchicum* were among the first to be used effectively against leukaemia. This plant is not recommended for domestic use.

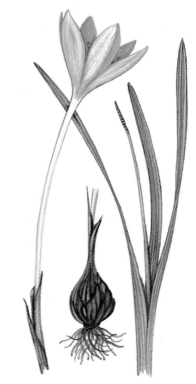

Saffron (Meadow) COLCHICUM AUTUMNALE

SAFFRON (Wild) or SAFFLOWER

It evacuates tough viscid phlegm, both upwards and downwards.

An annual plant growing two or three feet (61 or 91 cm) high with a whitish stem branching at the top. It has prickly leaves and saffron-coloured flowers.

Where to find it: Fields and gardens. It is cultivated in India.

Flowering time: Midsummer.

Astrology: It is saturnine.

Medicinal uses: It is a pretty strong cathartic and also clears the lungs and helps the phthisis. It is likewise serviceable against the jaundice.

Modern uses: The flowers are laxative and induce sweating. They are used as an infusion – ½ oz (14 g) to 1 pt (568 ml) of boiling water – for children's complaints, particularly measles, scarlet fever and eruptive skin diseases. The infusion also stimulates the menstrual flow.

The seed is laxative. Safflower oil, obtained from the seeds, is used for culinary purposes. It is also obtainable in capsules. Like Sunflower oil, it is rich in linoleic acid, an essential fatty acid.

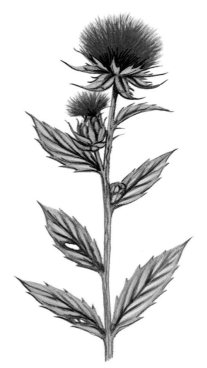

Saffron (Wild) or Safflower
CARTHAMUS TINCTORIUS

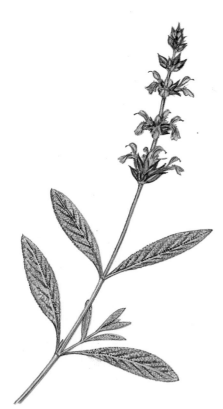

Sage (Common Garden) SALVIA OFFICINALIS

SALVIA OFFICINALIS

SAGE (Common Garden)

Good for the liver and to breed blood.

A shrubby plant with rough, wrinkled leaves, sometimes green and sometimes reddish purple. The flowers are a blueish-purple.

Where to find it: A common herb in the kitchen garden.

Flowering time: Early to late summer.

Astrology: Jupiter claims it.

Medicinal virtues: A decoction of the leaves and branches provokes the urine, brings down women's courses and expels the dead child.

It stays bleeding of wounds, and can be used to cleanse foul ulcers or sores. Three spoonfuls of the juice taken fasting, with a little honey, stops the casting of blood in those with consumption.

To make the pills, take two drams (3.5 g) each of Spikenard and Ginger and eight drams (14 g) of the Sage seed toasted at the fire. Make into a powder and add as much juice of Sage as needed to make into a mass of pills. Take a dram (1.7 g) of them every morning and night, fasting, and drink a little pure water after. They are profitable for pains in the head and joints and they help the falling-sickness, lethargy, lowness of spirits and the palsy.

The juice taken in warm water, helps hoarseness and cough. Drank with vinegar, it is good for the plague. Gargles are made with Sage, Rosemary, Honeysuckle and Plantain boiled in wine or water with honey or Alum added. Sage is boiled with other hot and comforting herbs to bathe the body and the legs in summertime, especially to warm cold joints or sinews, troubled with the palsy and cramp, and to comfort and strengthen the parts.

Modern uses: One of the best remedies for laryngitis, tonsillitis and sore throats. A teaspoonful of the dried leaves are infused in a cup of boiling water and the liquid used as a gargle. Alternatively half the water may be replaced by malt or cider vinegar. This may be taken internally as well as used as a gargle, as may the ordinary infusion.

The infusion sweetened with honey and taken in doses of 2 fl oz (56 ml) is anti-flatulent and mildly laxative. It also stimulates the menstrual flow.

TEUCRIUM SCORODONIA

SAGE (Wood)

The drink used inwardly, and the herb used outwardly, is found to be a sure remedy for the palsy.

A perennial belonging to the Nettle family. It grows to about two feet (61 cm) with square hairy stems and two leaves at every joint. The flowers are greenish-yellow and set in a slender spike.

Where to find it: Common in woodland, grassland and heaths. It is also found by the sides of roads and on hedge-banks.

Flowering time: Throughout the summer.

Astrology: The Sages are under Venus.

Medicinal virtues: A decoction provokes the urine and women's courses. It induces sweating, digests humours and discusses swellings and nodes in the flesh. It is therefore good against venereal disease.

A decoction of the green herb, made with wine, is a safe and sure remedy for those who by falls, bruises, or blows, suspect some vein to be inwardly broken, to disperse and void the congealed blood, and to consolidate the veins.

The juice of the herb, or the powder of it, is good for moist ulcers and sores in the legs to dry and heal them more speedily. It is no less effectual for fresh wounds.

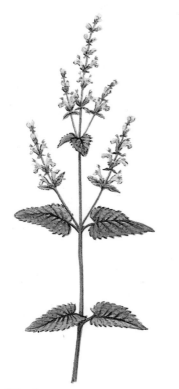

Sage (Wood) TEUCRIUM SCORODONIA

Modern uses: An infusion of the dried herb is taken in doses of 2 fl oz (56 ml) to improve appetite, to stimulate the menstrual flow and to produce sweating in feverish colds. In an infusion with Chickweed, it makes a good lotion for sore skin. The powdered herb is used in poultices for boils and ulcers.

HYPERICUM PERFORATUM

ST JOHN'S WORT

A tincture of the flowers in spirit of wine, is commended against the melancholy and madness.

A perennial plant growing to about two feet (61 cm) high with yellow flowers which yield a reddish juice like blood when bruised. Also called Perforate St John's Wort.

Where to find it: Shady woods and copses, meadows and by roadsides.

Flowering time: Midsummer.

Astrology: It is under the celestial sign of Leo and the dominion of the Sun.

Medicinal virtues: Aperient, detersive and diuretic. It is helpful against tertian and quartan agues, is alexipharmic and destroys worms. It is an excellent vulnerary plant. Outwardly it is of great service in bruises, contusions and wounds, especially in the nervous parts, if it be boiled in wine.

Made into an ointment, it dissolves swellings and closes up the lips of wounds. The decoction of the herb and flowers, but especially of the seeds, drunk in wine, with the juice of Knotgrass, helps all manner of vomiting and spitting of blood. It is also good for those who cannot make water, and are bitten or stung by venomous creatures. Two drams (3.5 g) of the seed made into powder and drank in broth, expels choler or congealed blood in the stomach. The seed taken in warm wine is recommended for sciatica, falling-sickness, and the palsy.

Modern uses: St John's Wort has an affinity for nerve endings and is used in all cases where there is nerve irritation, whether it be a tickly cough, referred pain, neuritis or neuralgia. It is expectorant, diuretic and sedative. In dry irritating coughs, it is combined with Colt's Foot and Marsh Mallow. It is usually added to all prescriptions where the condition is painful. For wounds and boils, the ointment, made by digesting the herb in white wax and straining, can be combined with ointment of Marsh Mallow. For skin diseases where there is inflammation, it is combined with Chickweed ointment. The infused oil made from the flowers is recommended as an application for external ulcers and wounds. Preparations are available from herbalists.

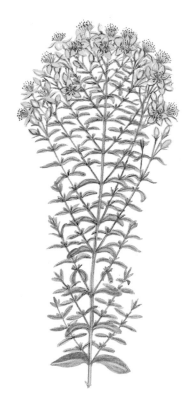

St John's Wort HYPERICUM PERFORATUM

SALSOLA KALI

SALTWORT

It opens stoppings of the liver and spleen, and wastes the hardness thereof.

An annual, growing with one upright, thick and almost transparent stalk, about a foot (30 cm) high. The stem produces swollen and fleshy leaves. The flowers are greenish-yellow, but insignificant.

Where to find it: On sandy shores at the coast.

Flowering time: Summer.

Astrology: Under the dominion of Mars.

Medicinal virtues: The powder or the juice, taken in drink, purges downwards and is effectual for the dropsy, to provoke urine, and to expel the dead child.

It must be used with discretion as a great quantity is hurtful and dangerous.

Modern uses: The juice has diuretic properties, but is rarely used in medicine. Its main use has been in the manufacture of soap and glass.

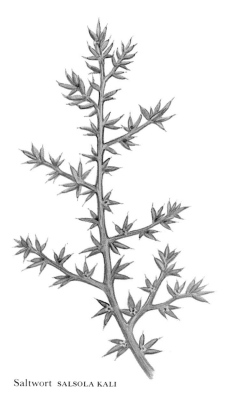

Saltwort SALSOLA KALI

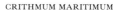

CRITHMUM MARITIMUM
SAMPHIRE (Rock or Small)
It is more agreeable as a pickle than useful as a medicine.

A succulent herb growing on rocks with thick, dull or blueish-green leaves and umbels of yellow flowers.

Where to find it: Fairly common at the coast where it grows on the cliffs, shingle and sandy shores.

Flowering time: Midsummer.

Astrology: A herb of Jupiter.

Medicinal virtues: It is well known that indigestion and obstructions are the cause of most of the diseases that the frail nature of man is subject to; both of which might be remedied by a more frequent use of this herb.

It is safe, pleasant to the taste and stomach. It provokes urine and helps to take away the gravel and stone engendered in the kidneys or bladder.

Modern uses: Not in general use as a medicine, but it is still pickled and eaten in seaside districts where it grows and where the people know its virtues. The leaves and stalks can be cooked and eaten like Asparagus.

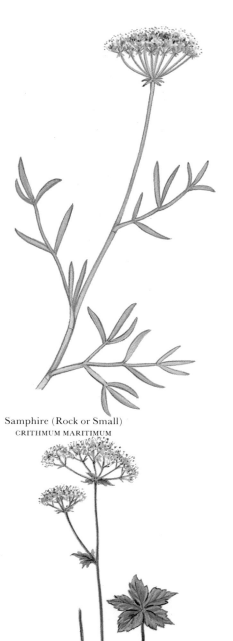

Samphire (Rock or Small)
CRITHMUM MARITIMUM

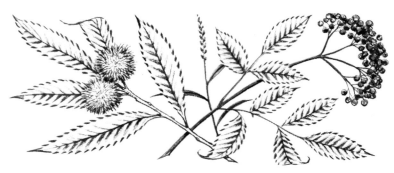

SANICULA EUROPAEA
SANICLE
It heals green wounds or any ulcers speedily.

A perennial growing two feet (61 cm) high, with finely dented leaves and pale pink or greenish-white flowers in umbels. The seeds are contained in round burs which cling to anything that comes into contact with them.

Where to find it: Woodland, thickets and shady moist places.

Flowering time: Early summer.

Astrology: Mars owns this herb.

Medicinal virtues: The decoction or powder taken in drink and the juice used outwardly dissipates evil humours. There is not found any other herb that can give such help when disease falls upon the lungs or throat.

Putrid malignant ulcers in the mouth, throat, and privities are healed by gargling with a decoction of the leaves and roots made into water, and a little honey put thereto.

It helps to stay women's courses, and all other fluxes of blood, from the mouth, in the urine or stool. It is healing to ulcerated kidneys, pains in the bowel, and gonorrhoea, or running of the reins, being boiled in wine or water and drunk.

Modern uses: An infusion of the whole herb in doses of 2 fl oz (56 ml) is useful in leucorrhoea and diarrhoea. It also stops internal haemorrhage. Used as a gargle, the infusion soothes sore throats; and used as a lotion, it heals septic wounds. As a blood purifier, it can be given in combination with other remedies, such as Red Clover.

Sanicle SANICULA EUROPAEA

SARSAPARILLA

Both leaves and berries, being drunk before or after taking any deadly poison, are an excellent antidote.

A perennial climber with prickly stems, large leaves, yellowish flowers and red or black berries.

Where to find it: There are several varieties, but the ones most used grow in the West Indies, America and India.

Flowering time: Late spring to late summer.

Astrology: Plant of Mars.

Medicinal virtues: If the juice of the berries be given to a new-born child, it shall never be hurt by poison. It is good against all venomous things. Twelve or sixteen berries, beaten to a powder, and given in wine, procure urine when it is stopped. The distilled water when drank has the same effect; and if the eyes be washed with it, they are thoroughly healed.

Sarsaparilla promotes sweating and is useful for catarrh. It expels wind from the stomach. It helps aches in the sinews or joints, running sores in the legs, phlegmatic swellings, tetters or ringworm, and spots on the skin. It has been found of service in venereal cases.

Infants infected by their nurses may be cured, even though they are covered with pustules and ulcers, by administering the powdered root with their food.

Modern uses: Sarsaparilla is used as a blood purifier and tonic, particularly in cases of rheumatism, gout and chronic skin disease. The variety from India has been used successfully against syphilis. The powdered root is taken in doses of 20 grains (1.3 g) or by infusion – 2 oz (56 g) to 1 pt (568 ml) of boiling water – the whole amount being taken in one day. The root of *Smilax officinalis* from tropical America contains the hormones testosterone, progesterone and cortin.

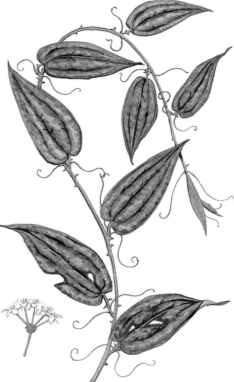

Sarsaparilla SMILAX

ALLIARIA PETIOLATA (= A. OFFICINALIS)

SAUCE-ALONE (Jack-by-the-Hedge or Common Garlic Cress)

The green leaves are held to be good to heal the ulcers in the legs.

A hedge plant also called Garlic Mustard with leaves resembling Nettles, although not prickly, and white flowers, which are followed by small pods containing blackish seeds.

Where to find it: By walls, hedges and paths.

Flowering time: Early to late summer.

Astrology: It is a herb of Mercury.

Medicinal virtues: It warms the stomach and helps digestion. The juice boiled with honey is good for a cough, to cut and expectorate tough phlegm. The seed bruised and boiled in wine is a good remedy for colicky wind or the stone, if drank warm. The leaves or the seed boiled and used in clysters eases the pain of the stone.

Modern uses: Not in general use, although commonly available. The juice of the leaves are diuretic and helpful in dropsy. The leaves are antiseptic and can be applied externally to leg ulcers. The plant is edible and has been eaten as a salad food. It has also been used in sauces, hence its common name. When bruised, the plant smells of Garlic.

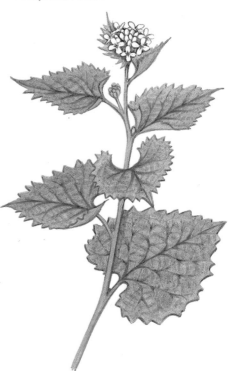

Sauce-alone (Jack-by-the-Hedge or Common Garlic Crests)
ALLIARIA PETIOLATA (=A. OFFICINALIS)

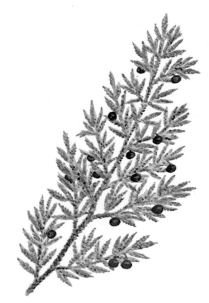

Savine JUNIPERUS SABINA

JUNIPERUS SABINA

SAVINE

It is a most powerful detersive, and has so violent an effect upon the uterine passages if used imprudently, that wicked women have employed it to very ill purposes.

This is a small evergreen shrubby tree, with branches set close together and clothed with narrow prickly leaves resembling Cypress. It produces small mossy green flowers succeeded by small, flattish, blackish-blue berries.

Where to find it: It is planted in gardens, but is indigenous to southern Europe and the northern states of the USA.

Flowering time: Summer.

Astrology: Under the dominion of Mars.

Medicinal virtues: It is a powerful provoker of the catamenia, causing abortion and expelling the birth. It is good to destroy worms in children, the juice being mixed with milk and sweetened with sugar. Beaten into a cataplasm with hog's lard, it cures children's scabby heads.

It is a fine opener of obstructions of any kind for jaundice, dropsy, scurvy and rheumatism. It deserves the regard of surgeons, as it is a very potent scourer and cleanser of old sordid stinking ulcers, either used in lotions, fomentations, ointments or the powder mixed with honey.

Modern uses: Savine is now considered to be unsafe for internal administration because its effects are unpredictable. It irritates the intestinal tract causing gastro-enteritis. It is definitely contra-indicated in pregnancy. It can be used externally in ointments to stimulate discharge from blisters, and to destroy warts.

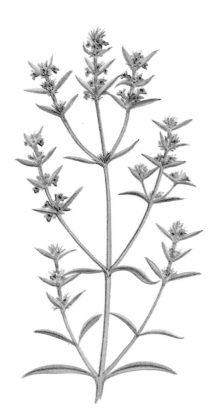

Savory (Summer) SATUREIA HORTENSIS

SATUREIA HORTENSIS

SAVORY (Summer)

It is much commended for pregnant women to take inwardly and to smell often unto.

Summer Savory is a hardy annual with small stringy roots and woody, hairy branches, eight or nine inches (20 or 23 cm) high. The flowers are white with a blush of pink or lilac.

Where to find it: It is grown in gardens, but often escapes and flourishes near gardens.

Flowering time: Early summer.

Astrology: Under Mercury.

Medicinal virtues: It expels tough phlegm from the chest and lungs, quickens the dull spirits in the lethargy, if the juice be snuffed up the nose. Dropped into the eyes it clears them of thin cold humours proceeding from the brain.

The juice heated with Oil of Roses, dropped into the ears, eases them of the noises in them and deafness. Outwardly applied as a poultice with Wheat flour, it eases the sciatica and palsied members. It eases the pain from stings of wasps and bees.

Modern uses: It is mainly used as a kitchen herb, but the dried tops are used as an expectorant and stomach medicine. Its aromatic properties make it a valuable addition to other medicines. It is indicated in the treatment of colic, flatulence, diarrhoea and frayed nerves. It also has a reputation as being aphrodisiac. The infusion of the dried tops – 1 oz (28 g) to 1 pt (568 ml) of boiling water – is given in doses of 2 fl oz (56 ml) three or four times a day.

SAVORY (Winter)

A good remedy for the colic and iliac passion.

This is a more woody, shrubby plant than Summer Savory, with leaves like Hyssop. The flowers are a pale pink or purple.

Where to find it: A cultivated herb, but sometimes found growing on old walls.

Flowering time: Midsummer to mid autumn.

Astrology: Under Mercury.

Medicinal virtues: Like Summer Savory it is carminative, and will expel wind from the stomach and bowels. It is also good for asthma and other affections of the chest. It opens obstructions of the womb and promotes menstrual evacuations.

Modern uses: Like Summer Savory it is mainly used as a culinary herb, particularly with beans. It is an intestinal antiseptic and has also been attributed with aphrodisiac qualities. An infusion is used to treat stomach pains and dyspepsia. It has similar properties to Summer Savory.

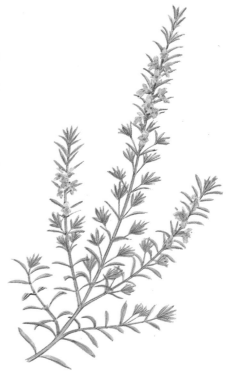

Savory (Winter) SATUREIA MONTANA

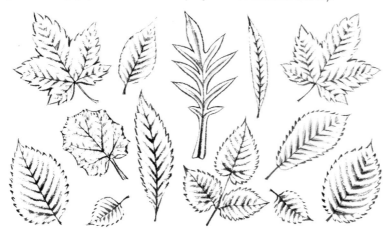

SAXIFRAGE (Great Burnet)

It has the properties of the Parsleys, but eases pains and provokes urine more effectually.

A perennial growing to about three feet (91 cm) with umbels of white flowers.

Where to find it: Edges of woods and hedgebanks.

Flowering time: Early summer.

Astrology: It is under the Moon.

Medicinal virtues: The root is good for the colic and expels wind. It is diuretic and useful against the stone, gravel and the scurvy. The roots or the seed are used in powder or in decoction to help the mother, procure the courses, remove phlegm and cure venom.

The juice of the herb dropped into bad wounds in the head, dries up their moisture and heals them.

Modern uses: The root is a powerful diuretic and useful to remove urinary tract stones. It is taken by decoction – 1 oz (28 g) of the root being boiled in 1½ pt (852 ml) of water until it measures 1 pt (568 ml) and taken in doses of 2 fl oz (56 ml).

The seeds are anti-flatulent and are powdered and given in water for colicky wind. Burnet Saxifrage, or Lesser Burnet, is more popular with herbalists.

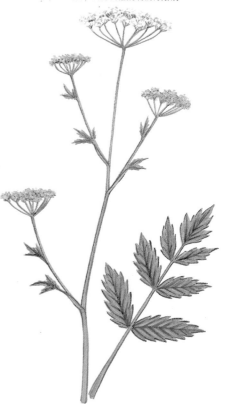

Saxifrage (Great Burnet) PIMPINELLA MAJOR

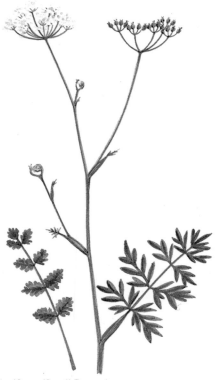

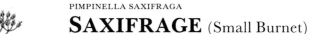

PIMPINELLA SAXIFRAGA

SAXIFRAGE (Small Burnet)

The root dried and powdered stops purgings.

This is a perennial, smaller and more slender than the previous variety, with reddish roots and stems, dented leaves and purple flowers in umbels.

Where to find it: Dry, grassy places, and in gardens. It likes a well-drained soil.

Flowering time: Early summer.

Astrology: It is under the dominion of the Moon.

Medicinal virtues: The whole plant is binding. The leaves put into wine give it a good flavour and the young shoots are eaten in salad. It is a promoter of sweat. A strong decoction of the root, or the juice of the leaves, is good to stop purgings.

Modern uses: It aids digestion and tones the stomach. An infusion of the leaves is generally used in combination with other stomach remedies like Meadowsweet and Centaury.

The fresh root is hot and peppery. It can be chewed to ease toothache. It is also useful to stop diarrhoea. A teaspoonful of the powdered root to a cup of boiling water, allowed to infuse and then drunk cold is good to cleanse the respiratory tract and stomach of mucus. It is diuretic and will expel stones from the bladder. The medicine can also be used as a gargle for sore throat and pharyngitis and applied to cuts and wounds to cleanse them and speed their healing.

Saxifrage (Small Burnet)
PIMPINELLA SAXIFRAGA

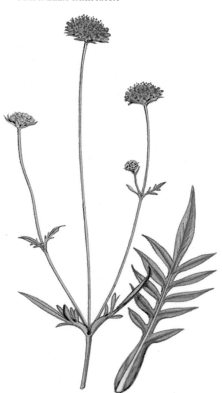

KNAUTIA ARVENSIS

SCABIOUS (Field)

It is effectual for all sorts of coughs, shortness of breath, and all other diseases of the chest and lungs.

The Field Scabious is a perennial growing three or four feet (0.9 to 1.2 m) high with soft, hairy whitish-green leaves and round heads of pale blue flowers.

Where to find it: Meadows, sunny banks and slopes, cornfields and hedgerows.

Flowering time: Early to late summer.

Astrology: A herb of Mercury.

Medicinal virtues: These are similar to the Lesser Field Scabious (*Scabiosa columbaria*), a description of which follows.

SCABIOSA COLUMBARIA

SCABIOUS (Lesser Field)

The herb bruised and applied, in a short time loosens and draws out any splinter, or broken bone lying in the flesh.

In appearance, it is similar to the Field Scabious, but smaller.

Where to find it: Dry pastures, cornfields.

Flowering time: Early to midsummer.

Astrology: Mercury owns this plant.

Scabious (Field) KNAUTIA ARVENSIS

Medicinal virtues: It ripens and digests cold phlegm, voiding it forth by coughing and spitting, and therefore is effectual for coughs and shortness of breath. It also ripens inward ulcers. If the decoction of the herb be taken in wine it is good for the pleurisy.

Four ounces (113 g) of the juice taken in the morning, fasting, with a dram (1.7 g) of mithridate, or Venice treacle, frees the heart from any infection of pestilence. After taking it, get a two hours' sweat in bed and repeat the medicine as often as necessary.

The fresh herb bruised and applied to any carbuncle or plague sore will dissolve and break it in three hours.

The decoction of the roots taken for forty days together, or a dram (1.7 g) of the powder of them taken in whey, helps those that are troubled with running or spreading ulcers, tetters or ringworms.

Drinking the juice or decoction helps scabs and breakings out of the itch. The juice made into an ointment is effectual for the same purpose. Made up with powder of Borax and Samphire, the juice cleanses the skin of freckles, pimples, morphew and leprosy. Washing the head with the decoction cleanses it from dandruff, scurf, sores and the itch.

Modern uses: Homoeopathic physicians make use of the Field Scabious for the treatment of chronic irritating skin diseases, such as eczema. The name of the plant 'scabious' is derived from the Latin *scabies*, which means itch. The plant is not popular with modern herbalists. For carbuncles, Slippery Elm and Marsh Mallow are preferred. For internal and external ulcers and pleurisy, Comfrey is used.

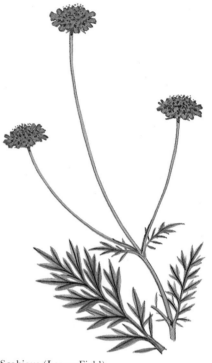

Scabious (Lesser Field)
SCABIOSA COLUMBARIA

CALYSTEGIA (= CONVOLVULUS) SEPIUM

SCAMMONY or GREAT WHITE BINDWEED

An extract made from the roots . . . hath a purgative quality.

This is a pernicious climbing, scrambling, perennial weed for the gardener. Its roots are larger than Couchgrass and spread underground to a great distance. The flowers are snowy white, some with a tint of purple or rose. Also known as Hedge Bindweed.

Where to find it: Hedges and banks.

Flowering time: Early summer to early autumn.

Astrology: Not assigned to any planet.

Medicinal virtues: This is the plant which produces Scammony, the gum resin used as a purgative. It does not grow as large in England as abroad. The juice of the root is hardened and is the Scammony of the shops. The best Scammony is black, resinous and shining when in the lump, but of a whitish ash-colour when powdered. It has a strong smell, but not a very hot taste, turning milky when touched by the tongue.

The smallness of the English root prevents the juice being collected as the foreign; but an extract made from the expressed juice of the roots has the same purgative quality, only to a lesser degree.

Modern uses: There are several Bindweeds, all of which have purgative properties. The Field Bindweed (*Convolvulus arvenis*) is not so active as *Calystegia sepium*. As a domestic medicine it is unreliable, since it is difficult to estimate dosage accurately and the resulting purging can be drastic. Scammony is the Syrian Bindweed (*Convolvulus scammonia*). It is from this and Jalap Bindweed that official purgatives have been prepared. Purgatives are not used by medical herbalists. The dose of the powdered root of Jalap Bindweed is 3–20 grains (0.2–2 g), and of the Syrian root 3–12 grains (195–780 mg). However, these are seldom used.

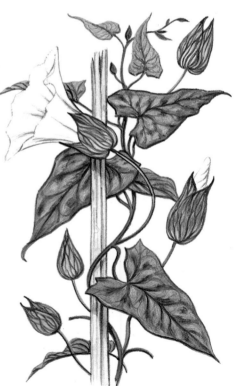

Scammony or Great White Bindweed
CALYSTEGIA (= CONVOLVULUS) SEPIUM

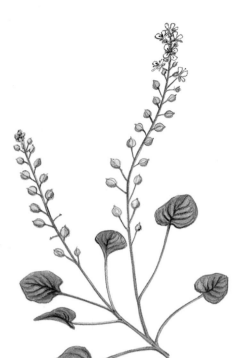

Scurvy-grass COCHLEARIA OFFICINALIS

COCHLEARIA OFFICINALIS

SCURVY-GRASS

The juice helps all foul ulcers and sores in the mouth when gargled therewith.

Also known as Spoonwort, it is a perennial with thick flat leaves and white or pink flowers. It grows between four and ten inches (10 and 25 cm) high.

Where to find it: Salt and brackish marshes and sea cliffs.

Flowering time: Late spring to late summer.

Astrology: A herb of Jupiter.

Medicinal virtues: A specific remedy against scurvy, purifying the juices of the body against that distemper. It clears the skin of scabs, pimples and foul eruptions. The juice is taken every morning, fasting. The decoction opens the liver and the spleen, bringing the body to a more livelier colour.

Modern uses: The plant contains vitamin C and the observation that it prevents scurvy was an accurate observation of the older herbalists. An infusion of the herb is taken in doses of 2 fl oz (56 ml). This is also used as a mouthwash.

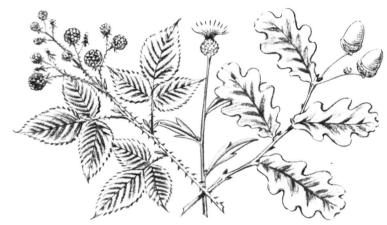

PRUNELLA VULGARIS

SELF-HEAL

A special remedy for inward and outward wounds.

This is a small, low, creeping herb, having many small roundish pointed leaves like Wild Mint, hairy stems and purplish-blue flowers.

Where to find it: Woodland and fields everywhere.

Flowering time: Early summer.

Astrology: Under Venus.

Medicinal virtues: It is taken in syrups for inward wounds and in unguents and plasters for outward wounds. It is like Bugle and answers the same purposes. It can be used with it or with Sanicle and other wound-herbs. It is good to wash wounds with it, or inject it into ulcers. Where sores, ulcers, inflammations or swellings need to be repressed, it will also be effectual. It stays the flux of blood from wounds and solders up their lips. It cleanses the foulness of sores and speedily heals them. It is a remedy for fresh wounds.

Anoint the temples and forehead with the juice and the Oil of Roses to remove headache. The same mixed with Honey of Roses, cleanses and heals ulcers in the mouth and throat and those in the secret parts.

Modern uses: Self-heal is a valuable astringent and styptic. An infusion of 1 oz (28 g) of herb in 1 pt (568 ml) of boiling water is taken in doses of 2 floz (56 ml) for internal bleeding. This is also useful for piles and leucorrhoea, taken internally or injected. As a gargle it eases a sore throat.

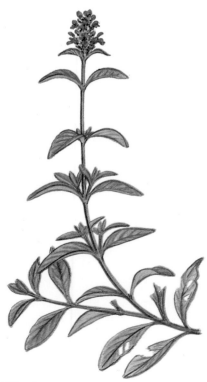

Self-heal PRUNELLA VULGARIS

SENNA (Red-flowered Bladder)

It cleanses and purifies the blood and causes a fresh and lively habit of the body.

A shrub with winged leaves, each being made up of six pairs of smaller leaves. The yellow flowers, produced in longish spikes at the tops of the branches, are moderately large and are striped with red.

Where to find it: It is a native of Eastern countries.

Flowering time: Summer.

Astrology: It is under Mercury.

Medicinal virtues: The leaves have a purging quality, but afterwards have a binding effect. It is corrected with Caraway seed, Aniseed, or Ginger and a dram (1.7 g) taken in wine, ale or broth, on an empty stomach comforts and cleanses the stomach and purges phlegm from the head and brain, lungs, heart, liver and spleen.

It strengthens the senses, procures mirth, and is good in chronic agues. The Common Bladder Senna (*Colutea arborescens*) works violently both upwards and downwards, offending the stomach and bowels.

Modern uses: In modern practice *Cassia angustifolia* is the variety of Senna used as a laxative. It is given with aromatic herbs, such as Ginger or Aniseed, to prevent griping pains. Both leaves and pods are used in over-the-counter pharmaceutical preparations. For domestic use, one teaspoonful of powdered Ginger is added to 2 oz (56 g) of Senna leaves in 1 pt (568 ml) of boiling water. Infuse for 20 minutes. The dose is 2 fl oz (56 ml).

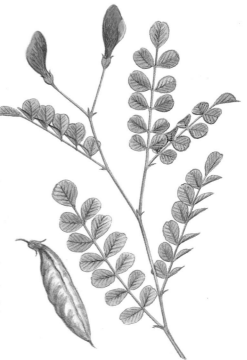

Senna (Red-flowered Bladder)
COLUTEA ORIENTALIS (= C. CRUENTA)

SHEPHERD'S PURSE

If bound to the wrists, or the soles of the feet, it helps the jaundice.

An annual growing to about 18 inches (46 cm) high. It has a small white root, pale-green, deeply cut leaves and very small white flowers. The seed cases are flat and triangular, almost in the shape of a heart.

Where to find it: A garden weed. Common on cultivated ground and found near paths.

Flowering time: All the year.

Astrology: It is under the dominion of Saturn.

Medicinal virtues: It helps all fluxes of blood, caused by inward or outward wounds. It is also used where there is flux of the belly and bloody flux, and spitting and voiding of blood. It will stop the terms in women. Made into a poultice, the herb helps inflammation and St Anthony's fire. The juice dropped into the ears, heals the pains, noise and matterings thereof. A good ointment may be made of it for all wounds, especially those of the head.

Modern uses: Shepherd's Purse is considered to be one of the best haemostyptic plants and, therefore, indicated for haemorrhages of all kinds both internal and external. Accurate diagnosis is, of course, important before administering this remedy internally.

It is given as an infusion, the whole dried herb being used in the ratio of 1 oz (28 g) to 1 pt (568 ml) of boiling water. The dose is 2 fl oz (56 ml). Its astringent properties make it useful to check diarrhoea. An ointment, made by digesting the herb in hot wax and straining, is useful for wounds and contusions. The herb is also diuretic and has been used with success for dropsy.

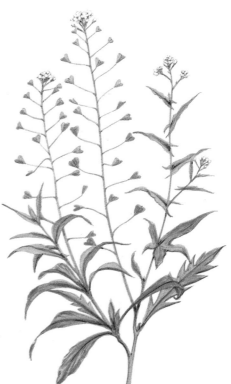

Shepherd's Purse CAPSELLA BURSA-PASTORIS

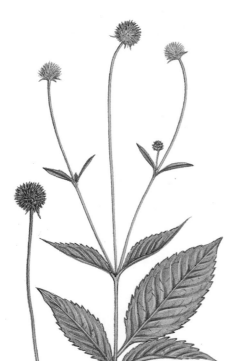

DIPSACUS PILOSUS
SHEPHERD'S ROD
Good against obstructions of the liver, and the jaundice.

A biennial, also known as Small Teasel. The lower leaves are large and rough, whereas the upper are attractive and deeply serrated. The flowers are a pale yellow and are followed by prickly heads of green and purple.

Where to find it: Damp woodland, ditches and hedgerows.

Flowering time: Late summer.

Astrology: It is a plant of Mars.

Medicinal virtues: The root is bitter and, given in strong infusion, it strengthens the stomach and creates an appetite. It is also a liver tonic.

Modern uses: It is not much used because it is not often found, growing only in scattered areas. The Common Teasel has similar virtues. See Teasel.

Shepherd's Rod DIPSACUS PILOSUS

POTENTILLA ANSERINA
SILVERWEED
This plant is of the nature of tansy and deserves to be universally known in medicine.

A perennial plant with a large stringy root, yellowish-green winged leaves divided into several deeply serrated segments opposite one another. The flowers are a beautiful shining yellow like large Buttercups and are on long slender stalks.

Where to find it: Common by roadsides, fields and dunes.

Flowering time: Late spring to late summer.

Astrology: Under Venus.

Medicinal virtues: The leaves are mildly astringent. Dried and given as a powder they cure agues and intermittent diseases. The usual dose is a tablespoonful every three or four hours. The roots are more astringent than the leaves, and are given in powder a scruple at a time, or more in obstinate purgings attended with bloody stools and immoderate menses. An infusion of the leaves stops the piles bleeding. Sweetened with a little honey, it is an excellent gargle for sore throats.

Modern uses: The plant is astringent, due to its tannin content. The infusion is taken internally and used as a lotion for piles. It is also anti-spasmodic and will relieve cramps in the stomach or abdomen. Looseness of the bowel is checked. Homoeopaths prescribe it for painful periods and inflammation of the stomach.

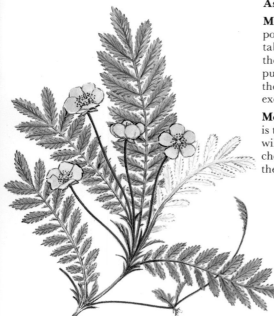

Silverweed POTENTILLA ANSERINA

SIMSON (Blue)

A remedy for disorders of the breast .

Also known as Blue Fleabane or Sweet Fleabane. The flowers are separate, one above another, on alternate sides of the stem. The leaves are a dull green and the flowers a purplish-blue and never spread wide open. It is a less attractive plant than the Common Fleabane, *Pulicaria dysenterica*.

Where to find it: Dry grassland, banks, dunes and walls.

Flowering time: Midsummer.

Astrology: Mars governs this plant.

Medicinal virtues: It is a sharp, acrid plant. Although a remedy for disorders of the chest arising from tough phlegm, it is one that should be cautiously tampered with.

Modern uses: Both this and Common Fleabane have fallen from use. The Canadian Fleabane is to be preferred, although that too is an unpleasant medicine. See Fleabane.

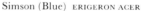

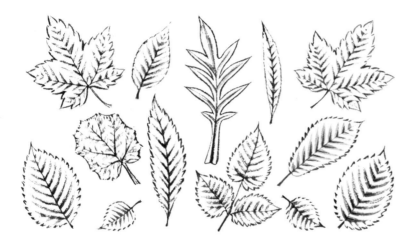

Simson (Blue) ERIGERON ACER

SIUM SISARUM

SKIRRET

The root . . . frees the bladder from slimy phlegm.

A root vegetable with a taste superior to Carrots. The roots are white inside and the flowers are white, too. The fruits are brown. It grows to about 18 inches (46 cm) and has serrated, sharp-pointed leaves.

Where to find it: A garden vegetable introduced into England from China in the reign of Henry VIII. Popular in Roman times. Rarely grown nowadays.

Flowering time: Early to midsummer.

Astrology: It is under Venus.

Medicinal virtues: The root is diuretic and cleansing, and useful for removing obstructions from the bladder. It is serviceable against dropsy by causing plenty of urine and helps liver disorders and the jaundice. The young shoots are a pleasant and wholesome food of easy digestion.

Modern uses: The root is not now used in herbal medicine, but when seeds are available they are sown in spring in fertile soil. The roots are ready in November and may be stored like other root vegetables. They are considered by some to be an excellent restorative for those suffering long illnesses and a useful item of diet in chest complaints.

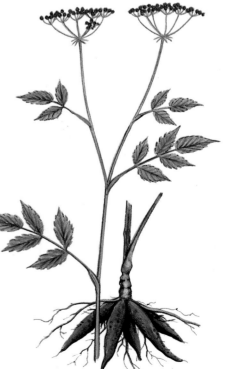

Skirret SIUM SISARUM

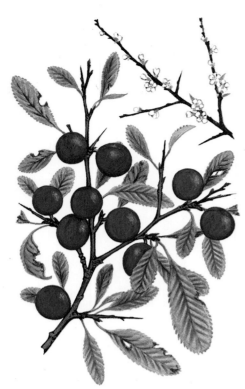

PRUNUS SPINOSA
SLOE BUSH

The juice expressed from the unripe fruit is a very good remedy for fluxes of the bowels.

This is a bush, also known as Blackthorn, whose tough branches are thorny and form a thick impenetrable barrier. Small white flowers appear before the leaves and these are followed by the fruit, which is the size of a small Damson.

Where to find it: Hedges and woodland.

Flowering time: Early spring.

Astrology: A saturnine plant.

Medicinal virtues: The fruit, or sloe, is chiefly used. It is astringent and binding and therefore good for all kinds of fluxes and haemorrhages. It is serviceable in washes for sore mouth and gums to fasten loose teeth.

A handful of the flowers infused makes an easy purge and excellent to di pel windy colic. The bark reduced to powder and taken in doses of two dr ims (3.5 g) has cured agues.

The juice may be reduced by gentle boiling to a solid consistence, in w ich state it will keep the year round. This is used for fluxes of the bowels.

Modern uses: *Prunus spinosa* provides the complete bowel medicine. The flowers are gently laxative and the fruits are binding. The fruits contain vitamin C and are used to make Sloe Gin. The flowers are also diuretic and an infusion – 1 oz (28 g) to 1 pt (568 ml) of boiling water – helps urinary tract disease such as cystitis and stones, and also rheumatism and gout. For diarrhoea, the fruits are picked just before they are ripe; they are dried and boiled for five to ten minutes and the liquid drunk. Take up to one cupful a day, regulating the dose as necessary.

Sloe Bush PRUNUS SPINOSA

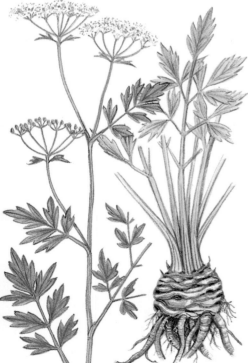

APIUM GRAVEOLENS
SMALLAGE

The leaves . . . eaten in the spring, sweeten and purify the blood, and help the scurvy.

A biennial, Smallage is also called Wild Celery. The roots are about a finger thick, wrinkled and grow deep in the earth. The stems are about three feet (91 cm) high with yellowish winged leaves, and it has umbels of small white flowers.

Where to find it: Marshes and damp land, especially near the sea.

Flowering time: Summer.

Astrology: It is under Mercury.

Medicinal virtues: The roots provoke the urine and are effectual where there is stoppage, or for removing stone and gravel. They also open obstructions of the liver and spleen, help dropsy and jaundice and remove female obstructions.

The leaves are of the same nature, and are eaten in the spring. The seeds are hot and carminative, and therefore good for the wind.

Modern uses: Although similar to Garden Celery, the wild variety has an unpleasant odour. The seeds and stems are mainly used to flavour other medicines, and as a tonic. It is normally prescribed as a fluid extract, the dose of which is three to seven drops every three or four hours. As a nerve tonic it is combined with Scullcap. For rheumatism and arthritis, combine with Damiana. The powdered seeds are used in doses of 20–60 grains (1.3 to 3.9 g) when the extract is not available.

Smallage APIUM GRAVEOLENS

ACHILLEA PTARMICA

SNEEZEWORT

The powder of the herb snuffed up the nose, causes sneezing, and cleanses the head of tough slimy humours.

A perennial also known as Bastard Pellitory. It has a long, slender fibrous root, woolly upright stems growing to about two feet (61 cm), and long narrow leaves finely serrated at the edges. The flowers are produced in a white umbel and are larger than the flowers of Yarrow.

Where to find it: Roadsides, damp meadows, marshes and by streams.

Flowering time: Midsummer.

Astrology: Not assigned to any planet.

Medicinal virtues: The root held in the mouth eases the toothache by evacuating the rheum. It can be used in salads.

Modern uses: Once a famous herbal medicine, Sneezewort was officially discarded by the medical profession 200 years ago. It is closely related to Yarrow (*Achillea millefolium*).

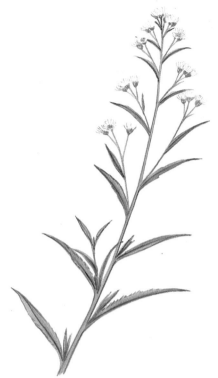

Sneezewort ACHILLEA PTARMICA

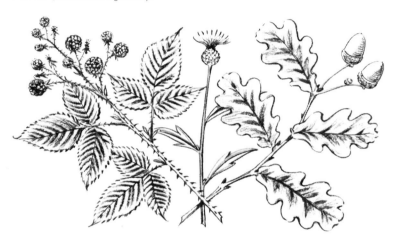

SAPONARIA OFFICINALIS

SOAPWORT

It cures gonorrhoea by taking the inspissated juice of it to the amount of half an ounce (14 g) a day.

A herbaceous perennial plant growing about two feet (61 cm) high with sharp-pointed leaves with large pale pink flowers.

Where to find it: Fairly common on roadsides, hedgerows, in watery places and near rivers.

Flowering time: Early summer.

Astrology: Venus owns this plant.

Medicinal virtues: The whole plant is bitter. Bruised and agitated with water, it raises a lather like soap, which washes greasy spots out of clothes. A decoction of it, applied externally, cures the itch.

Modern uses: Use cautiously because of its soapy taste and purgative properties. A decoction of the root is used as a wash to treat irritating skin conditions. Taken internally the expectorant properties help respiratory infections. The dose is 2–4 fl oz (56–114 ml) a day. This medicine is also useful in jaundice and for venereal disease.

Soapwort is not without side-effects including dry mouth, tremor and tongue paralysis, if allowed to macerate for too long. It is best to boil the root for a few minutes only and strain immediately.

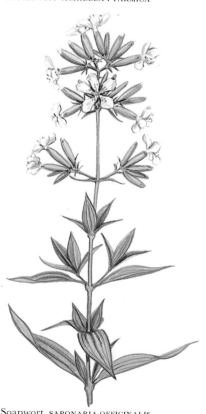

Soapwort SAPONARIA OFFICINALIS

SOLDIER (Common Water)

A specific against the king's-evil and scrofulous swellings.

An aquatic plant with a white fibrous root, long narrow leaves with small prickles along the edges, and large white flowers with a pretty tuft of yellow in the centre.

Where to find it: Ponds and ditches. The plant is normally submerged, but floats at the surface at flowering time.

Flowering time: Midsummer.

Astrology: A cold watery plant under the Moon in the celestial sign of Pisces.

Medicinal virtues: Used externally, it is cooling and repellant. It provokes the urine and is useful in hysteric disorders. A specific for scrofula.

Modern uses: A rare plant and therefore not much used in herbal medicine. However, where available, an ointment can be made by digesting the plant in wax and straining; it is good for wounds and inflammations.

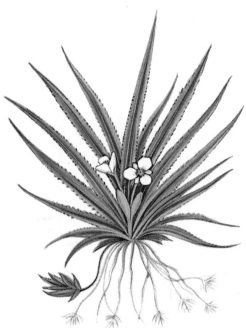

Soldier (Common Water)
STRATIOTES ALOIDES

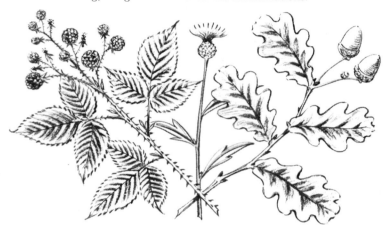

POLYGONATUM MULTIFLORUM

SOLOMON'S SEAL

It dispels congealed blood that comes of blows and bruises.

An attractive plant resembling Lily of the Valley. It grows to about 18 inches (46 cm) and bears white tubular flowers which droop from the stems in clusters.

Where to find it: A common garden plant, but found wild in woodland.

Flowering time: Late spring.

Astrology: Saturn owns this plant.

Medicinal virtues: The root heals wounds, sores and other injuries, if they are new, and restrains the flux of the old ones. It stays vomitings, bleedings and fluxes in man or woman. The roots bruised and applied fix joints that do not remain firm when set, and broken bones in any part of the body.

The decoction of the roots allowed to infuse overnight, strained and drank helps the broken bones of both men and beast. It also helps ruptures, if drank or applied outwardly to the place affected. The powdered root in broth does the same. It also takes away black and blue marks of bruises.

Modern uses: The root is a soothing, healing herbal medicine, with astringent and tonic properties. It is an excellent remedy for painful piles. A decoction of the root is made – 1 oz (28 g) to 1 pt (568 ml) of boiling water – and four or five tablespoonfuls injected into the rectum, several times a day. Taken internally it gives relief from neuralgia, and is useful for inflammation of the stomach and bowel and for diarrhoea. It is taken internally and used as a wash for erysipelas. The powdered roots are used in poultices for bruises.

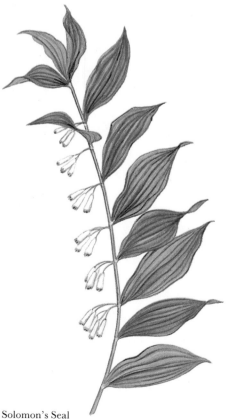

Solomon's Seal
POLYGONATUM MULTIFLORUM

SORREL (Common)

It quenches thirst and procures an appetite in fainting or decaying stomachs.

A perennial growing two or three feet (61 or 91 cm) high with smooth, succulent and tender leaves, a long slender stalk and a reddish spike of small flowers.

Where to find it: Roadsides, fields, meadows and woodland.

Flowering time: Late spring, early summer.

Astrology: Under Venus.

Medicinal virtues: It is useful to cool inflammations and the heat of the blood in pestilential or choleric agues, or sickness and fainting arising from the heart.

It resists putrefaction of the blood, kills worms and is a cordial to the heart. The seed is more effective because it is more drying and binding and thereby stays the fluxes of women's courses or flux of the stomach. The root in decoction or powder is effectual for all the foregoing purposes but also helps jaundice and expels gravel and stone from the reins and kidneys.

A decoction of the flowers helps black jaundice and inward ulcers in the body or bowel. A syrup made from the juice and Fumitory is a help to kill those sharp humours that cause the itch.

The juice with a little vinegar is used outwardly for the same and for tetters and ringworms.

Modern uses: The leaves are edible and may be added to salads to sharpen the taste. The plant contains oxalic acid which is contra-indicated in people with rheumatic complaints.

An infusion of the leaves – 1 oz (28 g) to 1 pt (568 ml) of boiling water – is used as a cooling drink in fevers. It is also laxative. A decoction of the root is prescribed for boils, eczema and acne. In making the decoction, the root is boiled for five to ten minutes and allowed to cool before being strained. It is taken internally – 2 fl oz (56 ml) three times a day – and used as a lotion.

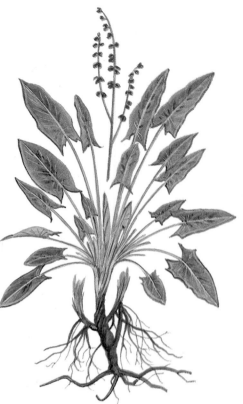

Sorrel (Common) RUMEX ACETOSA

OXYRIA DIGYNA (= O. RENIFORMIS)

SORREL (Mountain)

The leaves are as sour as the Common.

Mountain Sorrel is shorter and stouter than Common Sorrel, with blueish-green leaves and reddish-green flowers.

Where to find it: It grows in gardens, but is found wild in the mountainous regions of Europe, especially in damp rocky places and beside mountain streams.

Flowering time: Midsummer.

Astrology: Under Venus.

Medicinal virtues: May be used in place of Common Sorrel in both salads and as a medicine.

Modern uses: Not widely available and therefore only used by those familiar with it, mainly as a laxative. Its properties are similar to Common Sorrel.

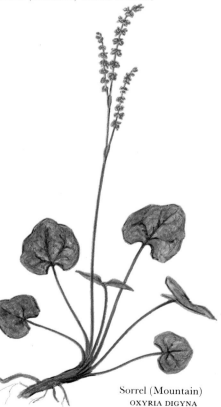

Sorrel (Mountain)
OXYRIA DIGYNA
(= O. RENIFORMIS)

SORREL (Sheep's)

Of great use against the scurvy if eaten in spring as salad.

An annual, also known as Field Sorrel, growing to about a foot (30 cm) high. It has narrow sharp-pointed leaves and spikes of green flowers turning to red.

Where to find it: Dry soils and pastures in most parts of the world.

Flowering time: Late spring.

Astrology: A plant of Venus.

Medicinal virtues: The leaves are cooling, allaying thirst and repressing bile. It is used as a cordial in fevers and to resist putrefaction. May be eaten in salad to prevent scurvy. The juice is frequently taken with other anti-scorbutic juices.

Modern uses: The leaves are used for their diuretic property. They may be eaten or given as an infusion – 1 oz (28 g) to 1 pt (568 ml) of boiling water – in doses of 2 fl oz (56 ml). Useful in fevers when it will also induce perspiration. The juice acts as a tonic to the kidneys and urinary tract, and is taken in doses of half to one teaspoonful.

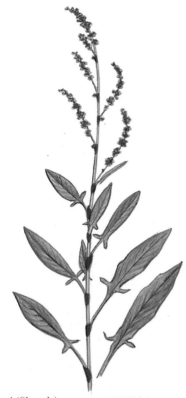

Sorrel (Sheep's) RUMEX ACETOSELLA

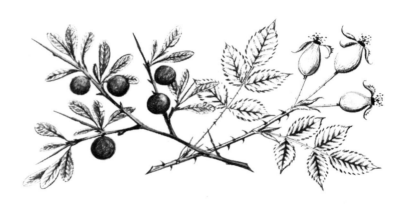

SORREL (Wood)

Excellent in any contagious sickness or pestilential fever.

A perennial, Wood Sorrel is a small plant with leaves in three parts, which often fold up. The flowers are bell-shaped and white with a dash of blue. Despite its name, the plant is not related to Sorrel, but is closely related to the Geranium family.

Where to find it: Moist and shady spots in woodland or beside hedges.

Flowering time: Mid to late spring.

Astrology: Under Venus.

Medicinal virtues: Similar to Sorrels, but is more effectual in hindering the putrefaction of the blood. It quenches the thirst, strengthens a weak stomach, stays vomiting and is excellent in fevers.

Modern uses: The plant is particularly rich in oxalic acid and potassium oxalate, which are not suitable for those with gouty or rheumatic tendencies. It can be injurious if prescribed injudiciously.

The leaves are used for their cooling action in fevers. The infusion – 1 oz (28 g) to 1 pt (568 ml) of boiling water – is also given for catarrh and urinary tract inflammation in doses of 2 fl oz (56 ml). Excessive or prolonged administration is not recommended. The infusion is used as lotion for skin infections. The juice is used as a gargle for mouth ulcers.

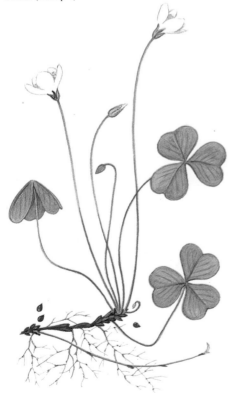

Sorrel (Wood) OXALIS ACETOSELLA

SOUTHERNWOOD

The seed bruised, heated in warm water, and drank, helps those that are troubled with cramps or convulsions of the sinews.

A perennial with woody stems, grey-green leaves and small yellow flowers. Also called Old Man's Tree, Boy's Love and Lad's Love.

Where to find it: A common garden plant, but a native of southern Europe.

Flowering time: Midsummer.

Astrology: A mercurial plant.

Medicinal virtues: The seed and dried herb kills worms in children. The herb bruised and applied draws out splinters and thorns from the flesh. The ashes mingled with salad oil, helps those that are bald, causing the hair to grow again on the head or beard.

A strong decoction of the leaves is a good worm medicine, but is disagreeable and nauseous. The leaves are a good ingredient in fomentations for easing pain, dispersing swellings, or stopping the progress of gangrenes.

Modern uses: The infusion of the dried herb – 1 oz (28 g) to 1 pt (568 ml) of boiling water – is taken in doses of 2 fl oz (56 ml) three times a day to promote menstruation. Combined with the infusion of Rosemary, it makes a good lotion, stimulating circulation in the scalp and encouraging the growth of healthy hair.

The powdered herb is given in teaspoonful doses in syrup twice a day to remove intestinal worms.

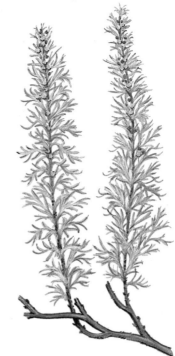

Southernwood ARTEMISIA ABROTANUM

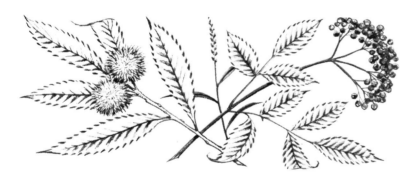

ARTEMISIA CAMPESTRIS

SOUTHERNWOOD (Field)

It is good in hysteric cases . . . and worthy of more esteem than it has.

A perennial, also known as Field Wormwood, it grows to about three feet (91 cm). The stalks are shrubby and branching. The leaves are grey-green and the small brown-yellow flowers appear in thick spikes at the top of the branches.

Where to find it: Heathland and by roadsides.

Flowering time: Midsummer.

Astrology: A mercurial plant.

Medicinal virtues: A powerful diuretic. The best way of using it is in a conserve made of the fresh tops, beaten up with twice their weight of sugar. Cut four ounces (113 g) of the leaves, beat them in a mortar with six ounces (170 g) of sugar till a paste is made. Take a piece of this about the size of a Nutmeg three times a day. It is a pleasant medicine and always disposes to sleep.

Modern uses: This plant has similar properties to Southernwood, but is not so strong in its action.

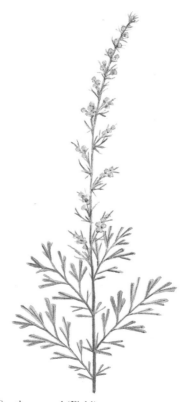

Southernwood (Field)
ARTEMISIA CAMPESTRIS

SOWBREAD

The juice is good against cutaneous eruptions.

This is a hardy Cyclamen, a perennial plant growing from a corm with reddish stems, dark-green leaves and pale purple or white flowers.

Where to find it: An alpine plant, occasionally found in hedgerows, but grown in gardens and as a pot plant.

Flowering time: Autumn.

Astrology: This is a martial plant.

Medicinal virtues: The root is very forcing, used to bring away the birth and the secundines. It also provokes the menses. The juice is commended against vertigo.

Modern uses: Cyclamen is used by homoeopathic physicians who make a tincture from the fresh corm. It is prescribed for uterine disease, rheumatism and migraine. The plant is not used by herbalists because it contains cyclamine, which is a drastic purgative. An ointment made from the corms and applied to the abdomen can cause vomiting; and applied over the bladder, it stimulates the flow of urine.

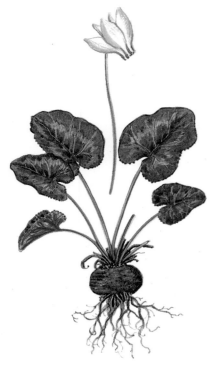

Sowbread CYCLAMEN HEDERIFOLIUM

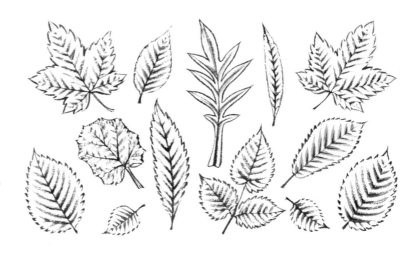

SOW-THISTLE (Common)

Good for the gravel and stoppage of urine.

A well-known perennial weed growing up to three feet (91 cm) high with a hollow stem and branches, full of milky juice. The numerous flowers are a pale lemon. Also known as the Smooth Sow-thistle.

Where to find it: A robust weed found in gardens and waste ground.

Flowering time: Summer.

Astrology: This is under Venus.

Medical virtues: It is cooling and good against obstructions. The young tops can be eaten in salad with oil and vinegar to ease the pain from scalding urine. The leaves act like Dandelion and are good for sediment in the bladder and retention of urine.

Modern uses: Seldom used, except as a food for rabbits. The young leaves may be eaten in salads. For inflammatory swellings, the leaves can be used in a poultice. Dandelion, which has similar properties, is more commonly used in modern practice.

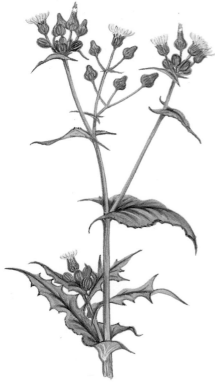

Sow-thistle (Common) SONCHUS OLERACEUS

SONCHUS ARVENSIS

SOW-THISTLE (Tree)

The milky juice is useful in deafness.

A perennial growing to three feet (91 cm) high with a tender, hollow stalk, yellowish-green leaves and large orange flowers. The leaves and stalk run with milk when crushed. Also called the Perennial Sow-thistle.

Where to find it: Cornfields, marshes, beside streams.

Flowering time: Late summer.

Astrology: It is under Venus.

Medicinal virtues: Its virtues lie chiefly in its milky juice, which is useful in deafness, either from accidental stoppage, gout or old age. Four spoonfuls of the juice of the leaves, two of salad oil and one of salt are shaken together and some cotton dipped into it and put into the ears. By doing this you may expect a good degree of recovery.

Modern uses: Little used, but like Common Sow-thistle the leaves may be used in poultices for application to inflammatory swellings, such as boils and other skin eruptions, and also as an application to haemorrhoids.

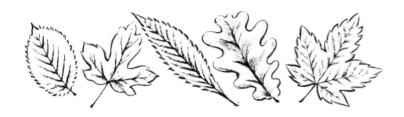

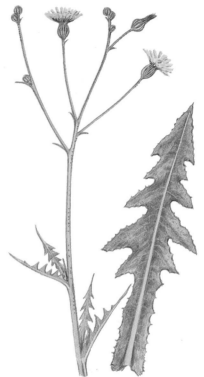

Sow-thistle (Tree) SONCHUS ARVENSIS

SONCHUS PALUSTRIS

SOW-THISTLE TREE (Marsh)

The milk taken from the stalks is beneficial for those who are short-winded.

This is a giant Thistle growing to about eight feet (2.4 m) high. The leaves are soft and tender and shaped like arrow-heads at their base. The numerous light yellow flowers stand in a broad clustering head. Also called the Marsh Sow-thistle.

Where to find it: Marshes, fens and beside streams.

Flowering time: Late summer.

Astrology: It is under Venus.

Medicinal virtues: The whole plant has an insipid taste. It is cooling and binding and eases pains. It will cool a hot stomach. The herb boiled in wine, and drank, stays the dissolution of the stomach. The milk taken from the stalks is beneficial to the short-winded.

A decoction of the leaves and stalks causes an abundance of milk in nursing mothers and their children to be well-coloured. The juice or distilled water is good for hot inflammations, wheals, eruptions, heat of the skin or itching haemorrhoids.

The juice boiled in a little oil of bitter almonds in the peel of a Pomegranate and dropped into the ears is a sure remedy for deafness or singing in the ears.

Modern uses: This plant is now very rare and thus little used in medicine. An infusion of Nettles helps milk production in nursing mothers. Pilewort or Comfrey are effective for haemorrhoids. No remedies should be introduced into the ears without adequate diagnosis.

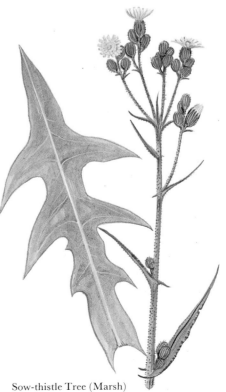

Sow-thistle Tree (Marsh)
SONCHUS PALUSTRIS

MEUM ATHAMANTICUM

SPIGNEL (Broad-leaved)

An excellent plant in disorders of the stomach . . .

A perennial aromatic herb, Spignel grows about a foot (30 cm) high with a few small leaves and umbels of white flowers. It is also known as Baldmony.

Where to find it: Grassy, mountain areas in rich, damp soil.

Flowering time: Early to midsummer.

Astrology: Under the dominion of Mercury in Cancer.

Medicinal virtues: Excellent for want of appetite and digestion, belchings, eructations, colic, gripes, urine retention and wind and pain in the stomach. The powdered root, given with loaf sugar, and the infusion taken in water, white wine or beer, evening and morning for several days, also brings down the menses and lochia and facilitates the expulsion of birth and afterbirth.

Modern uses: This has never been a common wild herb and is, therefore, little used, except as a vegetable by mountain folk. The root is comparable to Angelica or Lovage. The plant is a member of the Parsnip family. It can be cultivated in rock gardens or on banks. Herbalists tend to use remedies such as Fennel, Aniseed or Angelica for flatulence and other simple digestive problems.

Spignel (Broad-leaved)
MEUM ATHAMANTICUM

ARALIA RACEMOSA

SPIKENARD

It helps loathings, swellings or gnawings in the stomach.

Grows from three to six feet (0.9 to 1.8 m) high, with large leaves and small greenish flowers produced in clusters.

Where to find it: It is a native of India, but is also common in North America, Japan and New Zealand.

Flowering time: Mid to late summer.

Astrology: Not assigned to any planet.

Medicinal virtues: The powdered root is used. It is good to provoke urine and ease pains caused by stone in the reins and kidneys. The powder is drunk in cold water.

It helps the jaundice and those who are liver-grown. It makes a good ingredient in mithridate and other antidotes against poison.

Pregnant women are forbidden to take it inwardly. The oil is good to warm cold places and to digest crude and raw humours. It works powerfully on old cold griefs of the head and brain, stomach, liver, spleen, reins and bladder.

It purges the brain of rheum, being snuffed up the nostrils. It comforts the brains and helps cold pains in the head and the shaking palsy. Two or three spoonfuls help passions of the heart, swoonings and the colic.

Modern uses: The root is dried and powdered for use. The plant also contains an oil and a resin. It is used in much the same way as Sarsaparilla, previously described. An infusion is taken as a blood purifier in syphilitic, rheumatic and skin diseases. It is often combined in equal parts with Dandelion, Burdock and Yellow Dock. In making the infusion, use only ½ oz (14 g) of powder to 1 pt (568 ml) of boiling water.

A useful remedy for pectoral complaints, it can be made into a syrup and flavoured with Peppermint. It is particularly recommended for coughs and colds. Herbalists use a specially prepared fluid extract, of which the dose is 30–60 drops.

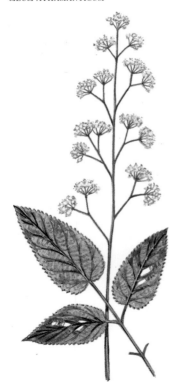

Spikenard ARALIA RACEMOSA

SPINACIA OLERACEA

SPINACH

Useful to temper the heat and sharpness of the humours.

The well-known vegetable, with broad sharp-pointed leaves and spikes of tiny green flowers.

Where to find it: Mainly grown in gardens in all temperate regions, but may be found wild near to places where it has been cultivated.

Flowering time: Late spring to early autumn.

Astrology: Not assigned to any planet.

Medicinal virtues: It is more used as food than for medicine and is much eaten as boiled salad. It cools and moistens and promotes the urine flow.

Modern uses: Still mainly used for food. The leaves are rich in minerals, particularly iron and calcium, and are recommended for anaemic persons. It also supplies vitamin A, C and K and folic acid. It is best grown organically, as chemical fertilisers tend to lower the vitamin content. A food for convalescence and for growing children.

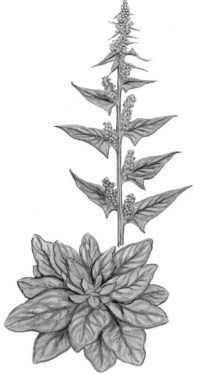

Spinach SPINACIA OLERACEA

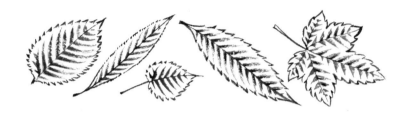

URGINEA (= SCILLA) MARITIMA

SQUILL

Taken internally in doses of a few grains, it promotes the expectoration and the urine.

A perennial plant with an Onion-like bulb, full of thick juice. It grows two or three feet (61 or 91 cm) high with bright green, pointed leaves some two feet (61 cm) long. The small white flowers are produced in longish spikes. Also called Sea Onion.

Where to find it: It prefers dry, sandy sites and flourishes on the Italian and Spanish coasts and other parts of the Mediterranean; but it can be cultivated in gardens.

Flowering time: Midsummer.

Astrology: A hot, biting martial plant.

Medicinal virtues: The root is bitter to the taste and so acrid that it will blister the skin if it is handled too much. In large doses it causes vomiting and sometimes purging.

It is a certain diuretic in dropsical cases and an expectorant in asthmatical ones, especially where the lungs or stomach are oppressed by tough viscid phlegm, or injured by the imprudent use of opiates.

Being disagreeable in taste, it is given in pill form, made from the powdered root beaten into a mass, with the addition of syrup or mucilage of gum arabic.

Modern uses: Still a valuable remedy for coughs and catarrh. A small amount is added to many over-the-counter lung mixtures. It is soothing to mucous membranes and cheeks excessive mucous secretion. It is also expectorant and diuretic. There are several official BPC preparations containing it. It is dangerous in overdosage and therefore not recommended for domestic use. In the form of a pill, the dosage of Squill is only one to three grains (65–200 mg).

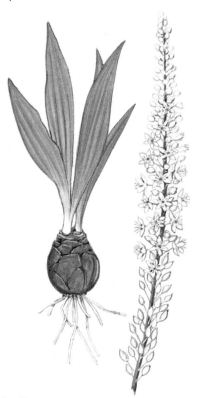

Squill URGINEA (= SCILLA) MARITIMA

STAVES-ACRE

The powder is used to kill lice.

This is closely related to the Larkspur and grows about four feet (1.2 m) high. The lower leaves are large and round but divided into sharp-pointed segments. The blue flowers are produced in a spike at the top of the stem and are followed by seed pods. Also called Housewort.

Where to find it: Is cultivated in gardens, but comes originally from warmer climes, such as Greece and Italy.

Flowering time: Midsummer.

Astrology: Not assigned to any planet.

Medicinal virtues: Only the seed is used. It is seldom taken inwardly, being of a hot burning taste. Sometimes it is used in masticatories and gargarisms for the toothache.

The seed is given in small doses against rheumatic and venereal disorders, but they cause vomiting and purging and it is better to omit their use internally. Chewed in the mouth, they largely expel watery humours from adjacent parts and are of service in disorders of the head.

Modern uses: The seeds are poisonous and should not be administered internally. They are used to make lotions and ointments for killing head lice and other parasites. Homoeopathic physicians prescribe pills made from the plant for impotency. These are prepared pharmaceutically and are safe to take. All Larkspurs are poisonous and ingestion of the seeds can cause paralysis of the nervous system.

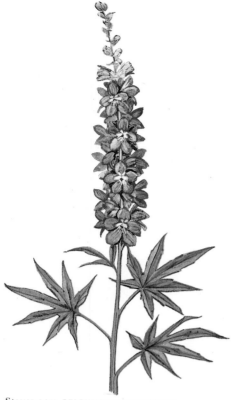

Staves-acre DELPHINIUM STAPHISAGRIA

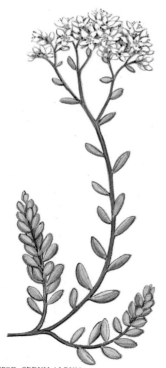

Stonecrop SEDUM ALBUM

SEDUM ALBUM

STONECROP

It stops bleeding, both inwardly and outwardly.

A perennial, also known as the Small Houseleek and White Stonecrop. It grows with trailing branches with flat whitish-green leaves and white star-like flowers.

Where to find it: Rocks and walls and roofs of houses.

Flowering time: Early to midsummer.

Astrology: It is under the dominion of the Moon.

Medicinal virtues: Very good to stay defluxions. It helps cankers and fretting sores and ulcers. It resists pestilential fevers and is good for tertian agues. Bruised and applied outwardly, it helps the king's-evil and other knots or kernels in the flesh and also the piles. But it should be used with caution when given internally. The juice causes vomiting. Under proper management, it is an excellent medicine in scorbutic cases.

Modern uses: An uncommon herb found only in scattered areas and therefore it has not gained a place in modern herbal medicine. Those that are familiar with its virtues have used it as a food by pickling it, but it is not recommended for domestic use because of its emetic properties and there is some possibility of confusion with another Stonecrop, *Sedum acre*, which has been used as an abortefacient. See Houseleek (Wall Pepper).

STORAX TREE

It heals, mollifies and digests.

This tree grows like the Quince tree in size and shape. The leaves are long and round, white underneath and stiff. The white flowers are followed by berries. The bark contains a gum. There are other similar varieties.

Where to find it: It prefers hotter climates such as in Cyprus and Syria. It will grow elsewhere, but is unlikely to produce any gum.

Flowering time: Spring. The berries appear in early autumn.

Astrology: This is a solar plant.

Medicinal virtues: Only the gum is used. It is good for coughs, catarrhs, distillations of rheum and hoarseness. It resists cold poisons.

Modern uses: A stimulating expectorant, Storax is a balsam obtained by slitting the bark of the tree. It acts in a similar way to other balsams and is mainly used for asthma, bronchitis and catarrh. It is an ingredient of Friar's Balsam. Ointments containing Storax are used for the treatment of scabies and ringworm. It is seldom available except as an ingredient of pharmaceutical preparations.

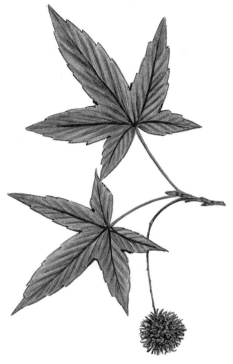

Storax Tree STYRAX OFFICINALIS

STRAWBERRIES

The juice or water is singularly good for hot or inflamed eyes, if dropped into them, or bathed therewith.

Strawberries are the well-known fruits produced by cultivated and wild low-growing perennial creeping plants.

Where to find it: Outside of gardens, they are found in woods and shady places, hedgerows and roadsides.

Flowering time: Late spring to midsummer.

Astrology: Venus owns the herb.

Medicinal virtues: The berries cool the liver, blood and spleen, or a hot choleric stomach. They refresh and comfort fainting spirits and quench the thirst. They are good for inflammations, but it is best to refrain from them in a fever, lest they putrefy in the stomach and increase the fits.

The roots and leaves boiled in wine and water, and drank, cool the liver and blood and assuage inflammation in the reins and bladder, provoke urine and allay heat and sharpness. This drink also stays the bloody flux and women's courses and helps the swelling of the spleen.

The water of the berries, distilled, is a remedy and cordial in the panting and beating of the heart, and good for the jaundice. The juice can be dropped into foul ulcers or used as a wash, or the decoction of the herb and root, cleanses and helps to cure them.

Lotions and gargles for sore mouths, or ulcers in the mouth, or privy parts are made with the leaves and roots.

Modern uses: The leaves are astringent and may be used in the form of an infusion – 1 oz (28 g) to 1 pt (568 ml) of boiling water – to check simple diarrhoea. This infusion is also diuretic and is useful in the treatment of urinary tract inflammation. A decoction of the roots has similar properties. An ounce (28 g) of root is boiled for about ten minutes in a pint of water and strained. This also makes a useful gargle for a sore throat and a vaginal douche to check simple discharges.

The fruits are rich in vitamin C and iron and make a pleasant supplement for the anaemic.

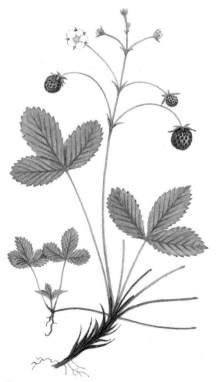

Strawberries FRAGARIA VESCA

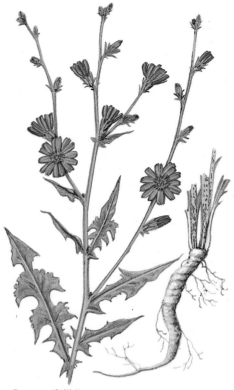

Succory (Wild) CICHORIUM INTYBUS

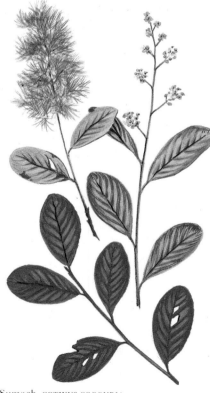

Sumach COTINUS COGGYRIA
(= RHUS COTINUS)

CICHORIUM INTYBUS

SUCCORY (Wild)

Effectual for sore eyes that are inflamed, or for nurses' breasts that are pained by the abundance of milk.

A perennial, also known as Chicory, of which there are garden varieties. It is a member of the Dandelion family and has leaves which are much indented. The flowers are sky blue and are produced in groups of two or three.

Where to find it: A common plant on waste ground and roadsides.

Flowering time: Midsummer to early autumn.

Astrology: It is under Jupiter.

Medicinal virtues: A handful of the leaves or roots, boiled in wine or water, and drank, drives forth choleric and phlegmatic humours, opens obstructions of the liver, gall and spleen, helps the jaundice, the heat of the reins and of the urine.

A decoction made of the wine, and drank, is effectual against lingering agues. A dram (1.7 g) of the seed, powdered, and drank in wine before the fit of the ague, helps to drive it away.

The distilled water of the herb and flowers has similar properties and is good for hot stomachs and in pestilential agues. It is also good for swooning and passions of the heart, for heat and headache in children, and for the blood and liver.

The juice, or the bruised leaves applied outwardly, allays swellings, inflammations, St Anthony's fire, wheals and pimples, especially if used with a little vinegar.

Modern uses: The swollen roots of the plant, which contain Chicory, are dried and ground and added to coffee. The root is laxative and diuretic. One ounce (28 g) is boiled in one pint (568 ml) of boiling water and taken as required. It is an effective remedy for liver complaints, especially jaundice, and for rheumatic conditions. Like Dandelion root, it stimulates the flow of bile. This helps digestion.

The young leaves can be eaten, although the Chicory most used as a salad vegetable is actually Garden Endive.

COTINUS COGGYRIA (= RHUS COTINUS)

SUMACH

The seeds dried, and reduced to a powder and taken in small doses, stop purgings and haemorrhages.

A hardy shrub with winged leaves growing in pairs and small purple flowers produced on long, thick, woolly spikes.

Where to find it: A native of warm climates, particularly of southern Europe, but grows well in colder areas where it has been introduced.

Flowering time: Summer.

Astrology: It is under the dominion of Jupiter.

Medicinal virtues: The young shoots taken by infusion strengthen the stomach and bowels. The bark of the roots and the powdered seeds stop purgings and haemorrhages.

Modern uses: The sweet Sumach (*Rhus aromatica*), from Canada and the United States, is now more popular with herbalists. This is an ornamental shrub growing to four feet (1.2 m) high. The bark of the root is used for its astringent and diuretic properties. It is indicated in diabetes and where there is an excessive output of urine. For incontinence in the aged and enuresis in children, the infusion of 1 oz (28 g) of root-bark to 1 pt (568 ml) of boiling water is taken in doses of 1–2 fl oz (28–56 ml). It will also check diarrhoea, vaginal discharge and dysentery.

Smooth Sumach (*Rhus glabra*) is also used. The bark is astringent and antiseptic, and the berries are diuretic. The bark is indicated for chronic diarrhoea and rectal bleeding. An infusion of the leaves or berries is helpful where there is bladder inflammation. For diabetes the infusion is combined in equal parts with leaves of Blueberry (*Vaccinium myrtillus*). For diarrhoea, combine with Blackberry root.

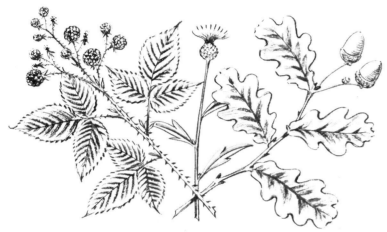

DROSERA ANGLICA

SUNDEW

Some authors tell us that a water distilled from this plant is highly cordial and restorative; but it is more than probable that it never deserved the character given of it in that respect.

A perennial, now known as Great Sundew, which catches and digests insects. It grows to about ten inches (25 cm) high with club-shaped, hollow leaves, full of red hairs. The leaves stay moist on the hottest day. The stalks bear small whitish buds which are the flowers and which afterwards contain the seeds.

Where to find it: In bogs and wet places in woods.

Flowering time: Early summer.

Astrology: The Sun rules it, and it is under the sign of Cancer.

Medicinal virtues: The leaves, bruised and applied to the skin, will erode it and bring out inflammations not easily removed. The juice destroys warts and corns if a little be frequently applied to them.

Modern uses: This is a fairly rare plant, except for some parts of Scotland and Ireland. Herbalists, therefore, use the Common or Round-leaved Sundew (*Drosera rotundifolia*). This is quite commonly found in Europe, the United States, South America and China, in bogs, wet moors and heathland, but is expensive to buy.

• The plant contains a natural antibiotic and is regarded as a specific for whooping cough, but also useful for chronic bronchitis, asthma and laryngitis. Drosera controls the spasms of whooping cough and can be administered as a prophylactic when an epidemic is threatened. Best results are obtained by using a fluid extract or tincture prepared by a herbalist. Five to ten drops are taken in water three or four times a day. Homoeopathic pills in various strengths are also available and have similar indications.

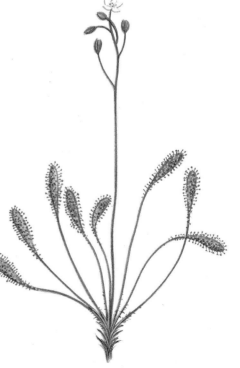

Sundew DROSERA ANGLICA

SUN SPURGE

It provokes lust and heals numbness and stiffness of the privities proceeding from cold, by anointing.

Sun Spurge belongs to a group of poisonous plants, some of which have been used medicinally, and are known as spurges. This plant has finely toothed, oval leaves and the root has many fibres. It produces small yellowish-green flowers.

Where to find it: A native of Africa, but it grows in meadows elsewhere.

Flowering time: Early summer to early autumn.

Astrology: It is under Mars.

Medicinal virtues: A plaster made of one part Sun Spurge to 12 parts oil, plus a little wax, heals all aches of the joints, lameness, palsies, cramps and shrinking of the sinews. Mixed with Oil of Bay and bear's grease, it cures scurvy and scalds in the head and restores lost hair. Applied with oil to the temples, it heals the lethargy, and by putting it to the nape of the neck, prevents the apoplexy. Mixed with vinegar it removes all blemishes in the skin, or with other ointments, heals the parts that are cold, and heals the sciatica.

Taken inwardly, it frets the entrails, and scorches the whole body. For that reason it must be beaten small and tempered with something that lubricates and allays its heat, and then it purges water and phlegm.

Pills of Sun Spurge help dropsy, pains in the loins and guts, but should only be given in desperate cases, as it operates violently. The oil of the plant snuffed up the nose purges the head of phlegm and is good in old and cold pains of the joints, liver and spleen.

Modern uses: Owing to the poisonous nature of the Spurge family, they are not used in modern practice. Most of them taken internally are purgative or emetic.

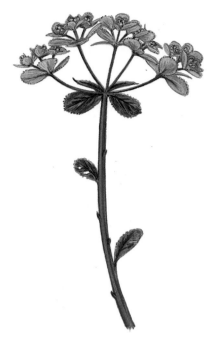

Sun Spurge EUPHORBIA HELIOSCOPIA

SWALLOW-WORT

Its root is a counter-poison, both against the bad effects of poisonous herbs, and the bites and stings of venomous creatures.

An herbaceous plant with stringy roots, tough stems about two feet (61 cm) high and bunches of star-shaped flowers, white or a dull red in colour. The seeds are in pods containing a silky down.

Where to find it: A cultivated plant for the herbaceous border, but found wild in Syria, although it is a native of the United States and Canada where it is a common roadside weed.

Flowering time: Early summer.

Astrology: Jupiter owns this plant.

Medicinal virtues: The root is the only part used. It is helpful against malignant pestilential fevers, which it carries off by sweat. It is also good against the dropsy and jaundice.

Modern uses: The root has analgesic properties and is powdered and administered by infusion for asthma and fevers accompanied by much mucus. It helps expectoration, giving relief from coughing and reduces pain. The juice is applied to warts. The young shoots of the plant can be eaten like Asparagus.

The name Swallow-wort is also applied to *Asclepius tuberosa*, which has similar properties, but is generally known to herbalists as Pleurisy Root because of its specific action on the lungs. It is also a native of the United

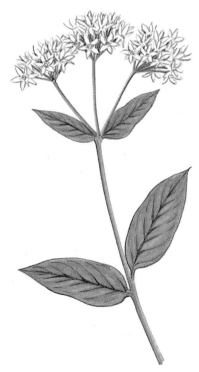

Swallow-wort ASCLEPIAS SYRIACA

States and Canada. The root is powdered and 1 oz (28 g) is infused in 1½ pt (1.1 l) of boiling water and given in doses of 2 fl oz (56 ml) three or four times a day. It reduces the pain in pleurisy and helps breathing. Overdoses cause vomiting and purging.

The fluid extract is best combined in equal parts with composition essence, available from herbalists, and taken in teaspoonful doses in warm water sweetened with honey.

ACER PSEUDOPLATANUS

SYCAMORE TREE

The fruit makes the belly soluble, but troubles it and gives little nourishment.

Also known as the Great Maple and, in Scotland, the Plane Tree. It is a hardy, fast-growing tree reaching a height of 50 feet (15 m) or more in 50 years. The leaves are five-lobed – pointed at the ends and indented at the edges. It bears characteristic winged fruit following the appearance of the hanging racemes of flowers. The whole tree is full of juice.

Where to find it: It grows wild in Europe, but is often planted near farmhouses for the protection it gives from winds. It is found in woods, hedges and gardens and at the roadside.

Flowering time: Mid spring to early summer.

Astrology: It is under the particular influence of Venus.

Medicinal virtues: The juice, or milk, is taken from the tree by piercing the bark, and dried. It is then made into troches and applied to tumours which it softens and dissolves. It also solders together the lips of fresh wounds. The fruit can be applied as a plaster to achieve the same effect.

Modern uses: The juice has been used to make wine. Sugar is also obtainable from the sap by distillation. It is not used in medicine at the present time, but several related trees of the Maple family are of value. See Maple Tree.

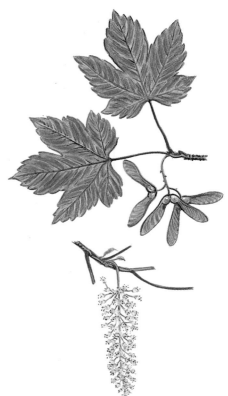

Sycamore Tree ACER PSEUDOPLATANUS

TANACETUM VULGARE

TANSY

The distilled water cleanses the skin of all discolourings, as morphew, sunburns, pimples and freckles.

A perennial related to the Dandelion, growing to about three feet (91 cm) high with large, bright yellow flowers. The leaves are winged.

Where to find it: Most frequently found on high ground, in dry pastures and in hedgerows.

Flowering time: Mid to late summer.

Astrology: This is under Venus.

Medicinal virtues: It is an agreeable bitter, a carminative and a destroyer of worms. The powder of the flowers is taken night and morning in doses of six to twelve grains (390–780 mg). The leaves are astringent and vulnerary and will stop all kinds of fluxes. The powdered herb is taken in distilled water for the whites in women. Boiled in water and drank it eases the griping pains of the bowels and is good for the sciatica and aching joints. The same boiled in vinegar, with honey and Alum, and gargled, eases toothache and helps sore gums.

Modern uses: It is used for expelling worms in children. An infusion of the dried herb – 1 oz (28 g) to 1 pt (568 ml) of boiling water – is taken night and morning on an empty stomach, in teacupful doses. It promotes menstruation and, for this, the infusion is given in doses of 2 fl oz (56 ml), three times a day before food. It is not recommended in pregnancy. The dried flowers and seeds are a useful remedy for gout. Infuse half a teaspoonful in hot water for each dose.

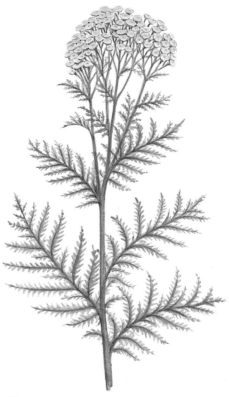

Tansy TANACETUM VULGARE

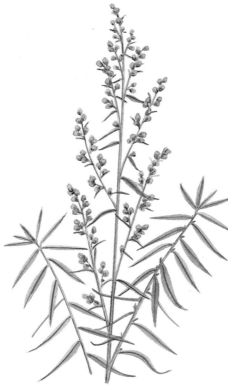

ARTEMISIA DRACUNCULUS

TARRAGON

An infusion of the young tops increases the urinary discharge.

A shrubby plant with woody stems growing about three feet (91 cm) high and clothed with narrow green leaves two inches (5 cm) long. The greenish flowers are small and inconspicuous.

Where to find it: Tarragon is cultivated in the herb garden. It was originally from Siberia and north-west America.

Flowering time: Mid to late summer.

Astrology: A martial plant.

Medicinal virtues: The leaves are drying and good for those with the flux or any discharge. An infusion of the young tops gently promotes the menses.

Modern uses: The plant is still mainly grown for its leaves, which are used in salads and for seasoning and in the manufacture of Tarragon vinegar. It stimulates the appetite and digestive processes. To make Tarragon vinegar, the fresh leaves are simply infused in white vinegar for several hours and strained for use.

An infusion of the leaves – 1 oz (28 g) to 1 pt (568 ml) of boiling water – eases intestinal distention and flatulence. Take in doses of 2 fl oz (56 ml).

Tarragon ARTEMISIA DRACUNCULUS

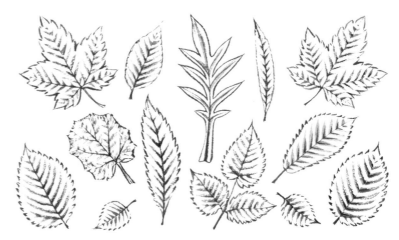

CAMELLIA THEA

TEA

Strong tea is prejudicial to those with weak nerves.

An evergreen shrub growing about eight feet (2.4 m) high with oblong leaves and white flowers like that of the Dog Rose. It produces a berry.

Where to find it: Tea is cultivated in China, Japan, Ceylon and India.

Flowering time: Varies depending on where it is grown.

Astrology: Not assigned to any planet.

Medicinal virtues: The leaves are dried and roasted, then rolled. Green tea is diuretic and gently astringes the fibres of the stomach, toning it and improving digestion. A strong solution is salutory for headache and sickness due to inebriation.

Modern uses: Tea contains tannin, which is astringent and helps to check a loose bowel. It is, therefore, not suitable for those with constipation. It also contains caffeine, which is stimulating to the nervous system. Used moderately, it is sedative and relaxing, but taken to excess will cause sleeplessness and nervous and digestive disturbances. It is used so extensively domestically that it is rarely used as a medicine.

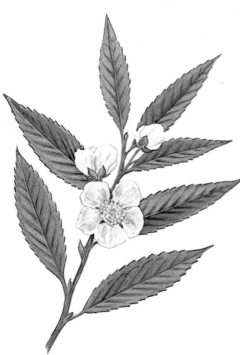

Tea CAMELLIA THEA

DIPSACUS FULLONUM (=D. SYLVESTRIS)

TEASEL

The water found in the hollow of the leaves is commended as a cosmetic to render the face fair.

A biennial growing to five or six feet (1.5 or 1.8 m) high with a rigid, prickly stem and prickly leaves. The flowers are pink to violet.

Where to find it: Roadsides, edges of fields and woods and the banks of streams.

Flowering time: Mid to late summer.

Astrology: Under the dominion of Venus.

Medicinal virtues: The roots are said to have a cleansing property. A decoction of them in wine is applied to the rhagades or clefts of the fundament and for a fistula therein. It is also used to take away warts. The water held by the leaves is used to cool inflammations of the eyes.

Modern uses: A tincture made from the fresh plant while in flower is prescribed by homoeopathic physicians for anal fistula and inflammation of the skin.

Teasel DIPSACUS FULLONUM (= D. SYLVESTRIS)

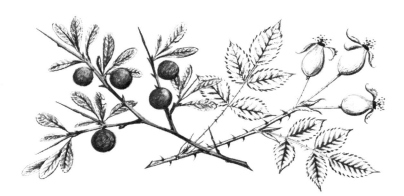

DATURA STRAMONIUM

THORN-APPLE

An ointment made from the leaves is cooling and repelling.

An annual growing to about three feet (91 cm) high. It has large, broad, sharp-pointed leaves. The large flowers are white and trumpet-shaped.

Where to find it: It grows in most parts of the world. It is common on both cultivated and waste ground.

Flowering time: Midsummer to mid autumn.

Astrology: It is governed by Jupiter.

Medicinal virtues: The juice pressed out of the fresh plant and reduced to an extract, has been taken in doses of half a grain (32 mg) up to a dram (1.7 g), in 24 hours, for epileptic disorders, convulsions and madness.

Modern uses: The whole plant is extremely poisonous and acts in a similar way to Belladonna. It is used in medicine for its narcotic, anti-spasmodic and analgesic properties.

The leaves are dried and powdered and used in doses of one-tenth of a grain (6.5 mg) to five grains (325 mg) for spasmodic asthma. It is added to medicinal powders for asthma and to Tobacco used for asthma cigarettes. The leaves can be burned and the smoke inhaled to relieve asthma.

The seeds have similar properties, but are usually made in fluid extracts or tinctures. Dosage is very small, being only one or two drops of the fluid extract and five of the tincture. An ointment is prepared to ease the pain of neuralgia and muscular rheumatism.

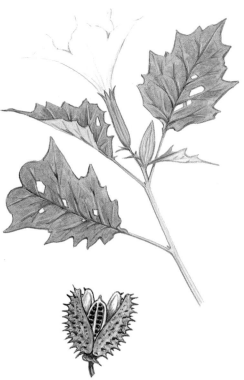

Thorn-apple DATURA STRAMONIUM

191

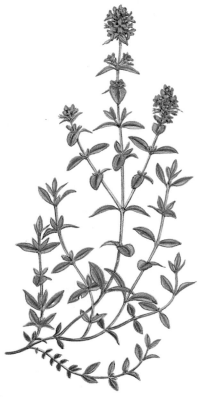

Thyme THYMUS VULGARIS

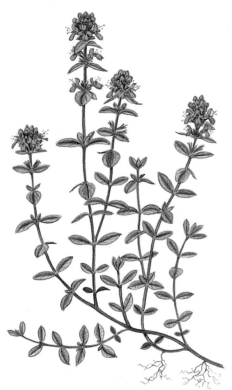

Thyme (Wild) THYMUS SERPYLLUM

THYMUS VULGARIS

THYME

It purges the body of phlegm, and is an excellent remedy for shortness of breath.

This is Garden Thyme, a low-growing shrub with fibrous roots and woody stalks. The dusky green leaves are short, broad and pointed. The numerous flowers are small and pink.

Where to find it: Cultivated in herb gardens for culinary use.

Flowering time: Early summer.

Astrology: A notable herb of Venus.

Medicinal virtues: It strengthens the lungs and is a good remedy for chin-cough in children. It kills worms in the belly, provokes the terms and gives safe and speedy delivery to women in labour. It helps to bring away the afterbirth.

An ointment made of it takes away hot swellings and warts, helps sciatica and dullness of the sight, and takes away pains and hardness of the spleen. It is excellent for those troubled with gout and also to anoint swollen testicles. It eases pains in the loins and hips. Taken inwardly, the herb comforts the stomach and expels wind.

Modern uses: Thyme is a natural antiseptic as it is rich in thymol. It relieves throat and bronchial irritation and the spasms of whooping cough. An infusion is made from the dried herb by adding 1 oz (28 g) to 1 pt (568 ml) of boiling water. The dose is 2 fl oz (56 ml) three or four times a day. Herbalists use a tincture in doses of 20–40 drops.

The infusion also improves appetite and relieves dyspepsia and gastritis. Oil of Thyme also reduces wind and colic and is taken in doses of 1–5 drops.

THYMUS SERPYLLUM

THYME (Wild)

An infusion of the leaves removes headache.

A low-growing perennial with small oval leaves. The flowers are produced in small loose spikes of a reddish-purple colour.

Where to find it: Sandy heaths, dry grassland and rocky ground.

Flowering time: Mid to late summer.

Astrology: It is under Venus.

Medicinal virtues: The whole plant is fragrant and yields an essential oil that is very heating. The infusion is excellent for nervous disorders. Drank as a tea it is a pleasant and effectual remedy for headache, giddiness and similar disorders. Good for headache due to inebriation. It is a certain remedy for that troublesome complaint, the nightmare.

Modern uses: The properties of Wild Thyme are similar to Garden Thyme, but not so effective. The herb is anti-spasmodic, carminative and tonic. It is a good remedy for flatulence. The infusion of 1 oz (28 g) of dried herb to 1 pt (568 ml) of boiling water is given in tablespoonful doses for whooping cough, sore throat and catarrh. It is best sweetened with honey or flavoured with liquorice. It may be combined with Linseed tea when a more demulcent remedy is required. Children should be given smaller, more frequent doses.

NICOTIANA TABACUM

TOBACCO

A slight infusion of the fresh gathered leaves vomits roughly.

Tobacco is an annual plant growing to about five feet (1.5 m) with large, dusky green leaves and pretty trumpet-shaped flowers of a reddish colour.

Where to find it: Cultivated throughout the world. It can be grown in the garden, but does best in warmer regions. It is a native of South America.

Flowering time: Midsummer.

Astrology: It is a hot martial plant.

Medicinal virtues: It is a good medicine for rheumatic pains. An ointment made of the leaves, with hog's lard, is used for painful and inflamed piles. The distilled oil dropped on cotton cures the toothache if applied. The powdered leaves, or a decoction of them, kills lice and other vermin. The smoke of Tobacco injected in the manner of a clyster is of efficacy in stoppages of the bowels, for destroying small worms and for the recovery of persons apparently drowned.

Modern uses: Tobacco was a medicinal herb of the Red Indians who taught the Spaniards how to use it. All parts of the plant contain nicotine which is toxic to the body. It is narcotic, sedative and emetic. The powdered leaves used as a snuff irritate the lining of the nose and cause sneezing. An ointment made from the leaves by simmering them in wax has been used as an application to ulcers and tumours, but there is a danger of the nicotine being absorbed through the skin and causing serious poisoning. Tobacco is not used in modern herbal practice. Smoking is associated with many diseases, including the two main causes of death, cancer and heart disease.

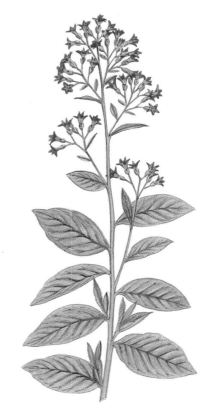
Tobacco NICOTIANA TABACUM

POTENTILLA ERECTA (= P. TORMENTILLA)

TORMENTIL

Excellent to stay all kinds of fluxes of blood or humours in man or woman, whether at nose, mouth or belly.

A plant with long narrow leaves, serrated at the ends. The flowers are small and yellow with four parts.

Where to find it: Grassland, mountains, heaths and bogs.

Flowering time: Early to midsummer.

Astrology: This is a herb of the Sun.

Medicinal virtues: The juice of the herb or root, or a decoction taken with treacle, and the person laid to sweat, expels venom or poison, or the plague, fever or other contagious diseases.

It is an ingredient in all antidotes or counter-poisons. The root taken inwardly is most efficacious to help any flux in the belly, stomach, spleen or blood. The juice opens obstructions of the liver and lungs and thereby helps the jaundice.

It is powerful in ruptures and bruises or falls, used outwardly or inwardly.

The root with Pellitory of Spain and Alum, put into the hollow of a tooth, assuages the pain and stays the flux of the humours which causes it. It is also an effectual remedy against outward wounds, sores and hurts, as well as inward, and is therefore a special ingredient in drinks for wounds, lotions and injections, for foul corrupt rotten sores and ulcers of the mouth, or the secret parts of the body.

Modern uses: The root contains tannin and if chewed occasionally it hardens the gums and keeps the mouth healthy. The astringency of the root is useful for simple diarrhoea. One ounce (28 g) of the root is infused in 1 pt (568 ml) of boiling water and given in doses of 2 fl oz (56 ml). The infusion may be used externally as a lotion for ulcers, as an injection for leucorrhoea and as a gargle for a sore throat. For a stronger medicine, the root is boiled in 1½ pt (852 ml) of water until it measure 1 pt (568 ml) and then strained for use.

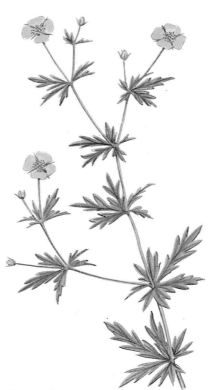
Tormentil POTENTILLA ERECTA
(= P. TORMENTILLA)

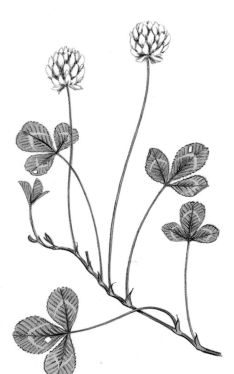

Trefoil TRIFOLIUM REPENS

TREFOIL

If the herb be made into a poultice, and applied to inflammations, it will ease them.

Formerly known as the Meadow Honeysuckle, this Trefoil is probably better known now as Clover. It is the white variety with leaves and flowers produced on long stalks.

Where to find it: Grassland, waste places and lawns.

Flowering time: Early summer.

Astrology: Mercury has dominion over it.

Medicinal virtues: The leaves and flowers are good to ease the pains of gout, if the herb be boiled and used as a clyster. Boiled in lard and made into an ointment, the herb is good to apply to the bites of venomous beasts. The decoction of the herb and flowers with the seed and root taken for some time helps those troubled with the whites.

The seed and flowers boiled in water and made into a poultice with some oil, and applied, helps hard swellings and imposthumes.

Modern uses: Herbalists now prefer to use Red Clover (*Trifolium pratense*). The blossoms purify the blood if infused and drunk like tea. They are also sedative and will relieve bronchial and irritating coughs. A poultice of the herb is applied to malignant tumours of the skin. Red Clover blossom tea is obtainable from herbalists and health food stores. One teaspoonful is used per cup of boiling water.

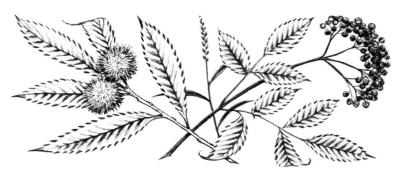

VALERIAN (Greek)

Epilepsies have been cured by the use of this herb.

Greek Valerian, also known as Jacob's Ladder, is a perennial with a thick, short, greyish root, long, broad main leaves followed by indented ladder-like secondary leaves, and drooping purplish-blue or white flowers. It belongs to the Phlox family.

Where to find it: Rarely found in the wild. The white variety is more commonly found in or near gardens.

Flowering time: Late spring to midsummer.

Astrology: It is under Mercury.

Medicinal virtues: It helps in nervous complaints, headaches, trembling, palpitations of the heart and the vapours. It is also good in hysteric cases. The whole plant is used and taken by infusion.

Modern uses: It is astringent and diaphoretic and similar in action to False Jacob's Ladder, or Abscess Root (*Polemonium reptans*). It is recommended in fevers and inflammatory disease of the lungs, such as bronchitis and pleurisy. Unfortunately the plant is rare and, therefore, not much used professionally. Where available, the dried herb is taken by infusion – 1 oz (28 g) to 1 pt (568 ml) of boiling water – in doses of 2 fl oz (56 ml).

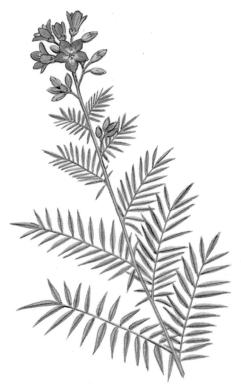

Valerian (Greek) POLEMONIUM CAERULEUM

VALERIAN (True Wild)

It is excellent against nervous affections.

It has a strong-smelling root, long, winged, hairy leaves and pinkish flowers.

Where to find it: High pastures and dry heathland.

Flowering time: Late spring.

Astrology: A herb of Mercury.

Medicinal virtues: An excellent medicine for loosening the bowel when other medicines fail. It is excellent for headaches, tremblings, palpitations, hysteric complaints and the vapours.

Modern uses: *Valeriana sylvestris* is very similar to *Valeriana officinalis*, the variety most used by herbalists, and is considered to be medically superior, but is otherwise similar in all respects. Valerian is an important remedy in modern herbal practice, being an effective nervine tonic. The root is dried and powdered and given as a tincture or by infusion. It eases pain and aids sleep and is tranquillising without having side-effects. It should be tried in all cases of neuralgia.

One ounce (28 g) of the powder is infused in 1 pt (568 ml) of boiling water and taken in doses of up to 2 fl oz (56 ml). The tincture made by herbalists is taken in doses of one or two teaspoonfuls three or four times a day.

For high blood pressure due to stress, combine in equal parts with Scullcap and Lime blossoms. For nervous conditions, combine with Scullcap and Mistletoe. The dose of the mixtures when infused is from one teaspoonful to 2 fl oz (56 ml).

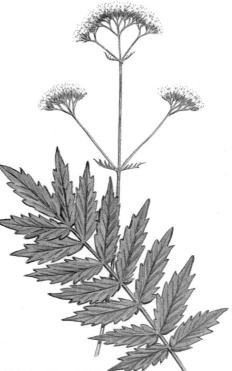

Valerian (True Wild) VALERIANA OFFICINALIS (= V. SYLVESTRIS)

VERVAIN (Common)

Used with lard, it helps swellings and pains in the secret parts.

A perennial growing to about 18 inches (46 cm) high with broad leaves at ground level a squarish stalk and long spike of lilac or pinkish-white flowers.

Where to find it: Waste ground, roadsides and dry grassland.

Flowering time: Midsummer.

Astrology: A herb of Venus.

Medicinal virtues: Excellent for the womb. It strengthens and remedies all cold distempers of it as Plantain does the hot.

It opens obstructions and is cleansing and healing. It helps the yellow jaundice, the dropsy and the gout. It kills and expels worms in the belly and causes a good colour in the face and body. It strengthens as well as corrects diseases of the stomach, liver and spleen.

It helps the cough, wheezings, shortness of breath and defects of the reins and bladder, expelling gravel and stone. Used with honey it heals old ulcers and fistulas in the legs.

Modern uses: As a nervine, it is combined with Mistletoe and Valeriana and given by infusion. On its own, it is a good remedy for coughs and colds, but may be combined with remedies such as Colt's Foot and Horehound. In the early stages of colds and fevers, the warm infusion will induce sweating and may be combined with Yarrow. Its astringent properties make it of use in acute diarrhoea.

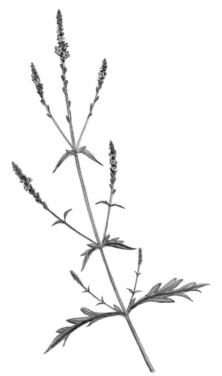

Vervain (Common) VERBENA OFFICINALIS

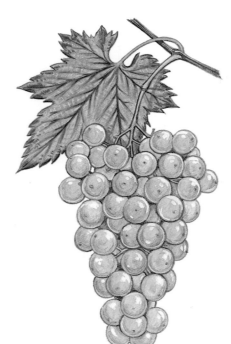

Vine Tree VITIS VINIFERA

VITIS VINIFERA

VINE TREE

The leaves of the English vine, boiled, make a good lotion for sore mouths.

This is the Grape Vine, one of the oldest cultivated plants. It is a long-lived climbing shrub cloaked in large, lobed leaves and clusters of small green or whitish flowers, which are followed by the grapes.

Where to find it: A native of southern Europe and Asia, but cultivated throughout the world by the wine industry.

Flowering time: Early to midsummer.

Astrology: A fine plant of the Sun.

Medicinal virtues: The dried fruit – currants and raisins – is good in coughs, consumptions and other disorders of the chest. The leaves boiled with Barley-meal and made into a poultice cools the inflammation of wounds.

The droppings of the Vine, when it is cut in the spring, boiled with sugar into a syrup, and taken inwardly, is excellent to stay women's longings when pregnant.

The ash of the burnt branches is used to make discoloured teeth white by rubbing them with it in the morning. Spirit of wine is the greatest cordial among the vegetables.

Modern uses: Grape juice is rich in vitamins and minerals particularly iron. It provides a source of instant energy and is ideal for convalescents. The grape is laxative and diuretic. Despite its sugar content, it is not fattening. Fasting, except for grape juice and grapes, has been recommended by naturopaths to clear many chronic diseases. Grapes are used in the treatment of poor blood circulation, low blood pressure, anaemia, liver congestion and skin blemishes.

VIOLA ODORATA

VIOLET

A fine, pleasing plant . . . of a mild nature, and in no way hurtful.

A perennial with heart-shaped leaves and large fragrant deep blue or purple flowers.

Where to find it: Warm, sunny banks and edges of woods.

Flowering time: Late winter to mid spring.

Astrology: A plant of Venus.

Medicinal virtues: It is used to cool any heat or distemperature of the body, such as eye inflammations, or hot swellings in the matrix or fundament. The leaves and flowers are taken by decoction and also used in a poultice. A dram (1.7 g) by weight of the powdered leaves or flowers purges the body of choleric humours if taken in wine. The powdered flowers taken in water relieves the quinsy and the falling-sickness in children. The flowers of White Violets ripen and dissolve swellings. Taken fresh, the flowers or herb are effectual in pleurisy and diseases of the lungs and help hoarseness, hot urine and pains in the back or bladder.

Modern uses: The leaves are antiseptic and are used internally and externally for the treatment of malignancies. Research is required in this area, but an infusion of the leaves appears to reduce pain in cancerous cases. A strong infusion is made by using 2 oz (56 g) of leaves to 1 pt (568 ml) of boiling water, which is left to stand overnight. It is then strained and taken in doses of 2 fl oz (56 ml) every two or three hours. The crushed leaves can be applied directly to the skin where an antiseptic is required. The flowers are expectorant and a syrup is made by adding honey to an infusion of them. This is an excellent remedy for coughs taken in dessertspoonful doses. The roots and leaves are also expectorant, but the root tends to be emetic and has been used as an alternative to Ipecacuanha. In combination with Vervain (*Verbena officinalis*), it is effective in whooping cough. Colt's Foot may also be added.

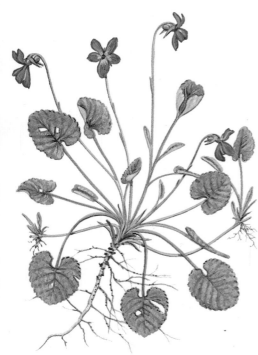

Violet VIOLA ODORATA

VIOLET (Water)

Some commend the herb as of great use against the king's-evil.

A perennial aquatic plant, resembling Yarrow, but is a member of the Primrose family. The root is a tuft of long, black and slender fibres which penetrate deep into muddy places. The leaves are beautifully pinnated and the pale lilac flowers with yellow eyes stand in little clusters.

Where to find it: Ponds and ditches.

Flowering time: Early summer.

Astrology: It is governed by Saturn.

Medicinal virtues: The leaves are cooling when externally applied, but they are more used by country people than by physicians. The flowers are considered to be specific against fluor albus and are frequently made into a conserve or decoction for that purpose; but it is a remedy that must be continued for some time. The herb has been commended for all scrofulous swellings.

Modern uses: It has always been used by those country people familiar with its virtues rather than by professional herbalists or physicians. The plant is fairly common and may deserve re-investigation. Leucorrhoea, a vaginal discharge, is the modern term of fluor albus. For this condition, there are a variety of remedies that can be tried including Marigold flowers, Cranesbill, Witch Hazel, Rasberry leaves and Tormentil.

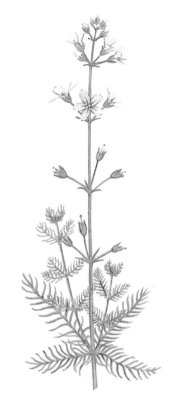

Violet (Water) HOTTONIA PALUSTRIS

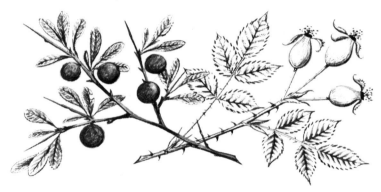

VIPER'S BUGLOSS

An especial remedy against both poisonous bites and poisonous herbs.

A showy biennial and a member of the Borage family. It grows two or three feet (61 or 91 cm) high with prickly stems and leaves. The purplish violet flowers stand in spikes at the top.

Where to find it: Dry soils, grassland, sea cliffs and dunes.

Flowering time: Early summer to early autumn.

Astrology: A herb of the Sun.

Medicinal virtues: The seed drank in wine produces an abundance of milk in nursing mothers. It also eases pains in the back, loins and kidneys. The distilled water of the flowering herb may be used inwardly or outwardly for the same purpose.

Modern uses: The herb stimulates kidney function, soothes inflammatory conditions and increases expectoration.

The lower leaves are made into an infusion – 1 oz (28 g) to 1 pt (568 ml) of boiling water – and used to produce sweating in fevers. This is also good for headaches, nervous conditions and to allay pain due to inflammation. The seeds are administered as a simple decoction to improve lactation, but alcoholic wines are contra-indicated in pregnancy and nursing mothers.

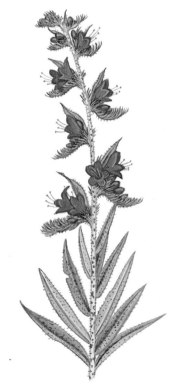

Viper's Bugloss ECHIUM VULGARE

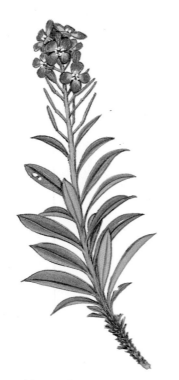

CHEIRANTHUS CHEIRI
WALLFLOWER (Common)

It is a singular remedy for gout and aches and pains in the joints and sinews.

A well-known garden plant. The cultivated varieties are biennial, whereas in the wild the Wallflower is perennial. The flowers are produced in spikes of yellow and are pleasantly scented. The seeds are small and flat and contained in long, slender, whitish pods.

Where to find it: It grows on rocks and walls.

Flowering time: Late spring, early summer.

Astrology: The Moon rules this herb.

Medicinal virtues: A conserve made of the flowers is used as a remedy both for the apoplexy and palsy. It also cleanses the blood, frees the liver and reins from obstructions, provokes women's courses, expels the secundine and the dead child.

It helps the hardness and pains of the mother and of the spleen. It stays inflammations and swellings and comforts and strengthens any weak part or bone out of joint.

Modern uses: Not used by professional herbalists at the present time. The plant is purgative and, therefore, dosage is critical. The plant produces an essential oil which is perfumed. The seeds and flowers are cardiotonic, containing a substance similar to Digitalis. They also increase urine production. Not recommended for domestic use.

Wallflower (Common) CHEIRANTHUS CHEIRI

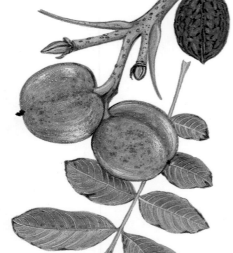

JUGLANS REGIA
WALNUT

An enemy to those that have the cough.

A large tree growing from 30 to 80 feet (9 to 24 m) high, valuable for its wood and fruit. The flowers are yellow-green, the male ones in hanging catkins, the female in short, erect spikes.

Where to find it: Gardens and woodland.

Flowering time: Late spring.

Astrology: A tree of the Sun.

Medicinal virtues: The bark is binding and drying and the young leaves are similar. Older leaves are heating and drying and harder of digestion. Taken with sweet wine, they move the belly downwards, but if they are old they grieve the stomach. They kill the worms in the stomach or belly. Taken with Onions, salt and honey they help the bites of mad dogs, or poisonous bites.

The juice of the green husks boiled with honey is an excellent gargle for sore mouths or heat and inflammations in the throat or stomach.

When the kernels grow old, they are more oily and unfit to be eaten, but are used to heal wounds of the sinews, gangrenes and carbuncles. If burned, the kernels are astringent and will stay laxes and women's courses.

Modern uses: Walnuts are a natural source of manganese. The dried leaves are astringent and used in the form of an infusion as a skin application – 1 oz (28 g) of the leaves to 1 pt (568 ml) of boiling water is allowed to stand for six hours and then strained. This is suitable for conditions such as eczema, herpes and ulcers. The powdered bark taken by infusion is laxative.

Walnut JUGLANS REGIA

TRITICUM
WHEAT
A poultice made of it with milk, eases pains and ripens tumours.

Wheat is the well-known cereal food derived from a perennial grass native to the Middle East.

Where to find it: Cultivated on farmland.

Flowering time: Summer.

Astrology: A plant of Venus.

Medicinal virtues: The pressed oil is used warm to heal tetters and ringworm. Wheat-bread poultices made with red wine and applied to hot, inflamed or blood-shot eyes, helps them. Applied for three days at a time, the poultices will heal kernels in the throat.

Wheat-flour mixed with the juice of Henbane, stays the flux of humours to the joints, if laid thereto. Mixed with the yolk of an egg, honey or turpentine it draws, cleanses and heals boils, plague sores or foul ulcers.

It is more useful as a food than as a medicine. A piece of toasted bread dipped in wine and applied to the stomach, is good to stay vomiting.

Modern uses: Bread poultices are excellent applied to painful swellings in the body. They are made by adding breadcrumbs to ½ pt (284 ml) of boiling water until the water appears to be absorbed. Then drain, but do not press, and spread on to a cloth.

Wheat germ oil is rich in vitamin E and improves circulation. It is available in capsules. The wheat germ itself is rich in vitamins and considered to be an excellent health food. Some people are allergic or hypersensitive to gluten, the protein in wheat, and suffer various diseases due to its ingestion. Conditions ranging from mild gastro-intestinal discomfort to coeliac disease and even mental imbalance are included in what is now termed glutenenteropathy.

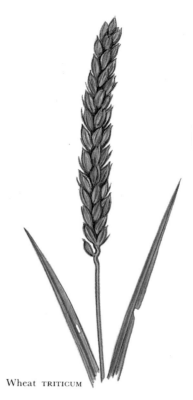

Wheat TRITICUM

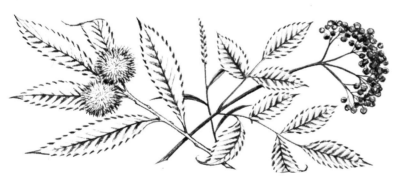

EPILOBIUM HIRSUTUM
WILLOWHERB (Hairy)
The root, dried and powdered, is good against haemorrhages.

A perennial growing to about three feet (91 cm) high with a thick, firm, upright stem. The leaves are long and hairy and the flowers large and purplish-pink. Also called the Great Willowherb.

Where to find it: Ditches, sides of streams, damp meadows, and hedgerows.

Flowering time: Midsummer.

Astrology: Under Saturn.

Medicinal virtues: This is cooling and astringent. The fresh juice or the powdered root is taken to stop internal haemorrhaging. They stop looseness of the bowel and other fluxes and also nocturnal pollutions.

Modern uses: This remedy has been discarded by professional herbalists as the use of the leaves has been associated with poisonings and convulsions. See Willowherb (Rosebay).

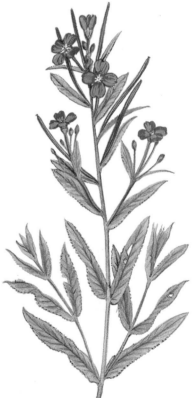

Willowherb (Hairy) EPILOBIUM HIRSUTUM

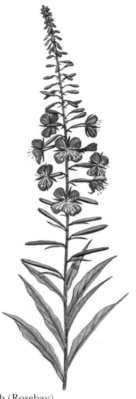

EPILOBIUM ANGUSTIFOLIUM

WILLOWHERB (Rosebay)

The most beautiful of all the willow herbs.

A perennial growing to five feet (1.5 m) with a large, spreading root and a thick, firm, upright stem. The first leaves are long and narrow, deep green on the upper side, silver-grey underneath. The large and beautiful pink-purple flowers are produced in a long deep red spike.

Where to find it: Damp meadows, rocks, roadsides, edges of woodland and waste ground.

Flowering time: Early summer to early autumn.

Astrology: Under Saturn.

Medicinal virtues: As for the previous Willowherb.

Modern uses: A decoction is made from the dried and powdered root for digestive disorders accompanied by diarrhoea. It is soothing and astringent. The dried leaves can be used as a tea and are also demulcent and astringing. The herb, dried and infused is indicated in the treatment of whooping cough and asthma.

Willowherb (Rosebay)
EPILOBIUM ANGUSTIFOLIUM

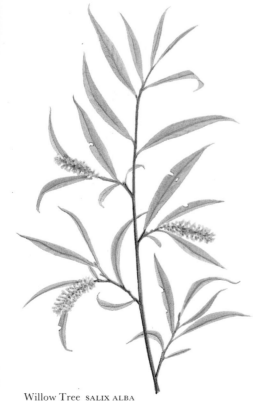

SALIX ALBA

WILLOW TREE

The leaves bruised with pepper, and drank in wine, help in the wind-colic.

A well-known tree from which cricket bats are made. It grows 60 to 70 feet (18 to 21 m) high has a rough bark and narrow, sharp-pointed leaves on its whitish-grey branches. It produces yellow male and green female catkins. Also called the White Willow.

Where to find it: Beside running streams and in other moist places.

Flowering time: Spring.

Astrology: The Moon owns it.

Medicinal virtues: The leaves, bark and seeds are used to staunch the bleeding of wounds and other fluxes of blood in man or woman. The decoction helps to stay vomiting and also thin, hot, sharp salt distillations from the head upon the lungs, causing consumption.

Water gathered from the Willow when it flowers, by slitting the bark, is good for dimness of sight or films that grow over the eyes. If drank it provokes the urine, and clears the face and skin from spots and discolourings. The decoction of the leaves, or bark in wine, takes away scurf and dandruff, if used as a wash.

Modern uses: The bark of the Willow contains salicin from which aspirin is derived. Herbalists use the bark and leaves as an astringent tonic and as a preventive treatment against diseases that are apt to recur, such as malaria.

The decoction, made by boiling 1 oz (28 g) of bark in 1½ pt (852 ml) of water until it measures 1 pt (568 ml) is given in doses of 1–2 fl oz (28–56 ml) for fevers, diarrhoea and dysentery. The powdered root can be taken in sweetened water in doses of one teaspoonful. An infusion of the leaves – 1 oz (28 g) to 1 pt (568 ml) of boiling water – is a useful digestive tonic.

Willow Tree SALIX ALBA

WINTERGREEN

A good vulnerary both for inward and outward wounds.

A perennial with a creeping root. The leaves resemble those of a Pear tree, although not so large. It grows to about ten inches (25 cm) and produces a spike of white flowers.

Where to find it: Woods, moors, rock ledges and dunes.

Flowering time: Early to late summer.

Astrology: A lunar plant.

Medicinal virtues: The leaves are the only part used. They are cooling and drying and a good vulnerary.

They are used for inward and outward wounds and haemorrhages, ulcers in the kidneys or bladder, and to prevent making bloody water and an excess of the catamenia.

Modern uses: The Common Wintergreen is now a rare plant and, therefore, not available for medicinal use. It should not be confused with *Gaultheria procumbens*, from which Oil of Wintergreen is produced. Another variety, the Large Wintergreen (*Pyrola rotundifolia*), which resembles Lily of the Valley, is also rare, but pockets of abundance are sometimes found in fenland and boggy soils throughout Europe, Asia and North America.

An infusion of the dried leaves is a good remedy for cystitis as it flushes the urinary tract and purifies it. The plant contains a natural antiseptic. The dose is 1 fl oz (28 ml), three times a day.

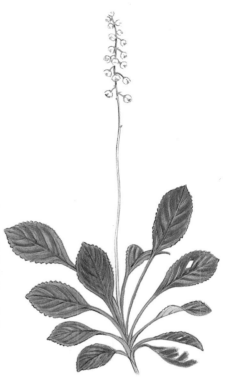

Wintergreen PYROLA MINOR

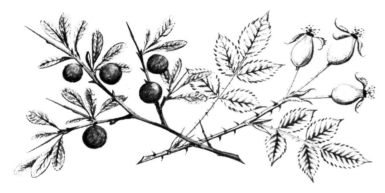

WOODRUFFE (Squinancy)

The green herb, bruised, heals fresh wounds and cuts.

Also known as Quinsy-wort and Squinancywort, it is a perennial, growing about a foot (30 cm) high with square and slender stalks and four or six narrow green leaves encircling every joint. The flowers are presented in an umbel and are pink or white and pleasant to smell.

Where to find it: Woodland, chalkland, dry pastures and dunes.

Flowering time: Late spring.

Astrology: It is ruled by Mars.

Medicinal virtues: The herb should be used fresh. It is good for jaundice, and all diseases of the stomach and liver. It opens obstructions and causes appetite.

Modern uses: An infusion of the plant was used as a gargle for quinsy, but the plant has become rarer and is not now used by herbalists. A related plant, the Sweet Woodruffe (*Asperula odorata*), has similar properties (see overleaf). A gargle for sore throat is best made from Sage. Use 1 oz (28 g) of the dried leaves to 1 pt (568 ml) of boiling water, infuse and strain, and it is ready for use.

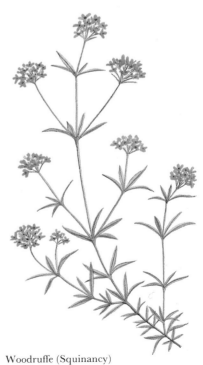

Woodruffe (Squinancy)
ASPERULA CYNANCHICA

WOODRUFFE (Sweet)

It is nourishing and restorative.

A perennial growing to about a foot (30 cm) high, with leaves encircling the stem at each joint. The flowers are small and white and very sweet smelling.

Where to find it: Woods and shady banks.

Flowering time: Mid spring to early summer.

Astrology: A plant of Mars.

Medicinal virtues: It opens obstructions of the liver and spleen and is said to be a provocative to venery. It is good for weak consumptive people.

Modern uses: The whole herb is used as an infusion to strengthen the stomach and remove obstructions from the biliary system. In Germany the fresh herb is infused cold in white wine to make a digestive tonic. The simple infusion – 1 oz (28 g) of the dried herb to 1 pt (568 ml) of boiling water – can also be taken for its tranquillising effects, and to treat insomnia and neuralgia. The dose is 1–2 fl oz (28–56 ml) three times a day.

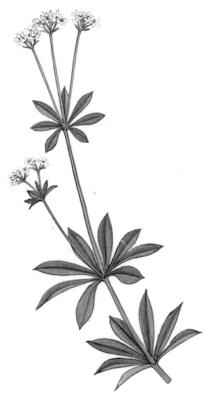

Woodruffe (Sweet) GALIUM ODORATUM
(= ASPERULA ODORATA)

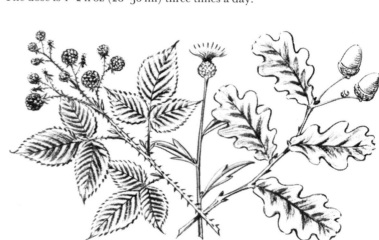

ERYSIMUM CHEIRANTHOIDES

WORMSEED (Treacle)

A poultice of the roots disperses hard tumours in any part of the body.

Also known as Treacle Mustard, it is an annual, about two feet (61 cm) high with long slender roots, long narrow leaves and small yellow flowers produced in a spike. The seed is borne in vessels resembling pea pods.

Where to find it: Waste ground.

Flowering time: Late spring, early summer.

Astrology: It is under the dominion of Mars.

Medicinal virtues: The whole plant has a hot taste and so have the seeds, which are good in rheumatic complaints. Small doses of the juice given in white wine promote the menses and hasten delivery of the child. In larger doses it is an excellent medicine for jaundice and dropsy.

Made into syrup with honey and a small quantity of vinegar, it is beneficial in asthmatic complaints. The seeds kill worms in the stomach and intestines and, in small quantities, are used for hysteric cases, but should be continued for some time.

Modern uses: The seeds are laxative in small doses – 10 grains (650 mg). They ease rheumatic conditions and kill intestinal worms. Overdosing must be avoided, because of purging.

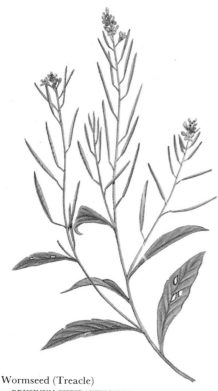

Wormseed (Treacle)
ERYSIMUM CHEIRANTHOIDES

WORMWOOD

Excellent for those with weakness of the stomach.

A perennial with a pale green, tough stalk growing to about three feet (91 cm) high. The leaves are pale green and the flowers are a pale olive colour at first but change to yellow-brown.

Where to find it: Waste places and roadsides.

Flowering time: Early to midsummer.

Astrology: This is governed by Mars.

Medicinal virtues: This is excellent for gout and gravel. The leaves and flowers are used.

Modern uses: The infusion of the dried herb – 1 oz (28 g) to 1 pt (568 ml) of boiling water – is taken in doses of 2 fl oz (56 ml) as a stomach tonic, to expel worms and to reduce temperature in fevers. It is considered to be one of the finest remedies for dyspepsia, gastro-intestinal pain and poor liver function.

It is also antiseptic and will promote menstruation. Wormwood is an ingredient of Vermouth. A liquor made from Absinthol, extracted from the plant, is soothing to the nervous system, but damaging if taken for a prolonged period. The infusions should also not be taken continuously.

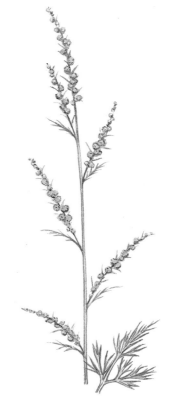

Wormwood ARTEMISIA ABSINTHIUM

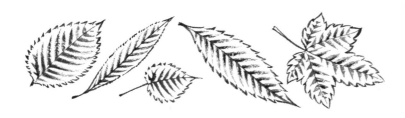

WORMWOOD (Roman)

The juice of the fresh tops . . . has been known singly to cure the jaundice.

This is smaller than the former variety with smaller and finer leaves. The flowers are more yellow in colour.

Where to find it: It prefers warmer climes, but will grow in gardens. It is found wild in southern Europe.

Flowering time: Midsummer.

Astrology: It is also a martial plant.

Medicinal virtues: It is excellent to strengthen the stomach. The juice of the fresh tops remove obstructions of the liver and spleen. Made into a light infusion, the flowering tops strengthen the digestion, correct acidity and supply gall where it is deficient.

One ounce (28 g) of the flowers and buds are placed in a vessel and 1½ pt (852 ml) of boiling water poured on them. This is allowed to stand all night. In the morning the clear liquor, with two spoonfuls of wine, is taken at three draughts at one and a half hour intervals.

Regularly observed for a week, this will cure all complaints arising from indigestion and wind.

An ounce (28 g) of the flowers steeped in a pint (568 ml) of brandy for six weeks will produce a tincture, of which a tablespoonful taken in a glass of water twice a day will give relief in gout and prevent an increase in the gravel.

Modern uses: The properties of Roman Wormwood are similar to the previous variety, but less strong. Continued use is not recommended, because of its effects on the nervous system.

Wormwood (Roman) ARTEMISIA PONTICA

ARTEMISIA MARITIMA

WORMWOOD (Sea)

A very noble bitter that succeeds in procuring an appetite, better than Common Wormwood, which is best to assist digestion.

A plant about two feet (61 cm) high, with a white stalk and irregular branches. The yellowish-brown flowers hang down from drooping shoots.

Where to find it: Coastal areas, salt marshes and sea walls.

Flowering time: Late summer, early autumn.

Astrology: A herb of Mars.

Medicinal virtues: The flowering tops and the young leaves and shoots possess all the virtues. The older leaves and the stalk should be thrown away as useless.

Boiling water poured upon it produces an excellent stomachic infusion, but the best way is to take it as a tincture made with brandy. For lighter complaints a conserve, as made of Field Southernwood, agreeably answers the purpose.

Hysteric complaints have been cured by the use of this tincture. In scurvy and in hypochondriacal disorders few remedies have greater effect than when this is taken in a strong infusion.

Modern uses: This possesses similar properties to the two former Wormwoods, but is not as potent as the first. It is usually used as a substitute for *Artemesia absinthium* by country people who realise its virtues. The flowering tops are collected and dried and given as an infusion for digestive problems. It is also useful for intermittent fever. Prolonged use is not recommended.

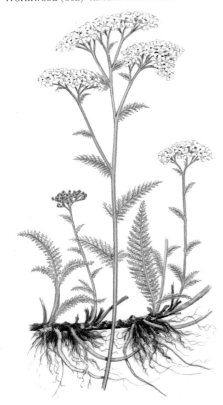

Wormwood (Sea) ARTEMISIA MARITIMA

ACHILLEA MILLEFOLIUM

YARROW

An ointment of the leaves cures wounds and is good for inflammations.

An upright, and not unhandsome plant, it is a common perennial of much more use than is generally known. Also called Milfoil (a thousand leaves) or Nosebleed, it grows up to two feet (61 cm) high and has many leaves which are divided into a multitude of parts. The flowers are white or pink with yellowish centres.

Where to find it: Roadsides, meadows, and waste ground.

Flowering time: Mid to late summer.

Astrology: It is under the influence of Venus.

Medicinal virtues: A decoction of it boiled with white wine is good to stop the running of the reins in men and whites in women. It restrains violent bleedings and is excellent for piles. A strong tea is made of the leaves and drunk frequently. In addition, a poultice made of equal parts of Yarrow and Toadflax is applied outwardly. This induces sleep, eases pain and reduces bleeding.

The ointment made from the leaves is applied to ulcers, fistulas and all such runnings as abound with moisture.

Modern uses: Still an important agent in herbal medicine. An infusion of the dried herb, combined with Elderflowers and Peppermint, is taken in doses of 2 fl oz (56 ml) with a teaspoonful of composition essence, available from herbalists, added to each dose. This is one of the best remedies for the common cold and influenza.

Yarrow induces sweating and contains cineol, a natural antiseptic. It also contains a substance which hastens the clotting time of the blood following injury, thus its common name of Nosebleed given it by country people is justly deserved. It regulates menstruation, reduces blood pressure and heals bleeding piles.

Yarrow ACHILLEA MILLEFOLIUM

YEW

It has very powerful poisonous qualities.

The Yew tree grows 40 to 50 feet (12 to 15 m) high. It has long, narrow leaves, tiny flowers and red or yellow berries.

Where to find it: Grows wild in Europe, the United States and Asia. It is commonly planted in cemeteries.

Flowering time: Early to mid spring.

Astrology: A tree of Saturn.

Medicinal virtues: It has no place among medicinal plants. The leaves and berries are poisonous to man and beast, although people have eaten the berries and survived.

Its deleterious powers seem to act on the nervous system, but it totally differs from Opium and all other sleepy poisons for it does not bring on lethargic symptoms, but penetrates and destroys the vital functions. Though it is sometimes given in obstructions of the liver and bilious complaints, there have been too few experiments with it to recommend it to be used without the greatest caution.

Modern uses: The whole of the tree is highly poisonous, with the berries and seeds being the most toxic. A specially prepared tincture is prescribed by homoeopathic physicians for rheumatism and arthritis. This is made from the leaves but is non-poisonous.

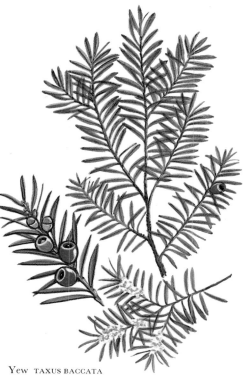

Yew TAXUS BACCATA

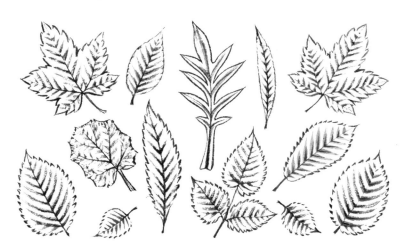

YUCCA or JUCCA

The raw juice is dangerous, if not deadly, and it is supposed that the Indians poisoned the heads of their darts with it.

The yucca is an evergreen plant with long strap-shaped leaves. It grows from four to eight feet (1.2 to 2.4 m) high and bears large white flowers.

Where to find it: The wild drier regions of North and Central America. It is also cultivated in gardens.

Flowering time: Midsummer.

Astrology: It is not assigned to any planet.

Medicinal virtues: It has no properties as yet known. In Virginia the roots are used for making bread. The juice is toxic.

Modern uses: The juice, which contains natural soaps, is used in tonics for the hair and scalp. It should not be taken internally.

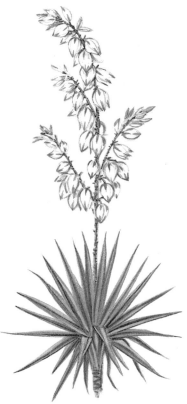

Yucca or Jucca YUCCA GLORIOSA

GLOSSARY

Ague: Malarial or intermittent fever.
Alexipharmic: A medicine neutralising a poison.
Alerative: Restoring normal body functions.
Anodyne: Relieving pain.
Apoplexy: Paralysis from rupture of a cerebral vessel.
Aromatic: A fragrant herb.
Astringent: Producing contraction of organic tissue, or arrest of a discharge.
Axungia: Lard.
Biles: Boils.
Blain: A blister or pustule.
Bloody flux: Dysentery.
Cachexia: Severe wasting as in terminal disease.
Cantharides: Dried and powdered beetle.
Carminative: A medicine that expels flatulence.
Casting: Vomiting.
Catamenia: Menstrual flow.
Cataplasm: Poultice.
Cathartic: A purgative medicine.
Cholagogue: A medicine to increase the flow of bile.
Cephalic: A medicine to clear the head.
Ceruse: Lead carbonate.
Choler: Bile.
Clysters: Enema or injection.
Courses: Menstrual flow.
Decoction: A medicine produced by boiling roots, bark, etc. in water.
Defluxion: Catarrh.
Deobstruent: An aperient.
Detersive: Cleansing medicine.
Diaphoretic: Inducing sweating.
Distemper: Ailment.
Distillation: A trickling discharge.
Diuretic: Increasing flow of urine.
Draught: A quantity of medicine taken in one dose.
Dropsy: Watery swelling in the tissues of cavities of the body.
Eczema: An irritating skin disease.
Electuary: A confection.
Excoriation: Abrasion.
Excrement: Faeces.

Falling-sickness: Epilepsy.
Febrifuge: A medicine that reduces fever.
Felon: Whitlow.
Fistula: Abnormal tube-like passage in the body.
Fluor albus: Whitish vaginal discharge.
Flux: Excessive flow of any body secretion.
Fundament: The anus.
Gall: Bile.
Gargarism: A gargle.
Gravel: Sand-like deposit in urine.
Hypochondrium: Upper part of abdomen.
Hypoglycaemic: Lowers blood sugar.
Humours: Any fluid of the body.
Imposthume: Purulent swelling or abscess.
Kernels: Hard swellings.
Kibes: Chilblains.
King's-evil: Constitutional condition with glanduar swellings and tendency to tuberculosis, scrofula.
Laxes: Looseness of the bowel.
Leprosy: Chronic infectious disease affecting the skin.
Lethargy: Drowsiness or sleeping sickness.
Leucorrhoea: Vaginal discharge.
Lochia: Vaginal discharge after labour.
Lye: An alkaline solution filtered from wood ashes, detergent.
Matrix: The womb.
Megrim: Migraine.
Mithridate: A medicine to protect against poison by giving gradually increasing doses of the toxic substance.
Morphy: Scleroderma, a chronic skin disease.
Olibanum: Frankincense, a gum resin.
Oxymel: A mixture of honey and vinegar.
Palsy: Paralysis.
Pectoral: A medicine for the chest.
Pestilence: Any deadly epidemic disease.

Phlegm: Mucous from the bronchial tubes.
Phthisis: Advanced or chronic tuberculosis in which wasting is marked.
Pin and web: Disease of the eye with film or excrescence.
Plague: An acute fever transmitted by the bites of fleas which have derived the infection from rats.
Posset: Drink made of hot milk, curdled with ale and flavoured with herbs and used as a cold remedy.
Psoriasis: A scaly skin disease.
Reds: Menstrual flow.
Reins: The kidneys, loins.
Rhagades: Fissures in the skin.
Rheum: Watery or catarrhal discharge.
St Anthony's fire: Erysipelas, an acute inflammatory disease involving the skin.
Schirrhi: Hard tumours.
Sciatica: Low back pain.
Scrofula: See King's-evil.
Scruple: Twenty grains.
Secundines: The afterbirth.
Simpler: A herb doctor.
Simples: Medicinal herbs.
Strangury: Painful urination drop by drop.
Stone: A stone-like concretion formed in the urinary tract or in the gall bladder.
Sudorific: Inducing sweating.
Styptic: An agent that checks haemorrhage.
Tetters: A form of herpes, ringworm or eczema.
Theriaca: Treacle or molasses.
Travail: Painful or laborious childbirth.
Troches: Lozenges.
Vapours: Low spirits, depression, hysteria.
Venery: Sexual intercourse.
Verdigris: Copper acetate, an astringent.
Vulnerary: Wound healer.
Wen: Sebaceous cyst.
Whites: Vaginal discharge.

ILLNESSES AND THEIR HERBAL CURES ACCORDING TO CULPEPER

Agues
Agrimony 10
Alder (Common) 12
Angelica 16
Archangel 17
Barberry 22
Barley 22
Betony (Wood) 27
Bilberries 28
Centaury 42
Chamomile 43
Cinquefoil 47
Colt's Foot 49
Fennel Flower 72
Feverfew 74
Fleur-de-lys (Garden or Blue) 79
Garlic 83
Hawkweed 91
Hellebore (Black) 93
Hemp 94
Houseleek 101
Juniper Tree 105
Lily (Water) 113
Lovage 116
Parnsip (Upright Water) 13
Pellitory of Spain 141
Pepper 143
Plantain (Ribwort) 146
Rue (Garden) 160
Saffron (Meadow) 161
St John's Wort 163
Senna (Red-flowered Bladder) 171
Silverweed 172
Sloe Bush 174
Sorrel (Common) 177
Stonecrop 184
Strawberries 185
Apoplexy
Lavender 110
Lily of the Valley 113
Lime Tree 114
Melilot 123
Pellitory of Spain 141
Sun Spurge 188
Wallflower (Common) 98
Appetite, loss of
Alder (Black) 12
Barberry 22
Chervil 44
Crosswort 51
Eglantine 65
Gentian (Autumn) 84
Goat's Beard 86
Gooseberry 88
Juniper Tree 105
Lady's Smock 108
Mallow (Common) 118
Mint (Garden or Spear) 125
Onion 135
Pepper 143
Plums 147
Shepherd's Rod 172
Sorrel (Common) 177
Spignel (Broad-leaved) 182

Woodruffe (Squinancy) 201
Wormwood (Sea) 204
Asthma
Flax 77
Horehound (White) 100
Knapwort (Harshweed) 106
Maidenhair (Common) 118
Rampion (Sheep's) 153
Rocket Cress 157
Savory (Winter) 167
Squill 183
Wormseed (Treacle) 202

Bites and stings
Aconite 9
Agrimony 10
Alexanders 14
Alkanet 14
Angelica 16
Ash Tree 19
Balm 21
Basil 23
Bay Tree 24
Beets 26
Bistort 29
Blackberry 30
Blue-bottle 31
Burdock (Greater) 35
Carduus Benedictus 39
Cleavers 48
Eglantine 65
Elder (Dwarf) 66
Garlic 83
Goat's Rue 86
Horehound (Black) 99
Hound's Tongue 101
Houseleek 101
Knotgrass 107
Lavender (Cotton) 110
Lichen (Dog) 112
Marsh Mallow 121
Mulberry Tree 129
Mustard (Black) 131
Nettle (Common) 132
Oak Tree 134
Plantain (Buck's Horn) 145
Rhubarb (Culinary or Tart) 156
St John's Wort 163
Sarsaparilla 165
Savory (Summer) 166
Swallow-wort 189
Trefoil 194
Viper's Bugloss 197
Walnut 198
Bladder infections
Hawkweed 91
Pine Tree 144
Skirret 173
Strawberries 185
Vervain (Common) 195
Violet 196
Bleeding, to stop
Adder's tongue 9
Amaranthus 15

Beans (Broad) 25
Betony (wood) 27
Buckthorn 33
Burnet 35
Cleavers 48
Clown's Woundwort 48
Green (Winter) 89
Hart's Tongue 90
Herb Robert 96
Horsetail 100
Hyacinth 102
Knapweed (Common) 106
Lady's Mantle 108
Loosestrife 115
Mint (Garden or Spear) 125
Moneywort 127
Plantain 145
Pomegranate Tree 148
Rose (Damask) 158
Sage (Common Garden) 162
Self-heal 170
Stonecrop 184
Sumach 186
Willow Tree 200
Yarrow 204
Bleeding, internal
Bistort 29
Bugle 34
Dove's-foot 63
Fleabane (Canadian) 78
Herb Robert 96
Moneywort 127
Sanicle 164
Self-heal 170
Bleeding at the mouth or nose
Adder's Tongue 9
Amaranthus 15
Archangel 17
Avens 20
Betony (Wood) 27
Bilberries 28
Bistort 29
Blackberry 30
Blue-bottle 31
Chestnut Tree 45
Clown's Woundwort 48
Comfrey 50
Dittany of Crete 59
Dock (Common) 60
Dog Rose 61
Fluellein 80
Holly 97
Houseleek 101
Knapweed (Common) 106
Knotgrass 107
Lady's Bedstraw 107
Loosestrife 115
Mulberry Tree 129
Mullein (Black) 129
Myrtle Tree 132
Oak Tree 134
Parsnip (Upright Water) 139
Peach Tree 140
Periwinkle (Great) 144

Plantain 145
Rhubarb (Culinary or Tart) 156
Rose (Damask) 158
Rue (Garden) 160
St John's Wort 163
Shepherd's Purse 171
Boils and abscesses
Barberry 22
Beans (Broad) 25
Carduus Benedictus 39
Clary 46
Cuckoo-pint 52
Mushroom (Garden) 130
Wheat 199
Bowel disorders
Agrimony 10
Chamomile 43
Cinquefoil 47
Cuckoo-pint 52
Fenugreek 72
Galingale 82
Hemp 94
Kidneywort 105
Lovage 116
Mallow (Common) 118
Mint (Water) 126
Mullein (Great) 130
Onion 135
Orpine 137
Plantain 145
Polypody 147
Rose (Damask) 158
Sanicle 164
Sumach 186
Teasel 191
Tobacco 192
Breasts, sore or swollen
Beans (Broad) 25
Borage 31
Comfrey 50
Henbane (Common) 95
Marsh Mallow 121
Mint (Pepper) 126
Mustard (Hedge) 131
Parsley (Common) 138
Quince Tree 151
Rice 157
Succory (Wild) 186
Breath, shortness of
Angelica 16
Balm 21
Bay Tree 24
Beans (French) 25
Betony (Wood) 27
Bryony 32
Butter-bur 37
Calamint 37
Catmint 40
Colt's Foot 49
Cuckoo-pint 52
Elecampane 67
Fennel 71
Fennel (Sow or Hog's) 71
Feverfew 74

Fig Tree 75
Fir Tree 76
Horehound (Black) 99
Horehound (White) 100
Hyssop 103
Juniper Tree 105
Knapwort (Harshweed) 106
Liquorice 115
Lungwort 116
Marsh Mallow 121
Masterwort 122
Mustard (Hedge) 131
Nettle (Common) 132
Peach Tree 140
Pellitory of the Wall 141
Rampion (Sheep's) 153
Rue (Garden) 160
Saffron 160
Scabious (Field & Lesser Field) 168
Sow-thistle Tree (Marsh) 181
Thyme 192
Vervain (Common) 195

Bruises
Alkanet 14
Archangel 17
Arssmart 18
Avens 20
Bay tree 24
Beans (Broad) 25
Betony (Water) 26
Bistort 29
Blue-bottle 31
Bugle 34
Caraway 38
Catmint 40
Comfrey 50
Cudweed 54
Daisy 54
Daisy (Little) 55
Devil's Bit 57
Dove's-foot 63
Fern (Royal) 73
Fig Tree 75
Hollyhocks 98
Knapweed (Common) 106
Knapwort (Harshweed) 106
Madder 117
Marjoram (Sweet) 120
Orpine 137
Parsley (Common) 138
Pennyroyal 142
Sage (Wood) 162
Solomon's Seal 176
Tormentil 193

Burns and Scalds
Alder (Common) 12
Archangel 17
Barberry 22
Beets 26
Elder (Dwarf) 66
Hemp 94
Houseleek 101
Ivy 104
Lady's Bedstraw 107
Lily (White Garden) 114
Onion 135
Orpine 137

Catarrh
Catmint 40
Hound's Tongue 101
Jessamine 104
Maidenhair (Common) 118
Myrtle Tree 132
Poppy (White or Opium) 149
Poppy (Wild) 150
Ragwort 153
Saraparilla 165

Storax Tree 185

Chest complaints
Agaric 10
Agrimony (Water) 11
Angelica 16
Avens 20
Bryony 32
Butcher's Broom 36
Elecampane 67
Fenugreek 72
Fig Tree 75
Fir Tree 76
Flax 77
Fleabane (Canadian) 78
Goat's Beard 86
Heart's Ease 92
Horehound (White) 100
Hyssop 103
Liquorice 115
Lungwort 116
Marjoram (Sweet) 120
Marsh Mallow 121
Mustard (Hedge) 131
Pennyroyal 142
Pepper 143
Rocket Cress 157
Rue (Garden) 160
Saffron 160
Savory (Winter) 167
Scabious (Field) 168
Simson (Blue) 173
Vine Tree 196

Chilblains
Beets 26
Kidneywort 105

Colds
Betony (Wood) 27
Catmint 40
Elder (Dwarf) 66
Feverfew 74
Jessamine 104
Masterwort 122
Mullein (Great) 130
Rose (Damask) 158
Yarrow 204

Colic
Agrimony 10
Angelica 16
Asparagus 20
Avens 20
Betony (Wood) 27
Caraway 38
Carrot (Wild) 39
Centaury 42
Dittany (White) 59
Eglantine 65
Elder (Dwarf) 66
Eryngo 69
Fern (Royal) 73
Flag (Yellow) 77
Flax 77
Galingale 82
Groundsel (Common) 90
Hawkweed 91
Hemp 94
Herb (True-love) 97
Holly 97
Juniper Tree 105
Lavender 110
Lettuce (Great Wild) 112
Mint (Water) 126
Mullein (Black) 129
Mullein (Great) 130
Mustard (Hedge) 131
Parsley (Rock or Milk) 139
Rue (Garden) 160
Sauce-alone 165
Savory (Winter) 167

Saxifrage (Great Burnet) 167
Sloe Bush 174
Spignel (Broad-leaved) 182
Spikenard 182

Constipation
Beans (French) 25
Beets 26
Buckthorn 33
Liquorice 115
Rose (Damask) 158
Valerian (True Wild) 195

Consumption
Bay Tree 24
Betony (Wood) 27
Chervil 44
Daisy (Little) 55
Elecampane 67
Flax 77
Fleabane (Canadian) 78
Goat's Beard 86
Horehound (White) 100
Juniper Tree 105
Lungwort 116
Marjoram (Common Wild) 120
Pellitory of Spain 141
Poppy (Wild) 150
Saffron 160
Sage (Common Garden) 162
Vine Tree 196
Willow Tree 200
Woodruffe (Sweet) 202

Convulsions
Asparagus 20
Bay Tree 24
Betony (Wood) 27
Bryony 32
Calamint 37
Centaury 42
Chickweed 45
Cowslip 51
Down or Cotton-thistle 64
Fleur-de-lys (Garden or Blue) 79
Garlic 83
Gentian (Autumn) 84
Gladwin 85
Heart's Ease 92
Hellebore (Black) 93
Honeysuckle 98
Juniper Tree 105
Lavender 110
Lettuce (Great Wild) 112
Lily of the Valley 113
Marsh Mallow 121
Mistletoe 127
Motherwort 128
Mullein (Great) 130
Southernwood 179
Thorn-apple 191

Coughs
Agrimony 10
Bay Tree 24
Betony (Wood) 27
Bilberries 28
Bryony 32
Calamint 37
Catmint 40
Chestnut Tree 45
Cinquefoil 47
Colt's Foot 49
Cuckoo-pint 52
Dog Rose 61
Elder (Dwarf) 66
Elecampane 67
Fennel (Sow or Hog's) 71
Fig Tree 75
Flax 77
Goat's Thorn 87
Hawkweed 91

Hazel Nut 92
Hemp 94
Honeysuckle 98
Horehound (Black) 99
Horehound (White) 100
Horsetail 100
Hyssop 103
Juniper Tree 105
Knapwort (Harshweed) 106
Liquorice 115
Lungwort 116
Mallow (Common) 118
Maple Tree 119
Marsh Mallow 121
Mullein (Black) 129
Mullein (Great) 130
Mustard (Hedge) 131
Onion 135
Peach Tree 140
Pellitory of Spain 141
Pellitory of the Wall 141
Pennyroyal 142
Pepper 143
Poppy (White or Opium) 149
Poppy (Wild) 150
Rattle Grass 154
Rocket Cress 157
Rose (Damask) 158
Rue (Garden) 160
Sage (Common Garden) 162
Sauce-alone 165
Scabious (Field) 168
Scabious (Lesser Field) 168
Storax Tree 185
Thyme 192
Vervain (Common) 195
Vine Tree 196
Walnut 198

Courses, women's
Adder's Tongue 9
Agrimony (Water) 11
Alehoof 13
Alexanders 14
Amaranthus 15
Anemone 15
Angelica 16
Balm 21
Bay Tree 24
Beets 26
Bilberries 28
Brook-lime 32
Bryony 32
Burnet 35
Butcher's Broom 36
Butter-bur 37
Calamint 37
Carrot (Wild) 39
Catmint 40
Celandine (The Greater) 41
Centaury 42
Chervil 44
Chestnut Tree 45
Clary 46
Comfrey 50
Cuckoo-pint 52
Cudweed 54
Devil's Bit 57
Elder 65
Elecampane 67
Eryngo 69
Feverfew 74
Flag (Yellow) 77
Flaxweed 78
Fluellein 80
Galingale 82
Garlic 83
Gentian (Autumn) 84
Golden Rod 87

Green (Winter) 89
Ground Pine (Common) 89
Hazel Nut 92
Hellebore (Black) 93
Holly 97
Hollyhocks 98
Hops 99
Horehound (Black) 99
Horehound (White) 100
Ivy 104
Juniper Tree 105
Knotgrass 107
Lavender 110
Loosestrife 115
Lovage 116
Lungwort 116
Lupin 117
Marjoram (Common Wild) 120
Masterwort 122
Mint (Garden or Spear) 125
Moneywort 127
Motherwort 128
Mugwort (Common) 128
Mulberry Tree 129
Mustard (Black) 131
Mustard (White) 132
Nettle (Common) 132
Nightshade (Common) 133
Oak Tree 134
Onion 135
Parsley (Rock or Milk) 139
Parsnip (Upright Water) 139
Pellitory of the Wall 141
Pennyroyal 142
Periwinkle (Great) 144
Plantain 145
Poppy (Wild) 150
Rattle Grass 154
Rue (Garden) 160
Sage (Common Garden) 162
Sage (Wood) 162
Sanicle 164
Saxifrage (Great Burnet) 167
Sorrel (Common) 177
Strawberries 185
Thyme 192
Wallflower (Common) 198
Walnut 198

Cramps
Asparagus 20
Bay Tree 24
Bryony 32
Calamint 37
Catmint 40
Centaury 42
Chamomile 43
Chickweed 45
Cowslip 51
Fennel 71
Fennel (Sow or Hog's) 71
Fleur-de-lys (Garden or Blue) 79
Garlic 83
Gentian (Autumn) 84
Gladwin 85
Honeysuckle 98
Juniper Tree 105
Lavender 110
Marsh Mallow 121
Masterwort 122
Motherwort 128
Mullein (Great) 130
Poppy (White or Opium) 149
Southernwood 179

Deafness
Alehoof 13
Angelica 16
Carduus Benedictus 39

Fig Tree 75
Henbane (Common) 95
Mallow (Common) 118
Sow-thistle (Tree) 181
Sow-thistle Tree (Marsh) 181
Digestion, poor
Angelica 16
Avens 20
Balm 21
Betony (Wood) 27
Burnet 35
Caraway 38
Clary (Wild) 47
Eglantine 65
Elecampane 67
Gentian (Autumn) 84
Goat's Beard 86
Hawkweed 91
Lady's Smock 108
Lettuce (Common Garden) 111
Lovage 116
Mallow (Common) 118
Mint (Garden or Spear) 125
Polypody 147
Rhubarb 155
Spignel (Broad-leaved) 182

Dropsy
Agrimony (Water) 11
Alder (Black) 12
Ash Tree 19
Bay Tree 24
Betony (Wood) 27
Bryony 32
Carrot (Wild) 39
Chamomile 43
Elder (Dwarf) 66
Eryngo 69
Flaxweed 78
Fleur-de-lys (Garden or Blue) 79
Galingale 82
Germander 84
Hawkweed 91
Hawthorn 91
Hyssop (Hedge) 103
Juniper Tree 105
Kidneywort 105
Laurel (Spurge) 109
Lavender 110
Lily (White Garden) 114
Madder 117
Marjoram (Common Wild) 120
Marjoram (Sweet) 120
Masterwort 122
Mezereon Spurge 124
Mustard (White) 132
Parsley (Common) 138
Parsley (Rock or Milk) 139
Pellitory of the Wall 141
Pennyroyal 142
Plantain 148
Saffron (Meadow) 161
Saltwort 163
Savine 166
Skirret 173
Smallage 174
Squill 183
Sun Spurge 188
Swallow-wort 188
Vervain (Common) 195
Wormseed (Treacle) 202

Ear problems
Agrimony 10
Alehoof 13
Arssmart 18
Bay Tree 24
Beets 26
Betony (Wood) 27

Calamint 37
Centaury 42
Cuckoo-pint 52
Daffodil 54
Elder (Dwarf) 66
Eryngo 69
Fennel (Sow or Hog's) 71
Fig Tree 75
Garlic 83
Hemp 94
Henbane (Common) 95
Horehound (White) 100
Knotgrass 107
Marjoram (Common Wild) 120
Marsh Mallow 121
Melilot 123
Mistletoe 127
Mustard (Hedge) 131
Poppy (White) 148
Rhubarb (Great Monk's) 156
Savory (Summer) 166
Shepherd's Purse 171
Eye problems
Adder's Tongue 9
Alehoof 13
Anemone 15
Angelica 16
Asparagus 20
Barley 22
Beans 25
Beets 26
Betony (Wood) 27
Blue-bottle 31
Borage 31
Caraway 38
Celandine (The Greater) 41
Centaury 42
Chickweed 45
Clary 46
Clary (Wild) 47
Crowfoot 52
Cucumber 53
Daisy 54
Elder 65
Elder (Dwarf) 66
Endive 68
Eyebright 70
Flaxweed 78
Fluellein 80
Fumitory 81
Hemlock 94
Henbane (Common) 95
Horehound (White) 100
Lily of the Valley 113
Lovage 116
Marsh Mallow 121
Meadowsweet 123
Melilot 123
Nightshade (Common) 133
Parsnip (Upright Water) 139
Pennyroyal 142
Pepper (Guinea) 143
Plantain 145
Poplar (White) 148
Rattle Grass 154
Savory (Summer) 166
Strawberries 185
Succory (Wild) 186
Teasel 191
Thyme 192
Wheat 199
Willow Tree 200

Falling-sickness
Betony (Wood) 27
Bryony 32
Cinquefoil 47
Cowslip 51

Dittany (White) 59
Fennel (Sow or Hogs) 71
Garlic 83
Heart's Ease 92
Hellebore (Black) 93
Hyssop 103
Juniper Tree 105
Lavender 110
Lily of the Valley 113
Lime Tree 114
Masterwort 122
Mistletoe 127
Mustard (Black) 131
Paeony 137
Pellitory of Spain 141
Plantain 145
Poplar (Black) 148
Rosemary 159
Sage (Common Garden) 162
Thorn-apple 191
Violet 196

Fevers
Barley 22
Blackberry 30
Blue-bottle 31
Borage 31
Butter-bur 37
Cinquefoil 47
Dandelion 56
Devil's Bit 57
Dittany (White) 59
Dog Rose 61
Elder (Dwarf) 66
Elecampane 67
Goat's Beard 86
Henbane (Common) 95
Lang de Boeuf 109
Laurel (Spurge) 109
Lily (White Garden) 114
Masterwort 122
Meadowsweet 123
Mustard (White) 132
Parsnip (Upright Water) 139
Quince Tree 151
Rhubarb 155
Sorrel (Sheep's) 178
Sorrel (Wood) 178
Stonecrop 184
Swallow-wort 188
Tormentil 193

Fluxes
Alder (Black) 12
Alkanet 14
Avens 20
Barley 22
Bilberries 28
Chestnut Tree 45
Cinquefoil 47
Comfrey 50
Dock (Common) 60
Eglantine 65
Flixweed or Fluxweed 80
Fluellein 80
Gall-oak 82
Green (Winter) 89
Hemp 94
Holly 97
Hollyhocks 98
Horestail 100
Hound's Tongue 101
Juniper Tree 105
Lady's Mantle 108
Lentils 111
Lettuce (Great Wild) 112
Lily (Water) 113
Loosestrife 115
Meadowsweet 123
Moneywort 127

Mulberry Tree 129
Mullein (Great) 130
Oak Tree 134
Orpine 137
Plantain 145
Plums 147
Poppy (Wild) 150
Quince Tree 151
Rattle Grass 154
Rhubarb (Culinary or Tart) 156
Rice 157
Rose (Damask) 158
Shepherd's Purse 171
Sloe Bush 174
Solomon's Seal 176
Sorrel (Common) 177
Stonecrop 184
Tansy 189
Tormentil 193
Wheat 199
Willowherb (Hairy) 199
Willow Tree 200

Flux of blood
Agrimony 10
Amaranthus 15
Balm 21
Barberry 22
Beets 26
Bilberries 28
Bistort 29
Blackberry 30
Burnet 35
Cinquefoil 47
Cleavers 48
Comfrey 50
Cudweed 54
Fig Tree 75
Fleabane (Small) 79
Gall-oak 82
Golden Rod 87
Hart's Tongue 90
Hollyhocks 98
Ivy 104
Juniper Tree 105
Knotgrass 107
Lily (Water) 113
Loosestrife 115
Moneywort 127
Myrtle Tree 132
Oak Tree 134
Orpine 137
Rattle Grass 154
Rhubarb (Great Monk's) 156
Sanicle 164
Shepherd's 171
Strawberries 185
Tormentil 193

Gangrenes
Bugle 34
Darnel 56
Hellebore (Black) 93
Nettle (Common) 132
Southernwood 179
Walnut 198
Gout
Alehoof 13
Angelica 16
Archangel 17
Asparagus 20
Balm 21
Barley 22
Beans (Broad) 25
Betony (Wood) 27
Centaury 42
Cinquefoil 47
Comfrey 50
Cuckoo-pint 52

Daisy 54
Dove's-foot 63
Elder (Dwarf) 66
Endive 68
Fennel 71
Germander 84
Gladwin 85
Goat's Rue 86
Goutweed 88
Ground Pine (Common) 89
Hellebore (Black) 93
Hemlock 94
Hemp 94
Henbane (Common) 95
Henry (Good) 95
Houseleek 101
Hyssop (Hedge) 103
Juniper Tree 105
Kidneywort 105
Mullein (Great) 130
Mustard (Black) 131
Pellitory of Spain 141
Plantain 145
Sow-thistle (Tree) 181
Thyme 192
Trefoil 194
Vervain (Common) 195
Wallflower (Common) 198
Wormwood 203
Wormwood (Roman) 203

Haemorrhoids
Catmint 40
Celandine (The Lesser) 41
Chickweed 45
Colt's Foot 49
Comfrey 50
Cuckoo-pint 52
Elder (Dwarf) 66
Figwort 76
Fleur-de-lys (Garden or Blue) 79
Garlic 83
Hound's Tongue 101
Juniper Tree 105
Kidneywort 105
Mulberry Tree 129
Mullein (Black) 129
Mullein (Great) 130
Pellitory of the Wall 141
Silverweed 172
Sow-thistle Tree (Marsh) 181
Stonecrop 184
Tobacco 192
Yarrow 204
Headaches
Bay Tree 24
Beets 26
Betony (Wood) 27
Burnet 35
Catmint 40
Fennel (Sow or Hog's) 71
Hops 99
Houseleek 101
Ivy 104
Lavender 110
Lettuce (Common Garden) 111
Marjoram (Common Wild) 120
Melilot 123
Mint (Garden or Spear) 125
Orach 136
Pellitory of Spain 141
Pennyroyal 142
Plantain 145
Sage (Common garden) 162
Self-heal 170
Succory (Wild) 186
Tea 190
Thyme (Wild) 192

Valerian (Greek) 194
Valerian (True Wild) 195
Heart disease
Borage 31
Burnet 35
Gentian (Autumn) 84
Green (Winter) 89
Lettuce (Common Garden) 111
Lily of the Valley 113
Motherwort 128
Mustard (Black) 131
Valerian (Greek) 194
Valerian (True Wild) 195
Hysteria
Dittany (White) 59
Horehound (Black) 99
Mint (Water) 126
Periwinkle (Great) 144
Saffron 160
Soldier (Common Water) 176
Valerian (Greek) 194
Wormseed (Treacle) 202

Impostumes
Agrimony (Water) 11
Arssmart 18
Barley 22
Beans (Broad) 25
Chickweed 45
Dill 58
Fenugreek 72
Flax 77
Garlic 83
Gladiole (Water) 85
Goat's Beard 86
Knotgrass 107
Lily (White Garden) 114
Marsh Mallow 121
Ragwort 153
Trefoil 194
Inflammations
Adder's Tongue 9
Alder (Common) 12
Alkanet 14
Arssmart 18
Barley 22
Beans 25
Brook-lime 32
Cherries (Winter) 43
Cinquefoil 47
Clary 46
Colt's Foot 49
Daffodil 54
Daisy 54
Dog's Grass 62
Endive 68
Flax 77
Gall-oak 82
Gladiole (Water) 85
Gooseberry 88
Green (Winter) 89
Groundsel (Common) 90
Hemlock 94
Hemp 94
Henbane (Common) 95
Herb True-love 97
Horsetail 100
Houseleek 101
Kidneywort 105
Lichen (Dog) 112
Marsh Mallow 121
Melilot 123
Mushroom (Garden) 130
Nightshade (Common 133
Nightshade (Deadly) 134
Oak Tree 134
Orpine 137
Plantain 145

Rhubarb (Great Monk's) 156
Shepherd's Purse 171
Sorrel (Common) 177
Sow-thistle Tree (Marsh) 181
Strawberries 185
Succory (Wild) 186
Sundew 187
Vine Tree 196
Wallflower (Common) 198
Yarrow 204
Itch
Agrimony (Water) 10
Alder (Black) 12
Alehoof 13
Barberry 22
Barley 22
Bay Tree 24
Beets 26
Borage 31
Carduus Benedictus 39
Chickweed 45
Dock (Common) 60
Fumitory 81
Heart's Ease 92
Hops 99
Horehound (White) 100
Lady's Bedstraw 107
Lavender (Cotton) 110
Marjoram (Common Wild) 120
Nettle (Common) 132
Oats 135
Plantain 145
Scabious (Field) 168
Soapwort 175
Sorrel (Common) 177

Jaundice
Agrimony 10
Alder (Black) 12
Alehoof 13
Alkanet 14
Arrach (Garden) 17
Ash Tree 19
Barberry 22
Bay Tree 24
Beets 26
Betony (Wood) 27
Bistort 29
Borage 31
Burnet 35
Calamint 37
Carduus Benedictus 39
Centaury 42
Chamomile 43
Cinquefoil 47
Cleavers 48
Dandelion 56
Dodder of Thyme 60
Elder (Dwarf) 66
Eryngo 69
Fennel 71
Flaxweed 78
Fleur-de-lys (Garden or Blue) 79
Fumitory 81
Garlic 83
Germander 84
Groundsel (Common) 90
Hellebore (Black) 93
Hemp 94
Hops 99
Horehound (White) 100
Hyssop 103
Hyssop (Hedge) 103
Lavender (Cotton) 110
Lichen (Dog) 112
Lungwort 116
Maidenhair (Common) 118
Maple Tree 119

Marjoram (Common Wild) 120
Mercury (French) 124
Mustard (Hedge) 131
Parsley (Common) 138
Parsley Piert 138
Parsley (Rock or Milk) 139
Peach Tree 140
Pennyroyal 142
Plantain 145
Rhubarb (Great Monk's) 156
Saffron (Wild) 161
Savine 166
Shepherd's Purse 171
Skirret 173
Smallage 174
Sorrel (Common) 177
Spikenard 182
Strawberries 185
Succory (Wild) 186
Swallow-wort 188
Vervain (Common) 195
Woodruffe (Squinancy) 201
Wormseed (Treacle) 202
Wormwood (Roman) 203

King's-evil
Archangel 17
Barley 22
Celandine (The Lesser) 41
Daisy (Little) 55
Eryngo 69
Figwort 76
Houseleek (Wall Pepper) 102
Kidneywort 105
Orchid 136
Ragwort 153
Rhubarb (Great Monk's) 156
Soldier (Common Water) 176
Stonecrop 184
Violet (Water) 197

Laxes
Alder (Black) 12
Barley 22
Beans (Broad) 25
Bilberries 28
Blackberry 30
Burnet 35
Cleavers 48
Dock (Common) 60
Dog's Grass 62
Flixweed or Fluxweed 80
Fluellein 80
Hart's Tongue 90
Hawthorn 91
Hazel Nut 92
Hemp 94
Horsetail 100
Ivy 104
Mint (Pepper) 126
Moneywort 127
Mulberry Tree 129
Mullein (Great) 130
Myrtle Tree 132
Rice 157
Willowherb (Hairy) 199
Walnut 198

Leprosy
Alkanet 14
Anemone 15
Barley 22
Bryony 32
Calamint 37
Darnel 56
Elm Tree 68
Fumitory 81
Hellebore (Black) 93
Oats 135

Pennyroyal 142
Scabious (Lesser Field) 168

Liver disorders
Agrimony 10
Agrimony (Water) 11
Alder (Black) 12
Balm 21
Barberry 22
Betony (Wood) 27
Bilberries 28
Burnet 35
Chickweed 45
Costmary 50
Cucumber 53
Daisy 54
Endive 68
Fleur-de-lys (Garden or Blue) 79
Goat's Beard 86
Gooseberry 88
Hart's Tongue 90
Hyssop (Hedge) 103
Kidneywort 105
Lettuce (Common Garden) 111
Lichen (Dog) 112
Maple Tree 119
Oak Tree 134
Orpine 137
Sage (Common Garden) 162
Shepherd's Rod 172
Skirret 173
Strawberries 185
Succory (Wild) 186
Sun Spurge 188
Vervain (Common) 195
Woodruffe (Squinancy) 201

Lung disorders
Agrimony (Water) 11
Alehoof 13
Angelica 16
Betony (Wood) 27
Bilberrues 28
Colt's Foot 49
Comfrey 50
Daisy (Little) 55
Elecampane 67
Fennel 71
Fenugreek 72
Fig Tree 75
Fir Tree 76
Flax 77
Goat's Beard 86
Heart's Ease 92
Horehound (White) 100
Hyssop 103
Knapwort (Harshweed) 106
Liquorice 115
Lovage 116
Lungwort 116
Maidenhair (Common) 118
Marsh Mallow 121
Masterwort 122
Moneywort 127
Mustard (Hedge) 131
Nettle (Common) 132
Orpine 137
Peach Tree 140
Pellitory of the Wall 141
Poppy (Wild) 150
Rocket Cress 157
Rue (Garden) 160
Saffron (Wild) 161
Sanicle 164
Scabious (Field) 168
Vervain (Common) 195
Violet 196

Measles
Alkanet 14

Goat's Rue 86
Saffron 160

Morphew
Alkanet 14
Bryony 32
Cucumber 53
Darnel 56
Dock (Common) 60
Fig Tree 75
Flaxweed 78
Hops 99
Lily (Water) 113
Madder 117
Scabious (Lesser Field) 168
Tansy 189

Mumps
Cudweed 54

Nausea
Mint (Pepper) 126

Nervous complaints
Knapwort (Harshweed) 106
Marjoram (Common Wild) 120
Mistletoe 127
Mustard (White) 132
Poppy (White or Opium) 149
Tea 190
Thyme (Wild) 192
Valerian (Greek) 194
Valerian (True Wild) 195

Obstructions
Alehoof 13
Angelica 16
Avens 20
Bay Tree 24
Beets 26
Betony (Wood) 27
Borage 31
Bryony 32
Butcher's Broom 36
Calamint 37
Celandine (The Greater) 41
Centaury 42
Dandelion 56
Dittany of Crete 59
Dodder of Thyme 60
Dog's Grass 62
Eryngo 69
Fennel 71
Flag (Yellow) 77
Flaxweed 78
Foxglove 80
Fumitory 81
Gentian (Autumn) 84
Germander 84
Hart's Tongue 90
Hemp 94
Honeysuckle 98
Hops 99
Horehound (Black) 99
Horehound (White) 100
Lavender 110
Lavender (Cotton) 110
Madder 117
Marjoram (Sweet) 120
Parsley (Common) 138
Parsnip (Upright Water) 139
Plantain 145
Rest-harrow 155
Saltwort 163
Scurvy-grass 170
Smallage 174
Sow-thistle (Common) 180
Succory (Wild) 186
Wallflower (Common) 198
Woodruffe (Squinancy) 201
Woodruffe (Sweet) 202

Wormwood (Roman) 203

Palsy
Bay Tree 24
Betony (Wood) 27
Bryony 32
Chickweed 45
Cowslip 51
Daisy 54
Fennel (Sow or Hog's) 71
Ground Pine (Common) 89
Juniper Tree 105
Lavender 110
Lily of the Valley 113
Mistletoe 127
Pellitory of Spain 141
Rosemary 159
Sage (Common Garden) 162
Sage (Wood) 162
St John's Wort 163
Savory (Summer) 166
Spikenard 182
Wallflower (Common) 198

Phthysis
Angelica 16
Chervill 44
Honeysuckle 98
Pellitory of Spain 141
Saffron (Wild) 161

Plague
Alehoof 13
Angelica 16
Avens 20
Bistort 29
Blue-bottle 31
Butter-bur 37
Carduus Benedictus 39
Chervil 44
Cuckoo-pint 52
Devil's Bit 57
Elecampane 67
Fumitory 81
Garlic 83
Ivy 104
Lily (White Garden) 114
Sage (Common Garden) 162
Scabious (Lesser Field) 168
Tormentil 193
Wheat 199

Quinsy
Blackberry 30
Cinquefoil 47
Cudweed 54
Hyssop 103
Lovage 116
Mushroom (Garden) 130
Orpine 137
Pepper 143
Pepper (Guinea) 143
Ragwort 153
Violet 196

Rein or kidney disorders
Amaranthus 15
Asparagus 20
Beans (French) 25
Bistort 29
Bryony 32
Clary 46
Comfrey 50
Dodder of Thyme 60
Eglantine 65
Eryngo 69
Fennel (Sow or Hog's) 71
Hawkweed 91
Kidneywort 105
Lavender (Cotton) 110

Lichen (Dog) 112
Liquorice 115
Maidenhair (Common) 118
Parsley (Rock or Milk) 139
Plantain 145
Sanicle 164
Strawberries 185
Succory (Wild) 186
Vervain (Common) 195
Wallflower (Common) 198
Yarrow 204

Rheumatic diseases
Angelica 16
Bay Tree 24
Germander 84
Ground Pine (Common) 89
Laurel (Spurge) 109
Mustard (White) 132
Orach 136
Pellitory of Spain 141
Savine 166
Staves-acre 184
Tobacco 192
Wormseed (Treacle) 202

Rickets
Down or Cotton-thistle 64

Ruptures
Avens 20
Betony (Wood) 27
Bistort 29
Calamint 37
Comfrey 50
Crosswort 51
Cudweed 54
Dove's-foot 63
Fern (Royal) 73
Gentian (Autumn) 84
Golden Rod 87
Hollyhocks 98
Horsetail 100
Juniper Tree 105
Lady's Mantle 108
Marsh Mallow 121
Solomon's Seal 176
Tormentil 193

St Anthony's Fire
Alkanet 14
Beets 26
Colt's Foot 49
Gooseberry 88
Hemlock 94
Houseleek 101
Kidneywort 105
Rue (Garden) 160
Shepherd's Purse 171
Succory (Wild) 186

Sciatica
Alehoof 13
Angelica 16
Archangel 17
Asparagus 20
Beans (Broad) 25
Centaury 42
Cinquefoil 47
Daisy 54
Darnel 56
Dittander (Karse) 58
Faverel (Wooly) 70
Fennel (Sow or Hog's) 71
Gladwin 85
Goutweed 88
Ground Pine (Common) 89
Hellebore (Black) 93
Henbane (Common) 95
Hyssop (Hedge) 103
Juniper Tree 105
Kidneywort 105

Madder 117
Mugwort (Common) 128
Mustard (Black) 131
Mustard (Hedge) 131
Mustard (White) 132
Pellitory of Spain 141
Poplar (White) 148
Radish (Wild or Horse) 152
Ragwort 153
Rue (Garden) 160
St John's Wort 163
Savory (Summer) 166
Sun Spurge 188
Tansy 189
Thyme 192

Scurvy
Dog Rose 61
Fir Tree 76
Ground Pine (Common) 89
Henry (Good) 95
Houseleek (Wall Pepper) 102
Juniper Tree 105
Lady's Smock 108
Mallow (Common) 118
Mustard (White) 132
Radish (Common Garden) 152
Radish (Wild or Horse) 152
Savine 166
Scurvy-grass 170
Sorrel (Sheep's) 178
Sun Spurge 188
Wormwood (Sea) 204

Shingles
Cinquefoil 47
Houseleek 101
Nightshade (Common) 133
Plantain 145

Skin diseases
Cucumber 53
Daisy (Little) 55
Lupin 117
Madder 117
Marsh Mallow 121
Rampion (Sheep's) 153
Scurvy-grass 170
Sun Spurge 188
Tansy 189

Smallpox
Alkanet 14
Bistort 29
Goat's Rue 86
Saffron 160

Spleen disorders
Agrimony (Water) 11
Alder (Black) 12
Alkanet 14
Archangel 17
Balm 21
Centaury 42
Dodder of Thyme 60
Fennel (Sow or Hog's) 71
Fern (Brake or Bracken) 73
Fern (Royal) 73
Fleur-de-lys (Garden or Blue) 79
Hawkweed 91
Ivy 104
Maple Tree 119
Melilot 123
Mustard (Black) 131
Nettle (Common) 132
Strawberries 185
Sun Spurge 188
Thyme 192
Vervain (Common) 195

Splinters
Agrimony 10
Archangel 17
Bryony 32

Clary 46
Darnel 56
Gladwin 85
Hawthorn 91
Mustard (Black) 131
Scabious (Lesser Field) 168
Southernwood 179

Spots and blemishes
Avens 20
Beans (Broad) 25
Bryony 32
Butter-bur 37
Centaury 42
Cowslip 51
Cucumber 53
Dock (Common) 60
Flaxweed 78
Garlic 83
Hops 99
Kidneywort 105
Lily (Water) 113
Lovage 116
Oats 135
Onion 135
Sarsaparilla 165
Scabious (Lesser Field) 168
Tansy 189
Willow Tree 200

Stomach disorders
Alder (Black) 12
Anemone 15
Ash Tree 19
Avens 20
Betony (Wood) 27
Caraway 38
Chervill 44
Clary (Wild) 47
Cucumber 53
Dog Rose 61
Endive 68
Fennel 71
Fern (Brake or Bracken) 73
Gentian (Autumn) 84
Gladwin 85
Goat's Beard 86
Gooseberry 88
Hart's Tongue 90
Horehound (Black) 99
Juniper Tree 105
Kidneywort 105
Lady's Smock 108
Lavender 110
Lovage 116
Marjoram (Common Wild) 120
Masterwort 122
Mint (Garden or Spear) 125
Mint (Pepper) 126
Mustard (Black) 131
Orpine 137
Parsley (Common) 138
Pear Tree 140
Pennyroyal 142
Pepper 143
Pepper (Guinea) 143
Poppy (Wild) 150
Rhubarb (Culinary or Tart) 156
Rose (Damask) 158
Rosemary 159
Saffron 160
Sauce-alone 165
Sorrel (Common) 177
Sorrel (Wood) 178
Sow-thistle Tree (Marsh) 181
Strawberries 185
Sumach 186
Tea 190
Vervain (Common) 195
Walnut 198

Woofruffe (Squinancy) 201
Wormwood (Sea) 204

Stones and gravel
Alkaret 14
Asparagus 20
Bay Tree 24
Beans 25
Beans (French) 25
Betony (Wood) 27
Birch Tree 28
Blackberry 30
Burnet 35
Carrot (Wild) 39
Cherries (Winter) 43
Columbine 49
Dittany (White) 59
Dog Rose 61
Dove's-foot 63
Dropwort 64
Elder (Dwarf) 66
Elecampane 67
Eryngo 69
Feverfew 74
Fir Tree 76
Flax 77
Fleur-de-lys (Garden or Blue) 79
Gentian (Autumn) 84
Goat's Beard 86
Golden Rod 87
Gooseberry 88
Groundsel (Common) 90
Hawthorn 91
Herb Robert 96
Hops 99
Horsetail 100
Juniper Tree 105
Kidneywort 105
Knotgrass 107
Lady's Bedstraw 107
Lady's Smock 108
Madder 117
Maidenhair (Common) 118
Mallow (Common) 118
Marsh Mallow 121
Masterwort 122
Mint (Garden or Spear) 125
Mint (Water) 126
Mugwort (Common) 128
Nettle (Common) 132
Parsley (Common) 138
Parsley Piert 138
Parsley (Rock or Milk) 139
Pellitory of the Wall 141
Pennywort (Common Marsh) 142
Plums 147
Radish (Common Garden) 152
Rest-harrow 155
Rhubarb (Great Monk's) 156
Samphire (Rock or Small) 164
Sauce-alone 165
Saxifrage (Great Burnet) 167
Sorrel (Common) 177
Sow-thistle (Common) 180
Spikenard 182
Vervain (Common) 195
Wormwood 203
Wormwood (Roman) 203

Strangury
Alexanders 14
Angelica 16
Asparagus 20
Burnet 35
Cherries (Winter) 43
Eglantine 65
Endive 68
Eryngo 69
Gladwin 85
Goat's Beard 86

212

Goat's Thorn 87
Groundsel (Common) 90
Horsetail 100
Juniper Tree 105
Knotgrass 107
Liquorice 115
Marjoram (Common Wild) 120
Mint (Garden or Spear) 125
Parsley Piert 138
Poplar (White) 148
Poppy (White or Opium) 149

Swellings
Arrach (Garden) 17
Arssmart 18
Balm 21
Brook-lime 32
Chamomile 43
Chickweed 45
Cinquefoil 47
Clary 46
Cleavers 48
Colt's Foot 49
Daffodil 54
Daisy 54
Devil's Bit 57
Dill 58
Endive 68
Fennel 71
Gall-oak 82
Garlic 83
Gladwin 85
Gooseberry 88
Hemlock 94
Herb Christopher 96
Herb True-love 97
Hyssop (Hedge) 103
Lily (White Garden) 114
Marsh Mallow 121
Mistletoe 127
Mullein (Great) 130
Mushroom (Garden) 130
Nightshade (Deadly) 134
Orchid 136
Plantain 145
Ragwort 153
Sage (Wood) 162
Sarsaparilla 165
Soldier (Common Water) 176
Southernwood 179
Succory (Wild) 186
Thyme 192
Trefoil 194
Violet 196
Wallflower (Common) 198

Tetanus
Jessamine 104

Tetters and ringworm
Barberry 22
Borage 31
Carduus Benedictus 39
Celandine (The Greater) 41
Darnel 56
Fumitory 81
Hops 99
Horehound (White) 100
Houseleek 101
Lichen (Dog) 112
Nightshade (Common) 133
Plantain 145
Plums 147
Sarsaparilla 165
Scabious (Lesser Field) 168
Sorrel (Common) 177
Wheat 199

Throat and mouth infections
Alehoof 13
Birch Tree 28

Cinquefoil 47
Cleavers 48
Columbine 49
Cuckoo-pint 52
Fig Tree 75
Fumitory 81
Hollyhocks 98
Honeysuckle 98
Hyssop 103
Knapweed (Common) 106
Lavender 110
Liquorice 115
Loosestrife 115
Marsh Mallow 121
Mint (Garden or Spear) 125
Mulberry Tree 129
Mullein (Great) 130
Mustard (Hedge) 131
Nettle (Common) 132
Nightshade (Common) 133
Oak Tree 134
Parsnip (Upright Water) 139
Peach Tree 140
Pepper 143
Plums 147
Poppy (Wild) 150
Quince Tree 151
Sage (Common Garden) 162
Sanicle 164
Silverweed 172
Sloe Bush 174
Vine Tree 196
Walnut 198
Wheat 199

Toothache
Alder (Black) 12
Angelica 16
Arssmart 18
Asparagus 20
Balm 21
Beets 26
Fennel (Sow or Hog's) 71
Fig Tree 75
Fleur-de-lys (Garden or Blue) 79
Hollyhocks 98
Lavender 110
Marjoram (Common Wild) 120
Mulberry Tree 129
Mullein (Great) 130
Pellitory of Spain 141
Pepper (Guinea) 143
Pomegranate Tree 148
Raspberry 154
Rest-harrow 155
Rhubarb (Great Monk's) 156
Rosemary 159
Sloe Bush 174
Sneezewort 175
Staves-acre 184
Tansy 189
Tobacco 192
Tormentil 193

Tumours
Alehoof 13
Archangel 17
Brook-lime 32
Celandine (The Lesser) 41
Clary 46
Devil's Bit 57
Dittander (Karse) 58
Endive 68
Flax 77
Gladwin 85
Groundsel (Common) 90
Herb Christopher 96
Herb True-love 97
Hound's Tongue 101
Jessamine 104

Lily (Water) 113
Lily (White Garden) 114
Marsh Mallow 121
Mayweed (Stinking) 122
Melilot 123
Mistletoe 127
Mullein (Great) 130
Nightshade (Deadly) 134
Orchid 136
Parsnip (Upright Water) 139
Sycamore Tree 189

Ulcers, sores, cankers and fistulas
Adder's Tongue 9
Agrimony 10
Alehoof 13
Alkanet 14
Anemone 15
Archangel 17
Arssmart 18
Asarabacca 18
Balm 21
Beets 26
Betony (Water) 26
Bistort 29
Blackberry 30
Borage 31
Bugle 34
Burdock (Greater) 35
Burnet 35
Butter-bur 37
Carduus Benedictus 39
Carrot (Wild) 39
Celandine (The Greater) 41
Chervil 44
Chickweed 45
Cinquefoil 47
Clown's Woundwort 48
Costmary 50
Crosswort 51
Cucumber 53
Daisy 54
Dandelion 56
Darnel 56
Dill 58
Dove's-foot 63
Elder (Dwarf) 66
Endive 68
Fenugreek 72
Fern (Brake or Bracken) 73
Fig Tree 75
Fir Tree 76
Flaxweed 78
Flixweed or Fluxweed 80
Fleur-de-lys (Garden or Blue) 79
Fluellein 80
Foxglove 80
Garlic 83
Green (Winter) 89
Hellebore (Black) 93
Hemlock 94
Herb Robert 96
Herb True-love 97
Horehound (Black) 99
Horehound (White) 100
Horsetail 100
Hound's Tongue 101
Houseleek 101
Ivy 104
Knotgrass 107
Lichen (Dog) 112
Lily (Water) 113
Lily (White Garden) 114
Lungwort 116
Lupin 117
Melilot 123

Mezereon Spurge 124
Mint (Garden or Spear) 125
Moneywort 127
Mustard (Hedge) 131
Nettle (Common) 132
Nightshade (Common) 133
Nightshade (Deadly) 134
Oats 135
Orpine 137
Parsnip (Upright Water) 139
Pellitory of the Wall 141
Pennyroyal 142
Plantain 145
Ragwort 153
Rattle Grass 154
Rest-harrow 155
Rhubarb (Great Monk's) 156
Rue (Garden) 160
Sage (Common Garden) 162
Sage (Wood) 162
Sanicle 164
Sarsaparilla 165
Sauce-alone 165
Scabious (Lesser Field) 168
Self-heal 170
Solomon's Seal 176
Sorrel (Common) 177
Stonecrop 184
Strawberries 185
Teasel 191
Tormentil 193
Vervain (Common) 195
Wheat 199
Wintergreen 201
Yarrow 204

Ulcers, mouth
Blackberry 30
Blue-bottle 31
Bugle 34
Daisy 54
Fumitory 81
Galingale 82
Golden Rod 87
Mustard (Hedge) 131
Pomegranate Tree 148
Ragwort 153
Sanicle 164
Scurvy-grass 70
Self-heal 170
Strawberries 185
Tormentil 193

Urine, bloody
Agrimony 10
Cherries (Winter) 43
Comfrey 50
Golden Rod 87
Plantain 145
Rhubarb (Culinary or Tart) 156
Wintergreen 201

Urine stoppage
Angelica 16
Asparagus 20
Bay Tree 24
Chives 46
Cowslip 51
Dog's Grass 62
Dropwort 64
Elder (Dwarf) 66
Elecampane 67
Germander 84
Gladwin 85
Goat's Beard 86
Hawkweed 91
Lavender 110
Marjoram (Sweet) 120
Pellitory of the Wall 141
Sow-thistle (Common) 180
Spignel (Broad-leaved) 182

Venereal disease
Araranthus 15
Bistort 29
Carduus Benedictus 39
Fir Tree 76
Golden Rod 187
Hops 99
Hound's Tongue 101
Laurel (Spurge) 109
Mezereon Spurge 124
Mint (Garden or Spear) 125
Sage (Woiod) 162
Sanicle 164
Sarsaparilla 165
Soapwort 175
Staves-acre 184
Vertigo
Bitter Sweet 30
Carduus Benedictus 39
Cowslip 51
Feverfew 74
Lily of the Valley 113
Lime Tree 114
Mistletoe 127
Sowbread 180
Vomiting/casting
Adder's Tongue 9
Bilberries 28
Bistort 29
Burnet 35
Calamint 37
Dill 58
Dog's Grass 62
Lady's Mantle 108
Mint (Garden or Spear) 125
Mint (Pepper) 126
Moneywort 127
Oak Tree 134
Peach Tree 140
Pennyroyal 142
Poppy (White or Opiuym) 149
Quince Tree 151
Raspberry 154
Rose (Damask) 158
St John's Wort 163
Solomon's Seal 176
Sorrel (Wood) 178
Tea 190
Wheat 199
Willow Tree 200

Warts and wens
Balm 21
Buckthorn 33
Celandine (The Greater) 41
Celandine (The Lesser) 41
Fig Tree 75
Figwort 76
Houseleek 101
Mercury (French) 124
Mugwort (Common) 128
Mullein (Great) 130
Poplar (Black) 148
Sundew 187
Teasel 191
Thyme 192

Whites
Adder's Tongue 9
Amaranthus 15
Archangel 17
Beets 26
Burnet 35
Comfrey 50
Eglantine 65
Fir Tree 76
Lavender (Cotton) 110
Lichen (Dog) 112
Mint (Garden or Spear) 125
Myrtle Tree 132
Oak Tree 134
Pomegranate Tree 148
Rosemary 159
Tansy 189
Violet (Water) 197
Yarrow 204
Wind
Alexanders 14
Angelica 16
Ash Tree 19
Bay Tree 24
Caraway 38
Carrot (Wild) 39
Catmint 40
Chervil 44
Devil's Bit 57
Dill 58
Dove's-foot 63
Elder (Dwarf) 66
Eryngo 69
Fennel 71
Fennel (Sow or Hog's) 71
Galingale 82
Hawkweed 91
Hemp 94
Juniper Tree 105
Lavender 110
Lovage 116
Marjoram (Common Wild) 120
Marjoram (Sweet) 120
Mayweed (Stinking) 122
Melilot 123
Mint (Pepper) 126
Mint (Water) 126
Oats 135
Parsley (Common) 138
Pellitory of the Wall 141
Pepper 143
Pepper (Gyinea) 143
Rosemary 159
Sarsaparilla 165
Sauce-alone 165
Savory (Winter) 167
Saxifrage (Great Burnet) 167
Sloe Bush 174
Smallage 174
Spignel (Broad-leaved) 182
Thyme 192
Wormwood (Roman) 203
Worms
Agrimony (Water) 11
Alkanet 14
Arssmart 18

Betony (Wood) 27
Bistort 29
Butter-bur 37
Centuary 42
Costmary 50
Cudweed 54
Devil's Bit 57
Dog's Grass 62
Dog's Tooth Violet 63
Eglantine 65
Fern (Brake or Bracken) 73
Fleur-de-lys (Garden or Blue) 79
Flixweed or Fluxweed 80
Garlic 83
Gentian (Autumn) 84
Goat's Rue 86
Groundsel (Common 90
Hemp 94
Hollyhocks 98
Hops 99
Horehound (Black) 99
Horehound (White) 100
Hyssop 103
Hyssop (Hedge) 103
Juniper Tree 105
Lavender (Cotton) 110
Motherwort 128
Mulberry Tree 129
Mustard (Hedge) 131
Nettle (Common) 132
Onion 135
Orchid 136
Peach Tree 140
Plantain 145
Radish (Wild or Horse) 152
St John's Wort 163
Savine 166
Sorrel (Common 177
Southernwood 179
Tansy 189
Thyme 192
Tobacco 192
Vervain (Common) 195
Wallflower (Common) 198
Wormseed (Treacle) 202
Wounds
Adder's Tongue 9
Alder (Common) 12
Alehoof 13
Alkanet 14
Archangel 17
Arssmart 18
Avens 20
Beans (Broad) 25
Betony (Water) 26
Blackberry 30
Blue-bottle 31
Burnet 35
Clown's Woundwort 48
Comfrey 50
Cowslip 51
Crosswort 51
Cudweed 54
Daffodil 54
Daisy 54
Daisy (Little) 55

Dittany of Crete 59
Dove's-foot 63
Eveweed or Double Rocket 69
Fern (Brake or Bracken) 73
Fern (Royal) 73
Fir Tree 76
Fleur-de-lys (Garden or Blue) 79
Foxglove 80
Germander 84
Gladiole (Water) 85
Gladwin 85
Golden Rod 87
Green (Winter) 89
Herb Robert 96
Herb True-love 97
Hollyhocks 98
Horsetail 100
Hound's Tongue 101
Knapweed (Common) 106
Knotgrass 107
Lady's Mantle 108
Lily (Water) 113
Loosestrife 115
Meadowsweet 123
Moneywort 127
Orpine 137
Pear Tree 140
Plantain 145
Plantain (Buck's Horn) 145
Plantain (Ribwort) 146
Ragwort 153
Sage (Common Garden) 162
Sage (Wood) 162
St John's Wort 163
Sanicle 164
Saxifrage (Great Burnet) 167
Self-heal 170
Shepherd's Purse 171
Solomon's Seal 176
Sycamore Tree 189
Tansy 189
Tormentil 193
Vine Tree 196
Willow Tree 200
Wintergreen 201
Yarrow 204
Wounds, inward
Agrimony 10
Alehoof 13
Avens 20
Betony (Water) 26
Bugle 34
Clown's Woundwort 48
Comfrey 50
Cudweed 54
Daisy 54
Dove's foot 63
Golden Rod 87
Lady's Mantle 108
Plantain 145
Palntain 'Buck's Horn) 145
Self-heal 170
Wintergreen 201
Wrinkles
Beans 25
Cowslip 51

ILLNESSES AND THEIR MODERN HERBAL CURES

Acne and spots
Burdock (Greater) 35
Elder 65
Figwort 76
Horsetail 100
Sorrel (Common) 177

Anaemia
Chervil 44
Nettle (Common) 132
Spinach 183
Strawberries 185
Vine Tree 196

Anorexia
Carduus Benedictus 39
Gentian (Autumn) 84
Appetite, loss of
Hops 99
Polypody 147

Rhubarb (Culinary or Tart) 156
Tarragon 190
Arthritis
Bryony 32
Golden Rod 87
Goutweed 88

Hyssop (Hedge) 103
Oats 135
Pepper (Guinea) 143
Pomegranate Tree 148
Poplar (Black) 148
Saffron (Meadow) 161
Smallage 174
Yew 205

Asthma
Anemone 15
Barley 22
Butter-bur 37
Colt's Foot 49
Daisy 54
Elecampane 67
Flixweed or Fluxweed 80
Germander 84
Hawkweed 91
Heart's Ease 92
Henbane (Common) 95
Honeysuckle 98
Horehound (White) 100
Masterwort 122
Mullein (Great) 130
Onion 135
Plantain (Ribwort) 146
Poppy (Wild) 150
Storax Tree 185
Sundew 187
Swallow-wort 188
Thorn-apple 191
Willowherb (Rosebay) 200

Baldness
Maidenhair (Common) 118
Southernwood 179

Biliousness
Barberry 22
Centaury 42

Bites and stings
Feverfew 74
Houseleek 101

Bladder sediment
Asparagus 20
Hart's Tongue 90
Onion 135
Plantain (Buck's Horn) 145

Bleeding, to stop
Avens 20
Clown's Woundwort 48
Holly 97
Hyacinth 102
Knotgrass 107
Periwinkle (Great) 144
Plantain (Ribwort) 146
Shepherd's Purse 171

Bleeding, internal
Bistort 29
Bugle 34
Dove's-foot 63
Fleabane (Canadian) 78
Herb Robert 96
Moneywort 127
Ploughman's Spikenard 146
Sanicle 164
Self-heal 170

Bleeding at the nose
Loosestrife 115
Yarrow 204

Bleeding, rectal
Amaranthus 15
Sumach 186

Blisters
Savine 166

Blood pressure, high
Chervil 44
Chives 46
Garlic 83

Horehound (Black) 99
Houseleek (Wall Pepper) 102
Hyssop 103
Lavender 110
Lime Tree 114
Nettle (Common) 132
Pomegranate Tree 148
Valerian (True Wild) 195
Yarrow 204

Boils and abscesses
Alehoof 13
Burdock (Greater) 35
Cudweed 54
Daisy (Little) 55
Fenugreek 72
Fig Tree 75
Figwort 76
Flax 77
Flixweed or Fluxweed 80
Hops 99
Ivy 104
Lily (Water) 113
Sage (Wood) 162
St John's Wort 163
Sorrel (Common) 177
Sow-thistle (Tree) 181

Bones, broken
Comfrey 50

Bowel disorders
Barley 22
Cinquefoil 47
Elm Tree 68
Fennel Flower 72
Flax 77
Peach Tree 140
Pennyroyal 142
Pennywort (Common Marsh) 142
Pepper (Guinea) 143
Pumpkin 151
Rhubarb (Culinary or Tart) 156
Silverweed 172
Sloe Bush 174
Solomon's Seal 176
Tea 190
Teasel 191

Bronchitis
Barley 22
Borage 31
Bryony 32
Chickweed 45
Colt's Foot 49
Comfrey 50
Cowslip 51
Cuckoo-pint 52
Daffodil 54
Dittander (Karse) 58
Elecampane 67
Elm Tree 68
Flax 77
Fluellein 80
Hart's Tongue 90
Hawkweed 91
Hollyhocks 98
Lungwort 116
Mullein (Great) 130
Mustard (Black) 131
Mustard (White) 132
Onion 135
Plantain (Ribwort) 146
Poplar (Black) 148
Poppy (Wild) 150
Storax Tree 185
Sundew 187
Thyme 192
Valerian (Greek) 194

Bruises
Elder 65
Fern (Royal) 73

Feverfew (Corn) 75
Knapweed (Common) 106
Marjoram (Sweet) 120
Solomon's Seal 176

Burns and scalds
Adder's Tongue 9
Flax 77
Goat's Thorn 87
Houseleek 101
Plantain (Ribwort) 146

Cancer
Carrot (Wild) 39
Down or Cotton-thistle 64
Hemlock 194
Mistletoe 127
Saffron (Meadow) 161
Violet 196

Catarrh
Archangel 17
Betony (Wood) 27
Dittander (Karse) 58
Down or Cotton-thistle 64
Eyebright 70
Fluellein 80
Heart's Ease 92
Holly 97
Honeysuckle 98
Jessamine 104
Knapweed (Common) 106
Lime Tree 114
Lungwort 116
Pear Tree 140
Poppy (Wild) 150
Pumpkin 151
Sorrel (Wood) 178
Squill 183
Storax Tree 185
Thyme (Wild) 192

Chest complaints
Bryony 32
Hyssop 103
Skirret 173
Spikenard 182

Childbirth/Pregnancy
Feverfew (Corn) 75
Raspberry 154

Cholera
Gall-oak 82

Circulatory problems
Chestnut Tree 45
Holly 97
Hyssop 103
Pepper (Guinea) 143

Colds
Borage 31
Butter-bur 37
Caraway 38
Carduus Benedictus 39
Colt's Foot 49
Elder 65
Garlic 83
Holly 97
Mallow (Common) 118
Sage (Wood) 162
Spikenard 182
Vervain (Common) 195

Colic
Calamint 37
Carrot (Wild) 39
Catmint 40
Mint (Garden or Spear) 125
Pennyroyal 142
Savory (Summer) 166
Saxifrage (Great Burnet) 167
Thyme 192

Colitis
Comfrey 50

Flax 77
Pear Tree 140

Constipation
Ash Tree 19
Asparagus 20
Buckthorn 33
Cherries (Winter) 43
Dock (Common) 60
Fern (Brake or Bracken) 73
Fig Tree 75
Fleur-de-lys (Garden or Blue) 79
Groundsel (Common) 90
Honeysuckle 98
Horehound (White) 100
Hyssop (Hedge) 103
Lichen (Dog) 112
Mulberry Tree 129
Mustard (White) 132
Peach Tree 140
Pear Tree 140
Plums 147
Polypody 147
Rhubarb (Great Monk's) 156
Saffron (Wild) 161
Sage (Common Garden) 162
Senna (Red-flowered Bladder) 171
Sorrel (Common) 177
Sorrel (Mountain) 177
Walnut 198
Wormseed (Treacle) 202

Consumption
Pine Tree 144

Convulsions
Jessamine 104
Paeony 137

Coughs
Agrimony 10
Calamint 37
Colt's Foot 49
Comfrey 50
Dropwort 64
Elecampane 67
Eryngo 69
Fir Tree 76
Flixweed or Fluxweed 80
Germander 84
Goat's Thorn 87
Hawkweed 91
Holly 97
Hollyhocks 98
Honeysuckle 98
Horehound (White) 100
Hyssop 103
Jessamine 104
Lady's Smock 108
Lettuce (Great Wild) 112
Lime Tree 114
Liquorice 115
Lungwort 116
Marjoram (Common Wild) 120
Maidenhair (Common) 118
Mallow (Common) 118
Mustard (Hedge) 131
Onion 135
Pine Tree 144
Polypody 147
Poppy (Wild) 150
St John's Wort 163
Squill 183
Swallow-wort 188
Trefoil 194
Vervain (Common) 195
Violet 196

Cramps
Clown's Woundwort 48
Pepper (Guinea) 143

Cuts and abrasions
Adder's Tongue 9

Crosswort 51
Fern (Royal) 73
Feverfew (Corn) 75
Knapweed (Common) 106
Saxifrage (Small Burnet) 168

Debility
Gentian (Autumn) 84
Diabetes
Beans (French) 25
Bilberries 28
Goat's Rue 86
Herb Robert 96
Knapwort (Harshweed) 106
Sumach 186
Diarrhoea
Amaranthus 15
Arssmart 18
Barberry 22
Barley 22
Betony (Wood) 27
Bilberries 28
Bistort 29
Blackberry 30
Dove's-foot 63
Elm Tree 68
Flag (Yellow) 77
Fleabane (Canadian) 78
Gall-oak 82
Herb Robert 96
Knotgrass 107
Lady's Mantle 108
Lily (Water) 113
Lime Tree 114
Lungwort 116
Meadowsweet 123
Mint (Water) 126
Nettle (Common) 132
Oak Tree 134
Orpine 137
Periwinkle (Great) 144
Plantain 145
Pomegranate Tree 148
Poplar (White) 148
Quince Tree 151
Raspberry 154
Rhubarb 155
Rhubarb (Culinary or Tart) 156
Rice 157
Sanicle 164
Savory (Summer) 166
Saxifrage (Small Burnet) 168
Shepherd's Purse 171
Sloe Bush 174
Solomon's Seal 176
Strawberries 185
Sumach 186
Tormentil 193
Vervain (Common) 195
Willowherb (Rosebay) 200
Willow Tree 200
Dropsy
Carrot (Wild) 39
Cleavers 48
Dandelion 56
Elm Tree 68
Flaxweed 78
Garlic 83
Holly 97
Lily of the Valley 113
Meadowsweet 123
Onion 135
Parsley (Common) 138
Pellitory of the Wall 141
Radish (Wild or Horse) 152
Rest-harrow 155
Sauce-alone 165
Shepherd's Purse 171

Dysentary
Amaranthus 15
Arssmart 18
Bilberries 28
Elm Tree 68
Fleabane (Small) 79
Gall-oak 82
Nettle (Common) 132
Poppy (Wild) 150
Poplar (White) 148
Quince Tree 151
Willow Tree 200
Dyspepsia
Alder (Common) 12
Alehoof 13
Angelica 16
Barberry 22
Blue-bottle 31
Caraway 38
Carduus Benedictus 39
Centaury 42
Gentian (Autumn) 84
Goat's Beard 86
Hops 99
Juniper Tree 105
Lichen (Dog) 112
Lime Tree 114
Meadowsweet 123
Plums 147
Savory (Winter) 167
Thyme 192
Wormwood 203

Earache
Chamomile 43
Mullein (Great) 130
Eczema
Arssmart 18
Birch Tree 28
Burdock (Greater) 35
Chickweed 45
Cleavers 48
Crowfoot 52
Dandelion 56
Dock (Common) 60
Figwort 76
Fir Tree 76
Fumitory 81
Golden Rod 87
Green (Winter) 89
Horsetail 100
Lavender 110
Nettle (Common) 132
Pine Tree 144
Scabious (Lesser Field) 168
Sorrel (Common) 177
Walnut 198
Epilepsy
Dittany (White) 59
Fennel 71
Hellebore (Black) 93
Kidneywort 105
Mistletoe 127
Nightshade (Common) 133
Paeony 137
Eye problems
Alehoof 13
Blue-bottle 31
Celandine (The Greater) 41
Clary (Wild) 47
Daisy (Little) 55
Elder 65
Eyebright 70
Herb Robert 96
Maidenhair (Common) 118
Melilot 123
Ragwort 153
Rose (Damask) 158

Fainting
Lavender 110
Fevers
Agrimony (Water) 11
Ash Tree 19
Avens 20
Balm 21
Borage 31
Butter-bur 37
Carduus Benedictus 39
Cherries (Winter) 43
Chestnut Tree 45
Devil's Bit 57
Fenugreek 72
Feverfew 74
Germander 84
Goat's Rue 86
Holly 97
Horehound (White) 100
Hyssop 103
Lovage 116
Lungwort 116
Mint (Water) 126
Motherwort 128
Mulberry Tree 129
Pennywort (Common Marsh) 142
Plums 147
Rice 157
Sorrel (Common) 177
Sorrel (Sheep's) 178
Swallow-wort 188
Valerian (Greek) 194
Vervain (Common) 195
Willow Tree 200
Wormwood 203
Flatulence
Angelica 16
Basil 23
Burnet 35
Caraway 38
Catmint 40
Chervil 44
Dill 58
Dropwort 64
Fennel 71
Juniper Tree 105
Lovage 116
Marjoram (Common Wild) 120
Masterwort 122
Melilot 123
Mint (Garden or Spear) 125
Mint (Pepper) 126
Pennyroyal 142
Pepper 143
Pepper (Guinea) 143
Rosemary 159
Saffron 160
Sage (Common Garden) 162
Savory (Summer) 166
Saxifrage (Great Burnet) 167
Tarragon 190
Thyme 192
Thyme (Wild) 192
Freckles
Alehoof 13
Elder 65

Gastro-intestinal disorders
Agrimony (Water) 11
Avens 20
Balm 21
Betony (Wood) 27
Burnet 35
Caraway 38
Clary 46
Dill 58
Dittany (White) 59
Dog's Mercury 62

Fennel Flower 72
Fenugreek 72
Feverfew (Corn) 75
Fumitory 81
Galingale 82
Golden Rod 87
Lady's Smock 108
Marsh Mallow 121
Oats 135
Peach Tree 140
Pennyroyal 142
Pepper 143
Polypody 147
Poplar (White) 148
Quince Tree 151
Rhubarb (Culinary or Tart) 156
Savory (Summer) 166
Savory (Winter) 167
Saxifrage (Small Burnet) 168
Silverweed 172
Solomon's Seal 176
Succory (Wild) 186
Tarragon 190
Thyme 192
Willowherb (Rosebay) 200
Woodruffe (Sweet) 202
Wormwood 203
Giddiness
Mint (Pepper) 126
Rue (Garden) 160
Gout
Ash Tree 19
Birch Tree 28
Bryony 32
Dandelion 56
Dock (Common) 60
Dog's Grass 62
Germander 84
Ground Pine (Common) 89
Nightshade (Deadly) 134
Primrose 150
Radish (Wild or Horse) 152
Saffron (Meadow) 161
Sarsaparilla 165
Sloe Bush 174
Sorrel (Wood) 178
Tansy 189

Haemorrhoids
Betony (Water) 26
Bistort 29
Catmint 40
Celandine (The Lesser) 41
Chestnut Tree 45
Chickweed 45
Figwort 76
Flaxweed 78
Gall-oak 82
Hemlock 94
Hound's Tongue 101
Houseleek 102
Houseleek (Wall Pepper) 102
Kidneywort 105
Knotgrass 107
Lungwort 116
Mayweed (Stinking) 122
Mullein (Great) 130
Oak Tree 134
Periwinkle (Great) 144
Plantain 145
Plantain (Ribwort) 146
Plums 147
Poplar (Black) 148
Self-heal 170
Silverweed 172
Solomon's Seal 176
Sow-thistle (Tree) 181
Yarrow 204

216

Hay fever
Eyebright 70
Onion 135
Headaches and migraine
Betony (Wood) 27
Butter-bur 37
Carduus Benedictus 39
Chamomile 43
Feverfew 74
Houseleek 101
Lime Tree 114
Poplar (White) 148
Primrose 150
Rosemary 159
Rue (Garden) 160
Sowbread 180
Viper's Bugloss 197
Heart disease
Butter-bur 37
Eryngo 69
Foxglove 80
Garlic 83
Hawthorn 91
Lavender 110
Lily of the Valley 113
Marsh Mallow 121
Mistletoe 127
Motherwort 128
Oats 135
Poppy (Wild) 150
Wallflower (Common) 198
Hiatus hernia
Comfrey 50
Hoarseness/Laryngitis
Mustard (Hedge) 131
Sage (Common Garden) 162
Sundew 187

Inflammations
Borage 31
Carduus Benedictus 39
Chickweed 45
Devil's Bit 57
Feverfew (Corn) 75
Nightshade (Common) 133
Nightshade (Deadly) 134
St John's Wort 163
Soldier (Common Water) 176
Sow-thistle (Common) 180
Teasel 191
Viper's Bugloss 197
Influenza
Colt's Foot 49
Holly 97
Yarrow 204
Insomnia
Catmint 40
Cowslip 51
Hops 99
Melilot 123
Mint (Pepper) 126
Poppy (Wild) 150
Primrose 150
Valerian (True Wild) 195
Woodruffe (Sweet) 202
Itch
Fir Tree 76
Ploughman's Spikenard 146

Jaundice
Barberry 22
Butcher's Broom 36
Centaury 42
Dodder of Thyme 60
Flaxweed 78
Parsley (Common) 138
Soapwort 175
Succory (Wild) 186

Kidney disorders
Agrimony (Water) 11
Alehoof 13
Beets 26
Bitter Sweet 30
Burdock (Greater) 35
Clary 46
Cucumber 53
Dodder of Thyme 60
Figwort 76
Fleabane (Canadian) 78
Holly 97
Lupin 117
Sorrel (Sheep's) 178

Leprosy
Pennywort (Common Marsh) 142
Leucorrhoea
Amaranthus 15
Archangel 17
Bistort 29
Dove's-foot 63
Flag (Yellow) 77
Gall-oak 82
Hyacinth 102
Lily (Water) 113
Oak Tree 134
Pomegranate Tree 148
Sanicle 164
Self-heal 170
Tormentil 193
Violet (Water) 197
Leukaemia
Saffron (Meadow) 161
Lice, head
Staves-acre 184
Liver disorders
Arssmart 18
Barberry 22
Celandine (The Greater) 41
Dodder of Thyme 60
Flaxweed 78
Fleur-de-lys (Garden or Blue) 79
Fumitory 81
Hart's Tongue 90
Hellebore (White) 93
Lichen (Dog) 112
Madder 117
Paeony 137
Poplar (White) 148
Radish (Common Garden) 152
Succory (Wild) 186
Vine Tree 196
Wormwood 203
Lumbago
Fern (Royal) 73
Lung disorders
Arssmart 18
Borage 31
Dittander (Karse) 58
Horehound (White) 100
Liquorice 115
Mullein (Black) 129
Mullein (Great) 130
Mustard (Black) 131
Valerian (Greek) 194

Malaria
Willow Tree 200
Mastitis
Figwort 76
Measles
Pennyroyal 142
Saffron (Wild) 161
Menopause
Balm 21
Motherwort 128

Menstrual problems
Agrimony (Water) 11
Amaranthus 15
Archangel 17
Balm 21
Butcher's Broom 36
Carduus Benedictus 39
Chamomile 43
Feverfew 74
Figwort 76
Flag (Yellow) 77
Germander 84
Golden Rod 87
Gooseberry 88
Ground Pine (Common) 89
Herb Christopher 96
Horehound (Black) 99
Jessamine 104
Lady's Mantle 108
Laurel (Spurge) 109
Lavender (Cotton) 110
Loosestrife 115
Lovage 116
Lupin 117
Madder 117
Marjoram (Sweet) 120
Masterwort 122
Mayweed (Stinking) 122
Mint (Water) 126
Motherwort 128
Mugwort (Common) 128
Parsley (Common) 138
Pennyroyal 142
Periwinkle (Great) 144
Ploughman's Spikenard 146
Raspberry 154
Rue (Garden) 160
Saffron 160
Saffron (Wild) 161
Sage (Common Garden) 162
Sage (Wood) 162
Silverweed 172
Tansy 189
Wormwood 203
Yarrow 204
Milk, to promote flow
Goat's Rue 86
Nettle (Common) 132
Viper's Bugloss 197

Nasal congestion
Eyebright 70
Nausea and vomiting
Balm 21
Golden Rod 87
Lavender 110
Mint (Garden or Spear) 125
Mint (Pepper) 126
Nervous complaints
Anemone 15
Catmint 40
Chamomile 43
Dandelion 56
Dittany (White) 59
Feverfew (Corn) 75
Gladwin 85
Hellebore (Black) 93
Hellebore (White) 93
Hemp 94
Herb Christopher 96
Jessamine 104
Lavender 110
Lime Tree 114
Mezereon Spurge 124
Mint (Pepper) 126
Mistletoe 127
Motherwort 128
Mugwort (Common) 128

Oats 135
Pear Tree 140
Primrose 150
Rue (Garden) 160
Savory (Summer) 166
Smallage 174
Valerian (True Wild) 195
Viper's Bugloss 197
Neuralgia/Neuritis
Butter-bur 37
Chamomile 43
Melilot 123
Nightshade (Deadly) 134
St John's Wort 163
Solomon's Seal 176
Thorn-apple 191
Valerian (True Wild) 195
Yew 205

Oedema/Water retention
Asparagus 20
Carrot (Wild) 39
Dandelion 56
Elder (Dwarf) 66
Galingale 82
Meadowsweet 123
Rest-harrow 155

Parkinson's disease
Henbane (Common) 95
Pharyngitis
Alder (Common) 12
Lungwort 116
Saxifrage (Small Burnet) 168
Pleurisy
Chickweed 45
Comfrey 50
Swallow-wort 188
Valerian (Greek) 194
Poison, to counteract
Devil's Bit 57
Prolapse
Myrtle Tree 132
Prostatis
Archangel 17
Hemlock 94
Pumpkin 151

Quinsy
Woodruffe (Squinancy) 201

Respiratory disorders
Agrimony (Water) 11
Burnet 35
Chestnut Tree 45
Colt's Foot 49
Daffodil 54
Elder (Dwarf) 66
Jessamine 104
Lungwort 116
Maidenhair (Common) 118
Marsh Mallow 121
Ploughman's Spikenard 146
Polypody 147
Saxifrage (Small Burnet) 168
Soapwort 175
Swallow-wort 188
Rhinitis
Onion 135
Rheumatic diseases
Arssmart 18
Ash Tree 19
Asparagus 20
Bay Tree 24
Beans (French) 25
Birch Tree 28
Bitter Sweet 30
Borage 31

Bryony 32
Chickweed 45
Crowfoot 52
Cucumber 53
Dandelion 56
Dock (Common) 60
Dog's Grass 62
Dog's Mercury 62
Fir Tree 76
Germander 84
Goutweed 88
Ground Pine (Common) 89
Holly 97
Hyssop (Hedge) 103
Lavender 110
Marjoram (Common Wild) 120
Meadowsweet 123
Mezereon Spurge 124
Mustard (Black) 131
Mustard (White) 132
Nightshade (Deadly) 134
Pepper (Guinea) 143
Poplar (Black) 148
Primrose 150
Radish (Wild or Horse) 152
Sarsaparilla 165
Sloe Bush 174
Smallage 174
Sorrel (Wood) 178
Sowbread 180
Spikenard 182
Succory (Wild) 186
Thorn-apple 191
Wormseed (Treacle) 202
Yew 205

Scalp disorders
Maple Tree 119
Rosemary 159
Southernwood 179
Yucca or Jucca 205
Scarlet fever
Saffron (Wild) 161
Sciatica
Bryony 32
Dodder of Thyme 60
Nightshade (Deadly) 134
Pine Tree 144
Scurvy
Brook-lime 32
Dog Rose 61
Eveweed or Double Rocket 69
Lady's Smock 108
Scurvy-grass 170
Sexual problems
Herb (True-love) 97
Hops 99
Jessamine 104
Lettuce (Common Garden) 111
Lily (Water) 113
Orchid 136
Rhubarb (Culinary or Tart) 156
Rhubarb (Great Monk's) 156
Staves-acre 184
Skin diseases
Agrimony 10
Angelica 16
Birch Tree 28
Bitter Sweet 30
Buckthorn 33
Chickweed 45
Cleavers 48
Crowfoot 52
Comfrey 50
Cucumber 53
Dock (Common) 60
Elder 65
Figwort 76

Fir Tree 76
Flaxweed 78
Heart's Ease 92
Hemlock 94
Herb Robert 96
Lavender 110
Lily (Water) 113
Mandrake 119
Mezereon Spurge 124
Pear Tree 140
Pine Tree 144
Plums 147
Rice 157
Saffron (Wild) 161
Sage (Wood) 162
Sarsaparilla 165
Scabious (Lesser Field) 168
Soapwort 175
Solomon's Seal 176
Sorrel (Wood) 178
Sow-thistle (Tree) 181
Spikenard 182
Storax Tree 185
Teasel 191
Vine Tree 196
Sprains
Elder 65
Figwort 76
Mandrake 119
Stones, urinary tract
Butcher's Broom 36
Elder 65
Dog Rose 61
Fleabane (Canadian) 78
Gooseberry 88
Knotgrass 107
Parsley (Common) 138
Parsley Piert 138
Pellitory of the Wall 141
Plantain (Buck's Horn) 145
Rest-harrow 155
Saxifrage (Great Burnet) 167
Saxifrage (Small Burnet) 168
Sloe Bush 174
Sunburn
Cowslip 51
Swellings
Borage 31
Chickweed 45
Daisy (Little) 55
Dog's Tooth Violet 63
Figwort 76
Hops 99
Sow-thistle (Common) 180
Wheat 199

Tetanus
Jessamine 104
Throat and mouth infections
Alder (Common) 12
Amaranthus 15
Bistort 29
Burnet 35
Cinquefoil 47
Fenugreek 72
Flixweed or Fluxweed 80
Gall-oak 82
Herb Robert 96
Horsetail 100
Knapwort (Harshweed) 106
Lily (Water) 113
Liquorice 115
Pellitory of Spain 141
Pomegranate Tree 148
Raspberry 154
Rest-harrow 155
Sage (Common Garden) 162
Scurvy-grass 170

Self-heal 170
Sorrel (Wood) 178
Strawberries 185
Thyme 192
Thyme (Wild) 192
Tormentil 193
Woodruffe (Squinancy) 201
Thrombosis
Melilot 123
Thrush
Plantain 145
Thyroid enlargement
Fleur-de-lys (Garden or Blue) 79
Tonsilitis
Bistort 29
Comfrey 50
Sage (Common Garden) 162
Toothache
Celandine (The Greater) 41
Chamomile 43
Feverfew (Corn) 75
Pellitory of Spain 141
Saxifrage (Small Burnet) 168
Tumours
Cleavers 48
Dog's Tooth Violet 63
Down or Cotton-thistle 64
Mistletoe 127
Pumpkin 151
Tobacco 192
Trefoil 194
Violet 196

Ulcers and sores
Adder's Tongue 9
Betony (Water) 26
Catmint 40
Chickweed 45
Comfrey 50
Dog's Tooth Violet 63
Down or Cotton-thistle 64
Fenugreek 72
Fern (Brake or Bracken) 73
Fleabane (Small) 79
Golden Rod 87
Herb Robert 96
Houseleek (Wall Pepper) 102
Ivy 104
Lily (Water) 113
Lily (White Garden) 114
Liquorice 115
Lupin 117
Plantain (Ribwort) 146
Ragwort 153
Sage (Wood) 162
St John's Wort 163
Sauce-alone 165
Teasel 191
Tobacco 192
Tormentil 193
Walnut 198
Urinary tract disorders
Agrimony (Water) 10
Beans (French) 25
Butter-bur 37
Cleavers 48
Dog's Grass 62
Dropwort 64
Eryngo 69
Flax 77
Horsetail 100
Juniper Tree 105
Lady's Bedstraw 107
Mallow (Common) 118
Marsh Mallow 121
Nettle (Common) 132
Parsley Pert 138
Peach Tree 140

Plantain (Duck's Horn) 145
Pumpkin 151
Ragwort 153
Rest-harrow 155
Rice 157
Sloe Bush 174
Sorrel (Sheep's) 178
Sorrel (Wood) 178
Strawberries 185
Sumach 186
Wintergreen 201
Urine stoppage
Eryngo 69
Pellitory of the Wall 141
Poplar (White) 148

Vaginal discharge
Hyacinth 102
Lily (White Garden) 144
Strawberries 185
Venereal disease
Mezereon Spurge 124
Sarsaparilla 165
Soapwort 175
Spikenard 182
Walnut 198

Warts/Corns
Buckthorn 33
Celandine (The Greater) 41
Crowfoot 52
Fig Tree 75
Houseleek 101
Savine 166
Swallow-wort 189
Whooping cough
Chestnut Tree 45
Cowslip 51
Cuckoo-pint 52
Daffodil 54
Fluellein 80
Henbane (Common) 95
Peach Tree 140
Pennyroyal 142
Poppy (Wild) 150
Sundew 187
Thyme 192
Thyme (Wild) 192
Violet 196
Willowherb (Rosebay) 200
Worms
Cucumber 53
Lavender (Cotton) 110
Lupin 117
Mulberry Tree 129
Pomegranate Tree 148
Pumpkin 151
Southernwood 179
Wormseed (Treacle) 202
Wormwood 203
Wounds
Adder's Tongue 9
Betony (Water) 26
Comfrey 50
Daisy (Little) 55
Fenugreek 72
Garlic 83
Green (Winter) 89
Herb Robert 96
Moneywort 127
Plantain (Ribwort) 146
Ragwort 153
St John's Wort 163
Sanicle 164
Saxifrage (Small Burnet) 168
Shepherd's Purse 171
Soldier (Common Water) 176

INDEX

Figures in italics refer to illustrations.

Aaron's Rod 130
Abscess Root 194
Acer 119, *119*
    pseudoplatanus 189, *189*
Achillea millefolium 175, 204,
    204
    ptarmica 175, *175*
Aconite 9, *9*, 97, 129
    Wholesome 9
Aconitum anthora 9, *9*
    napellum 9
Actaea alba 96
    spicata 96, *96*
Adder's Tongue 9, *9*, 50, 63
    American 63
Adiantum aureum 118
    capillus veneris 118, *118*
Aegopodium podagraria 88, *88*
Aesculus hippocastanum 44
Agaric 10, *10*
Agaricus 10, *10*
    campestris 130, *130*
    emeticus 10, 130
Agrimonia eupatoria 10–11, *10*
Agrimony 10–11, *10*, 12, 55
    Bastard 11
    Water 11, *11*
Ajuga chamaepitys 89, *89*
    reptans 33, *33*, 89
Alcea rosea 98, *98*
Alchemilla arvensis 138, *138*
    vulgaris 108, *108*
Alder, Black 12, *12*
    Buckthorn 12
    Common 12–13, *12*
Alecost 50
Alehoof 13, *13*
Alexanders 14, *14*
Alkanna tinctoria 14, *14*
Alkannet 14, *14*
All-good 95
Alliaria officinalis 165, *165*
    petiolata 165, *165*
Allium cepa 135, *135*
    sativum 83, *83*
    schoenoprasum 45, *45*
Alnus glutinosa 12–13, *12*
    nigra 12, *12*
Althaea officinalis 98, 121, *121*
    rosea 98, *98*
Alum 26, 33, 121, 162, 193
Amanita muscaria 10, 130
    phalloides 10, 130
Amara dulcis 30
Amaranthus 15, *15*
Amaranthus hybridus 15, *15*
    hypochondriacus 15, *15*
Amygdalus persica 140, *140*
Anacyclus pyrethrum 141, *141*

Anemone 15, *15*
    Wood 15
Anemone hepatica 112
    nemorosa 15, *15*
Anethum graveolens 58, *58*
Angelica 16, *16*, 43, 122, 182
    Wild 14
Angelica archangelica 16, *16*
Aniseed 14, 37, 40, 43, 71, 138,
    147, 171, 182
Annual Mercury 124
Anthemis cotula 122, *122*
    nobilis 42, *42*
    pyrethrum 141, *141*
Anthora 9
Aphanes arvensis 138, *138*
Apium graveolens 174, *174*
Apple, Crab 127
Aquilegia vulgaris 49, *49*
Arage 17
Aralia hispida 67
    racemosa 182, *182*
Archangel 17, *17*
Arctium lappa 34, *34*
Arctostaphylos uva-ursi 149
Armoracia rusticana 152, *152*
Arnica 9, 85
Arrach 136
    Garden 17, *17*
Arssmart 18
    Dead 18
    Hot 18
    Mild 18
Artemisia abrotanum 179, *179*
    absinthium 203, *203*, 204
    campestris 179, *179*
    dracunculus 190, *190*
    maritima 204, *204*
    pontica 203, *203*
    vulgaris 128, *128*
Arum maculatum 52–3, *52*
Asarabacca 18–19, *19*
Asarum europaeum 18–19, *19*
Asclepias syriaca 188–9, *188*
    tuberosa 187
Ash Tree 19, *19*, 59, 115,
    127
Asparagus 20, *20*, 35, 65, 164,
    188
    Garden 20
    Prickly 20
Asparagus officinalis 20, *20*
    sativus 20, *20*
Aspen, Common 149
    Quaking 149
Asplenium scolopendrium 90, *90*
    ruta muraria 118
    trichomanes 118
Asperula cynanchica 201, *201*
    odorata 201, 202, *202*

Astragalus gummifer 87, *87*
Atriplex hortensis 17, *17*
    patula 136, *136*
Atropa belladonna 134, *134*
    mandragora 119, *199*
Autumn Gentian 84
Avena sativa 135, *135*
Avens 20–1, *20*

Baldmony 182
Ballota nigra 99, *99*
Balm 21, *21*
    Lemon 21
    Sweet 21
Balmony 84
Balsam Herb 50
Balsamita major 50–1, *50*
    vulgaris 50–1, *50*
Baneberry 96
Barberry 22, *22*
Barley 22–3, *22*, 54, 71, 114,
    121, 144, 149, 196
Basil 23, *23*
    Garden 23
    Sweet 23
Bastard Agrimony 11
    Hemp 11
    Pellitory 175
Bay Tree 24, *24*, 135, 160
Beans 111, 121
    Broad 25, *25*
    French 25, *25*
    Kidney 25
Bedstraw 48
Beech 116
Beet 26, *26*, 147, 158
    Common Red 26
    Common White 26, 147
    Sea 158
Bellis perennis 55, *55*
Berberis vulgaris 22, *22*
Berula erecta 139, *139*
Beta 26, *26*
    altissima 158, *158*
    maritima 26
    vulgaris 26
Beth 63
Betonica aquatica 26–7, *26*
    officinalis 27, *27*
Betony 137
    Paul's 80, *80*
    Water 26–7, *26*
    Wood 27, *27*
Betula alba 28, *28*
    pendula 28–9, *28*
Bidens tripartita 11, *11*
Bilberries 28, *28*
    Black 28
    Red 28
Bindweed, Field 169

Great White 169
    Hedge 169
    Jalap 169
    Syrian 169
Birch Tree 28–9, *28*
    European 28
    Silver 28
Bishop's-leaves 26
Bistort 29, *29*
Biting Stonecrop 102
Bitter Sweet 30, *30*
Bittercress 108
    Large 108
Black Haw 128
    Pot-herb 14
Blackberry 30, *30*, 137, 187
    American 30
Blackthorn 174
Bladder Senna, Common 171
    Red-flowered 171
Blessed Thistle 31, 38
Bloodroot 29
Bloodwort 60
Bluebell 102
Blueberry 187
Blue-blow 31
Blue-bottle 31, *31*
Borage 31, *31*, 197
Borago officinalis 31, *31*
Borax 169
Boy's Love 179
Box Tree 28
Bracken 73
Brake 73
Bramble 30
Brassica nigra 131, *131*
Briar, Sweet 65
    Wild 61
Brimstone-wort 71
Bristly Ox-tongue 109
Broad Beans 25
Broad-leaved Dock 60
    Spignel 182
Brook-lime 32, *32*
Broom 22, 70, 89
    Butcher's 35
Brown-wort 26
Bruisewort 55
Bruscus 35
Bryonia dioica 32, *32*, 119
Bryony 32, *32*
    Common White 32
Buchu 138
Buck's Horn Plantain 145
Buckthorn 33, *33*
    Purging 33
Bugle 33, *33*, 170
    Brown 33
    Common 89
    Yellow 89

Bugloss, Spanish 14
  Viper's 197
Bull's Foot 49
Bur Marigold 11
Burdock 60, 70, 182
  Greater 34, 34
Burnet 34–5, 34, 138
  Salad 34
  Saxifrage 167
Burning Bush 59
Butcher's Broom 35, 35
Butomus umbellatus 85, 85
Butter-bur 36, 36
Buttercup 52, 172
  Field 52
Butter-flowers 52

Calamint 36–7, 37
Calamintha ascendens 36–7, 37
Calystegia sepium 169, 169
Camellia thea 190, 190
Camphire 111
Cannabis sativa 94, 94
Capsella bursa-pastoris 171, 171
Capsicum 38, 70, 143
Capsicum frutescens 143, 143
Caraway 37, 37, 138, 171
Carbenia benedicta 31, 38, 38
Cardamine amara 108
  pratensis 108, 108
Cardamom Aromatica 37
Carduus benedictus 38, 38
Carrot 14, 26, 53, 62, 119, 152,
  158, 173
  Wild 38–9, 38
Carthamus tinctorius 161, 161
Carum carvi 37, 37
Cassia angustifolia 171
Castanea sativa 44, 44
Catchweed 48
Catmint 39, 39
Cat's-foot 13
Cayenne 143
Celandine 13
  Greater 40, 40
  Lesser 40–1, 40
Celery 53, 152
  Garden 174
  Wild 174
Centaurea cyanus 31, 31
  jacea 106, 106
  nigra 106
  scabiosa 106, 106
Centaurium erythraea 41, 41
Centaury 41, 41, 168
  Great 85
Chamaemelum nobile 42, 42
Chamomile 13, 22, 40, 42, 42, 47,
  55, 74, 75, 121, 123, 130, 141
  Common 42
  German 75
  Roman 42
  Stinking 122
  Wild 75
Chamomilla recucita 75, 75
Cheese-rennet 107
Cheiranthus cheiri 198, 198
Chelidonium majus 40, 40
Chenopodium bonus-henricus 95, 95

Cherries, Winter 42–3, 42
Chervil 43, 43
Chestnut 44, 44
  Horse 44
  Sweet 44
Chickweed 44–5, 44, 162, 163
  Wintergreen 89, 89
Chicory 186
  Wild 68
Chillies 143
Chinese Lantern 42
Chives 45, 45, 83
Christ's Eye 47
Chrysanthemum leucanthemum
  54–5, 55
  parthenium 74, 74
Cicely, Sweet 43
Cichorium endivia 68, 68
  intybus 68, 186, 186
Cinquefoil 20, 46, 46
  Creeping 46
Clary 46–7, 46
  Garden 46
  Wild 47, 47
Cleavers 48, 48
Clot-bur 34
Clover 194
  King's 123
  Red 164, 194
Clown's Woundwort 48, 48
Cnicus benedictus 38, 38
Cochlearia armoracia
  152, 152
  officinalis 170, 170
Cohosh, White 96
Colchicum autumnale 161, 161
Colewort 20
Colt's Foot 13, 49, 49, 55, 67,
  86, 100, 103, 116, 129, 140,
  157, 163, 195, 196
Columbine 49, 49
Colutea arborescens 171
  cruenta 171, 171
  orientalis 171, 171
Comfrey 48, 50, 50, 51, 70, 73,
  80, 85, 169, 181
  Greater 31
  Middle 33
Confound, Middle 33
Conium maculatum 94, 94
Convallaria majalis 113, 113
Convolvulus arvensis 169
  sepium 169, 169
  scammonia 169
Conyza canadensis 78, 78
Coral Necklace 107
Cornflower 31
Corylus avellana 92, 92
Costmary 50–1, 50
Cotinus coggygria 186–7, 186
Cotton Lavender 110–11
Cotton-thistle 64, 64
Cottonweed 54
Cotyledon umbilicus 105, 105
Couchgrass 62, 70, 169
Cough-wort 49
Cowslip 51, 51, 150
  Jerusalem 116
Crab Apple 127

Cramp Bark 128
Cranesbill 29, 63, 197
  American Wild 63
Crataegus monogyna 91–2, 91
Creeping Cinquefoil 46
  Jenny 127
  Water Parsnip 139
Cress 103
  Garden 58
Crithmum maritimum 164, 164
Crocus 161
  Garden 160
Crocus sativus 160, 160
Crosswort 51, 51
  Common 51
Crowfoot 52, 52
Cruciata laevipes 51, 51
Cuckoo Flower 108
Cuckoo-pint 52–3, 52
Cucumber 53, 53
Cucumis sativus 53, 53
Cucurbita pepo 151, 151
Cudweed 54, 54
  Marsh 54
Cumin 24
Curled Dock 60
Cuscuta epithymum 60–1, 61
Cyanus 31
Cyclamen 180
Cyclamen hederifolium 180, 180
Cydonia oblonga 151, 151
Cynoglossum officinale 101, 101
Cyperus, Sweet 82
Cyperus 82
  esculentus 82
  longus 82, 82
  odoratus 82

Daffodil 54, 54
  Common 54
  Wild 54
Dahlia 64
Daisy 42, 54–5, 55, 74, 128
  Field 13
  Greater Wild 55
  Little 55, 55
  Ox-eye 55
  Small 55
Damask Prunes 147
  Rose 158–9
Dame's Violet 69
Damiana 174
Dandelion 41, 56, 56, 86, 91,
  180, 182, 186, 189
Daphne laureola 109, 109
  mezereum 124–5, 124
Darnel 56–7, 57
Datura stramonium 191, 191
Daucus carota 38–9, 38
Dead Arssmart 18
Dead-nettle 17, 128
  Red 17
  White 17
  Yellow 17
Deadly Nightshade 133, 134
Death Cap Mushroom 130
Delphinium staphisagria 184, 184
Descurainia sophia 80, 80

Devil's Bit 57, 57
  Scabious 153
Dictamnus albus 59, 59
Digitalis 198
Digitalis purpurea 80–1, 81
Dill 37, 58, 58, 71, 139, 160
Dipsacus fullonum 191, 191
  pilosus 172, 172
  sylvestris 191, 191
Dittander, Karse 58, 58
Dittany, of Crete 59, 59
  White 59, 59
Dock 29, 81, 156
  Broad-leaved 60
  Common 60, 60
  Common Wayside 60
  Curled 60
  Round-leaved 60
  Yellow 60, 182
Dodder 12
  of Thyme 60–1, 61
Dog Lichen 112
  Rose 61, 61, 65, 190
Dog's Grass 62, 62
  Mercury 62, 62, 124
  Tooth Violet 63, 63
Double Rocket 69, 69
Dove's-foot 63, 63
Down Thistle 64, 64
Draba incana 70, 70
Dragon-wort 29
Dropwort 64, 64
  Tubular Water 64
  Water 64
Drosera anglica 187, 187
  rotundifolia 187
Dwarf Elder 55, 66–7

Echium vulgare 197, 197
Eglantine 65, 65
Elder 12, 38, 43, 49, 65–6, 65,
  126, 204
  Common 65, 66
  Dwarf 55, 66–7, 66
Elecampane 67, 67
Elfwort 67
Elm Tree 68, 68
  Slippery 68, 113, 121, 169
Elymus agropyrum 62, 62
  repens 62, 62
Enchusa 14
Endive 12, 68, 68, 123
  Garden 186
Endymion non-scripta 102, 102
English
  Mandrake 119
  Serpentary 29
Epilobium angustifolium 200, 200
  hirsutum 199, 199
Equisetum arvense 100–101, 100
Erigeron acer 173, 173
  canadense 78, 78
Eryngium campestre 69
  maritimum 69, 69
Ervum lens 111, 111
Eryngo 69, 69
  Field 69
Erysimum cheiranthoides 202, 202
Erythraea centaurium 41, 41

Erythronium americanum 63
  dens canis 63, *63*
Eruca sativa 157, *157*
Eupatorium 11
Euphorbia helioscopia 188, *188*
Euphorbium 24
Euphrasia officinalis 70, *70*, 154
European Birch 28
Eveweed 69, *69*
Eyebright 70, *70*, 154

False Hellebore 93
  Jacob's Ladder 194
Faverel Wooly 70, *70*
Featherfew 74
Felon-wort 30
Fennel 12, 14, 37, 58, 70, 71, *71*,
  138, 139, 147, 182
  Flower 72, *72*
  Hog's 71, *71*, 139
  Sow's 71, *71*, 139
Fenugreek 22, 45, 72, *72*, 121
Fern 73, *73*
  Royal 73, *73*
Feverfew 74, *74*
  Corn 75, *75*
Few-leaved Hawkweed 91
Ficus carica 75, *75*
Fig Tree 75, *75*, 115
Figwort 76, *76*
  Water 26
Filaginella uliginosa 54, *54*
Filipendula ulmaria 123, *123*
  vulgaris 64, *64*
Fir Tree 76–7, *76*, 144
Five-leaved Grass 46
Five-fingered Grass 46
Flag, Blue 79
  Common Blue 79
  Yellow 77, *77*, 79, 85
Flax 77, *77*
  Dodder 60
Flaxweed 78, *78*
Fleabane 173
  Blue 173
  Canadian 78, *78*, 173
  Common 79, 173
  Small 79, *79*
  Sweet 173
Flea-worts 23
Fleur-de-lys 77, 103
  Blue 79, *79*
  Garden 79, *79*
Flixweed 80, *80*
Floramor 15
Flower-gentle 15
Flowering Rush 85
Flower-velure 15
Fluellein 80, *80*
Fluxweed 80, *80*
Fly Agaric 130
Foal's-wort 49
Foeniculum vulgare 71, *71*
Foxglove 80–1, *81*, 93, 103, 113
Fragaria vesca 185, *185*
Frangula alnus 12, *12*
Fraxinus excelsior 19, *19*
French Beans 25
  Mercury 124

Frog's-foot 52
Fumaria officinalis 81, *81*
Fumitory 31, 81, *81*, 177
Furze 22

Galega officinalis 86, *86*
Galingale 82, *82*
Galium aparine 48, *48*
  cruciata 51, *51*
  odoratum 200, *200*
  verum 107, *107*
Gallion 107
Gall-oak 82–3, *82*
Gallwort 78
Garlic 45, 83, *83*, 165
  Crests, Common 165
  Mustard 165
Gaultheria procumbens 89, 201
Gelwort 84
Gentian, Autumn 84, *84*
  Field 84
  Yellow 84
Gentiana amarella 84, *84*
  lutea 84
Gentianella amarella 84, *84*
  campestris 84
Geranium maculatum 63
  molle 63, *63*
  robertianum 96, *96*
German Chamomile 75
Germander 84–5, *84*
  Wall 84
Geum herbanum 20–1, *20*
  urbanum 20–1, *20*
Gill-creep-by-ground 13
Gill-go-by-ground 13
Ginger 147, 162, 171
Gladiole, Water 85, *85*
Gladwin 85, *85*
Glechoma hederacea 13, *13*
Glycyrrhiza glabra 115, *115*
Gnaphalium uliginosum 54, *54*
Goat-herb 88
Goat's Beard 86, *86*, 109
  Rue 86, *86*
  Thorn 87, *87*
Gold-cups 52
Golden Maidenhair 118
  Rod 87, *87*
Goldenseal 13, 73
Goldilocks 52
Goldknobs 52
Good Henry 95
  King Henry 95
Gooseberry 88, *88*
Goose-grass 48
Goutweed 88, *88*
Goutwort 88
Grape Vine 196
Grass, Dog's 62
  Five-fingered 46
  Five-leaved 46
Gratiola 103
Gratiola officinalis 103, *103*
Greek Hayes 72
  Valerian 194
Green, Winter 89, *89*
Ground Pine, Common 89, *89*
Ground-ivy 13, 49, 100, 118

Groundsel, Common 90, *90*
Guinea Pepper 143

Hairy Willowherb 199
Happy-major 34
Harshweed Knapwort 106
Hart's Tongue 90, *90*
Hart's-horn 33
Haw, Black 128
Hawkweed 91, *91*
  Few-leaved 91
  Mouse-eared 91
Hawthorn 81, 91–2, *91*, 127
Hay-maids 13
Hazel Nut 28, 92, *92*
Heart's Ease 16, 92, *92*
Heath 22
  Speedwell 80
Hedera helix 104, *104*
Hedge Bindweed 169
  Hyssop 103
  Mustard 80, 131
Hellebore, American 93
  Black 93, *93*
  False 93
  White 93, *93*
Helleborus niger 93, *93*
Helminthia echioides 109, *109*
Hemlock 43, 83, 94, *94*, 133
  Great 43, 94
  Water 64
Hemp 94, *94*
  Bastard 11
  Indian 94
  Water 11
Henbane 83, 133, 199
  Common 95, *95*
Henry, Good 95, *95*
Herb Bennet 20
  Christopher 96, *96*
  Paris 97
  Robert 96, *96*
  True-love 97, *97*
  Twopence 127
Herb-carpenter 33
Hesperis matronalis 69, *69*
Hieracium murorum 91, *91*
Hipatorium 11
Hoar-strange 71
Hoar-strong 71
Hog's Fennel 71, 139
Holly 97, *97*
  Sea 69
Hollyhocks 98, *98*
Holm 97
Holy Thistle 38
Honeysuckle 98, *98*, 162
  Meadow 194
  Perfoliate 98
Hops 12, 99, *99*
Hordeum vulgare 22–3, *22*
Horehound 13, 49, 67, 85, 86,
  103, 129, 157, 195
  Black 99, *99*
  Common 100
  White 99, 100, *100*
Horse Chestnut 44
  Parsley 14
  Radish 152

Horse-hoof 49
Horsetail 9, 31, 100–101, *100*
Hot Arssmart 18
Hottonia palustris 197, *197*
Hound's Tongue 101, *101*
Houseleek 101, *101*, 184
  Small 102, 184
  Wall Pepper 102, *102*
Housewort 154, 184
Hulver-bush 97
Humulus lupulus 99, *99*
Hurtsickle 31
Hyacinth 102, *102*
  Wild 102
Hyacinthoides non-scripta 102, *102*
Hydrastis canadensis 73
Hydrocotyle asiatica 142
  vulgaris 142, *142*
Hyoscyamus niger 95, *95*
Hypericum perforatum 163, *163*
Hyssop 24, 59, 91, 103, *103*
  Hedge 103, *103*
Hyssopus officinalis 103, *103*

Ilex aquifolium 97, *97*
Illecebrum verticillatum 107, *107*
Imperatoria ostruthium 122, *122*
Indian Hemp 94
  Pennywort 142
  Poke 93
Inula conyza 146, *146*
  helenium 67, *67*
Ipecacuanha 19, 69, 136, 157,
  196
Iris 77, 85
  Common 85
  Garden 79
  Stinking 85
Iris foetidissima 85, *85*
  germanica 79, *79*
  pseudacorus 77, *77*, 79
  versicolor 79
Iron Root 136
Ivy 104, *104*

Jack-by-the-hedge 165
Jack-go-to-bed-at-noon 86
Jacob's Ladder 194
  False 194
Jalap Bindweed 169
Jasione montana 153, *153*
Jasmine, White 104
Jasminum officinale 104, *104*
Jerusalem Cowslip 116
Jessamine 104, *104*
Jucca 205, *205*
Juglans regia 198, *198*
Juniper Tree 105, *105*, 138
Juniperus communis 105, *105*
  sabina 166, *166*
Jura 56

Karse Dittander 58
Kidney Beans 25
Kidneywort 105, *105*
King's Clover 123
Knapweed, Black 106
  Brown 106
  Common 106, *106*
  Greater 106

Knapwort, Harshweed 106, *106*
Knautia arvensis 168, *168*
Knee-holly 35
Kneeholm 35
Kneehulver 35
Knitbone 50
Knotbone 107, *107*, 163

Lactuca sativa 111, *111*
  virosa 112, *112*
Lad's Love 179
Lady's Bedstraw 107, *107*
  Mantle 108, *108*
  Smock 108, *108*
Lamium 17, *17*
Lang de Boeuf 109, *109*
Laurel, Spurge 109, *109*
Laurus nobilis 24, *24*
Lavender 27, 66, 110, *100*
  Cotton 110–11, *110*
Lavandula angustifolia 110, *110*
  officinalis 110, *110*
Leeks 83
Lemon Balm 21
Lens culinaris 111, *111*
Lentils 111, *111*
Leonurus cardiaca 128, *128*
Lepidium sativum 58, *58*
Lettuce, Common Garden 111, *111*
  Great Wild 112, *112*
  Prickly 112
  Salad 111
Lettuce-opium 112
Leucanthemum vulgare 54–5, *55*
Levisticum officinale 116, *116*
Lichen, American 112
  Dog 112, *112*
Lilium candidum 114, *114*
Lily, Madonna 114
  Meadow 114
  of the Valley 81, 113, *113*, 176, 201
  Water 113, *113*
  White 130
  White Garden 114, *114*
Lime Tree 114, *114*, 127, 195
Linaria vulgaris 78, *78*
Linden Tree 114
Linseed 22, 45, 77, 115, 121, 130, 192
Linum usitatissimum 77, *77*
Liquorice 115, *115*
Liverwort 112
Lluellin 80, *80*
Lobelia 70, 77
Lolium temulentum 56–7, *57*
Long Pepper 120, 143
Lonicera periclymenum 98, *98*
Loosestrife 115, *115*, 127
  Yellow 115
Lords and Ladies 52
Lovage 116, *116*, 182
Love in a Mist 72
Love Lies Bleeding 15
Lungwort 116–17, *116*, 129, 157
Lupin 117, *117*
  White 117

Lupinus albus 117, *117*
Lysimachia nummularia 127, *127*
  vulgaris 115, *115*, 127

Mace 50
Madagascar Periwinkle 144
Madder 117, *117*
Madonna Lily 114
Maidenhair, Common 118, *118*
  Fern 118
  Golden 118
  True 118
  White 118
Maidenhead 115
Maid-hair 107
Mallow 63, 147
  Common 118, *118*
  Common Marsh 98
  Marsh 29, 45, 48, 49, 100, 121, *121*, 138, 163, 169
  Wild 147
Malva sylvestris 118, *118*
Mandragora officinarum 119, *119*
Mandrake 119, *119*, 133
  American 119
  English 119
Mangel Wurzel 158
Maple Tree 119, *119*, 127, 189
  American Sugar 119
  Great 189
  Red 119
Marguerite 54
Marigold 73, 128, 197
  Bur 11
Marjoram 130
  Common Wild 120, *120*
  Field 120
  Sweet 59, 120–1, *120*
  Wild 59, 120
Marrubium vulgare 100, *100*
Marsh Cudweed 54
  Mallow 29, 45, 48, 49, 98, 100, 121, *121*, 138, 163, 169
  Pennywort, Common 142
  Sow Thistle 181
  Sow-thistle Tree 181
  Woundwort 48
Masterwort 122, *122*
Matricaria chamomilla 75, *75*
May Blossom 91
Mayweed Scented 75
  Stinking 122, *122*
Meadow Honeysuckle 194
  Lily 114
  Pimpernel 34
  Saffron 161
Meadowsweet 86, 123, *123*, 168
Melilot 22, 123, *123*
  Ribbed 123
Melilotus officinalis 123, *123*
Melissa calaminta 36–7, *37*
  officinalis 21, *21*
Mentha aquatica 126, *126*
  piperita 126, *126*
  pulegium 142, *142*
  spicata 125, *125*
  viridis 125, *125*
Mercurialis annua 62, *62*
  perennis 62, *62*

Mercury 95
  Annual 124
  Dog's 124
  French 124, *124*
Meum athamanticum 182, *182*
Mezereon Spurge 124–5, *124*
Middle Comfrey 33
  Confound 33
Mild Arssmart 18
Milfoil 204
Milk Parsley 139
Mint 142
  Garden 125, *125*
  Pepper 126, *126*
  Spear 125, *125*, 126
  Water 126, *126*
  Wild 170
Mistletoe 127, *127*, 195
Moneywort 127, *127*
Monk's Rhubarb 156
Mortal 30
Morus alba 129
  nigra 129, *129*
Motherwort 128, *128*, 150
Mountain Sorrel 177
  Spinach 17
Mouse-eared Hawkweed 91
Mugwort
  Common 128, *128*
Mulberry 30, 129, *129*
  Common Black 129
  Common White 129
Mullein 129
  Black 129, *129*
  Dark 129
  Great 130, *130*
  White 129
Mushroom, Death Cap 130
  Garden 130, *130*
  Poison 130
Mustard 80, 95
  Black 131, *131*
  Hedge 80, 131, *131*
  Treacle 202
  White 132, *132*
Myrrhis odorata 43, *43*
Myrtle 23, 132, *132*
  Flag 77
  Grass 77
Myrtus communis 132, *132*

Naked Ladies 161
Narcissus pseudonarcissus 54, *54*
Nasturtium 58
Navelwort 105
Nepeta cataria 39, *39*
Nettle 61, 99, 181
  Common 132–3, *133*
  Stinging 17, 132
Nicotiana tabacum 192–3, *193*
Nigella sativa 72, *72*
Nightshade 42, 49, 133
  Black 133
  Common 96, 133, *133*, 134
  Deadly 133, 134, *134*
  Woody 30
Noon Flower 86
Norway Pine 144
  Spruce 76

Nosebleed 204
Nymphaea alba 113, *113*
  odorata 113, *113*

Oak 116, 127
  Common 82
  Gall- 82–3, *82*
  Lungs 116
  Tree 134, *134*
  Oats 135, *135*
Ocymum basilicum 23, *23*
Oenanthe aquatica 64
  crocata 64
  fistulosa 64
Old Man's Tree 179
One-berry 97
Onion 45, 83, 135, *135*
  Sea 183
Ononis spinosa 155, *155*
Onopordum acanthium 64, *64*
Ophioglossum vulgatum 9, *9*, 63
Opium Poppy 149
Orach 17, 136, *136*
Orache 136
Orchanet 14
Orchid 136, *136*
Orchis 136, *136*
Origanum 24
Origanum dictamnus 59, *59*
  majorana 59, 120–1, *120*
  vulgare 59, 120, *120*
Orpine 137, *137*
Oryza sativa 157, *157*
Osmunda regalis 73, *73*
Osterick 29
Oxalis acetosella 178, *178*
Ox-eye Daisy 54
Ox-tongue, Bristly 109
Oxyria digyna 177, *177*
  reniformis 177, *177*

Paeonia officinalis 137, *137*
Paeony 137, *137*
Pansy, Wild 92
Papaver rhoeas 150, *150*
  somniferum 149, *149*
Paprika 143
Parietaria officinalis 141–2, *141*
Paris quadrifolia 97, *97*
Parsley 121, 138, 147, 167
  Common 138
  Horse 14
  Milk 139, *139*
  Piert 138, *138*, 142
  Rock 139, *139*
  Wild 14
Parsnip 14, 37, 86, 119, 182
  Creeping Water 139
  Great Water 139
  Lesser Water 139
  Upright Water 139, *139*
Pasque Flower 15
Passions 29
Patience, Dock 156
  Great Garden 156
Paul's Betony 80, *80*
Peach 22, 140, *140*
Peachwort 18
Peagle 51

Pear Tree 89, 140, *140*
  Wild 140, *140*
Pedicularis sylvatica 154
Pellitory, Bastard 175
  of Spain 120, 141, *141*, 193
  of the Wall 141–2, *141*
Peltigera canina 112, *112*
Pennyroyal 59, 142, *142*
  Wall 105
Pennywort 105
  Common Marsh 142, *142*
  Indian 142
Pepper 143, *143*
  Black 143
  Guinea 143, *143*
  Long 143
  White 143
Peppermint 38, 59, 66, 125, 126, 182, 204
Pepper-wort 58, 102
Perennial Sow-thistle 181
Perfoliate Honeysuckle 98
Perforate St John's Wort 163
Periwinkle, Great 144, *144*
  Madagascar 144
  Small 144
Personata 34
Petasites hybridus 36, *36*
Petroselinum crispum 138, *138*
  sativum 138, *138*
Pettigree 35
Pettinugget 107
Peucedanum officinale 71, *71*, 139
  ostruthium 122, *122*
  palustre 139, *139*
Phaseolus vulgaris 25, *25*
Phyllitis scolopendrium 90, *90*
Physalis alkekengi 42–3, *42*
Picea abies 76–7, *76*
Picris echioides 109, *109*
Pilewort 40, 101
Pimpernel, Meadow 34
  Water 32
Pimpinella major 167, *167*
  saxifraga 168, *168*
Pine Tree 144, *144*
  Norway 144
  Scots 144
Pinus picea 76–7, *76*
  sylvestris 76, 144, *144*
Piper nigrum 143, *143*
Piss-a-beds 56
Plane Tree 189
Plantago coronopus 145, *145*
  lanceolata 146, *146*
  major 145, *145*, 146
Plantain 29, 31, 80, 145, *145*, 162, 195
  Buck's Horn 145, *145*
  Ribwort 146, *146*
Pleurisy Root 187
Ploughman's Spikenard 146, *146*
Plums 147, *147*
Podophyllum peltatum 119
Poison Mushroom 130
Polemonium caeruleum 194, *194*
  reptans 194
Polygonatum multiflorum 176, *176*
Polygonum 18, *18*

aviculare 107
  bistorta 29, *29*
  hydropiper 18
  persicaria 18
Polypodium vulgare 147, *147*
Polypody 147, *147*
Pomegranate 23, 125, 148, *148*, 181
Poplar, Black 148, *148*, 149
  White 148–9, *149*
Poppy 66, 123
  Opium 149, *149*
  Red 149, 150
  White 149, *149*
  Wild 150, *150*
Populus alba 148–9, *149*
  nigra 148, *148*, 149
  tremula 149
  tremuloides 149
Potentilla anserina 172, *172*
  erecta 193, *193*
  reptans 46, *46*
  tormentilla 193, *193*
Pot-herb, Black 14
Prickly Asparagus 20
  Lettuce 112
Primrose 51, 119, 150, *150*, 197
Primula veris 51, *51*
  vulgaris 150, *150*
Prince's Feather 15
Prunella vulgaris 170, *170*
Prunes, Damask 147
Prunus domestica 147, *147*
  persica 140, *140*
  spinosa 174, *174*
Pteridium aquilinum 73, *73*
Pteris aquilina 73, *73*
Pulicaria dysenterica 79, *79*, 173
Pulmonaria officinalis 116, *116*
Pulsatilla vulgaris 15
Pumpkin 53, 151, *151*
Punica granatum 148, *148*
Purging Buckthorn 33
Pyrola minor 201, *201*
  rotundifolia 201
Pyrus cydonia 151, *151*
  pyraster 140
  sativa 140, *140*

Quaking Aspen 149
Quercus infectoria 82–3, *82*
  robur 134, *134*
Quickthorn 91
Quince Tree 23, 151, *151*, 185
Quinsy-wort 201

Radish 57
  Common Garden 152, *152*
  Horse 152, *152*
  Wild 152, *152*
Ragwort 153, *153*
Rampion, Sheep's 153, *153*
Ranunculus acris 52
  auricomus 52, *52*
  ficaria 40–1, *40*
Raphanus sativus 152, *152*
Raspberry 154, *154*, 197
Rattle Grass 154, *154*
  Red 154
  Yellow 154

Redshank 18
Rest-harrow 155, *155*
  Spiny 155
Rhamnus catharticus 33, *33*
Rheum palmatum 155, *155*
  rhaponticum 156, *156*
Rhinanthus 154, *154*
  minor 154
Rhubarb 75, 155, *155*
  Culinary 156, *156*
  Great Monk's 156, *156*
  Garden 155, 156
  Monk's 156
  Tart 156, *156*
Rhus aromatica 187
  cotinus 186–7, *186*
  glabra 187
Ribbed Melilot 123
Ribes uva-crispa 88, *88*
Ribwort Plantain 146
Rice 157, *157*
Rock Samphire 164
  Parsley 139
Rocket Cress 157, *157*
  Garden 157
Roman Chamomile 42
  Wormwood 203
Root of Scarcity 158, *158*
Rosa canina 61, *61*, 158
  damascena 158–9, *158*
  rubiginosa 65, *65*
  rubra 158
Rose, Christmas 93
  Damask 158–9
  Dog 61, 65, 158, 190
  Garden 61
  Red 44, 66, 111, 158
  White 158
  Wild 158
Rosebay Willowherb 200
Rosemary 66, 159, *159*, 162, 179
  Wild 107
Rosmarinus officinalis 159, *159*
Round-leaved Dock 60
  Sundew 187
Royal Fern 73
Rubia tinctorum 117, *117*
Rubus fructicosus 30, *30*
  idaeus 154, *154*
  villosus 30
Rue 22, 103
  Garden 160, *160*
  Goat's 86
Rumex acetosa 177, *177*
  acetosella 178, *178*
  alpinus 156, *156*
  crispus 60
  obtusifolius 60, *60*
Ruscus 35
Ruscus aculeatus 35, *35*
Ruta graveolens 160, *160*

Safflower 161, *161*
Saffron 140, 160, *160*
  Meadow 161, *161*
  Wild 161, *161*
Sage 46, 47, 130, 162
  Common Garden 162, *162*
  Wood 162–3, *162*

St James's Wort 9, 41, 153, 163, *163*
  Perforate 163
Salad Burnet 34
  Lettuce 111
Salix alba 200, *200*
Salsola kali 163, *163*
Saltwort 163, *163*
Salvia officinalis 162, *162*
  sclarea 46–7, *46*
  verbenaca 47, *47*
Sambucus ebulus 66–7, *66*
  nigra 65–6, *65*
Samphire 169
  Rock 164, *164*
  Small 164, *164*
Sanders 111
  White 111
Sanguisorba 34
Sanguisorba minor 34–5, *34*
Sanicle 164, *164*, 170
Sanicula europaea 164, *164*
Santolina chamaecyparissus 110–11, *110*
Saponaria officinalis 175, *175*
Sarsaparilla 125, 165, *165*, 182
Satan's Apple 119
Satureia hortensis 166, *166*
  montana 167, *167*
Sauce-alone 165, *165*
Savine 166, *166*
Savory, Summer 166, *166*, 167
  Winter 167, *167*
Saxifrage 138
  Burnet 167
  Great Burnet 167, *167*
  Lesser Burnet 167
  Small Burnet 168, *168*
Scabiosa columbaria 168–9, *169*
  succisa 57, *57*
Scabious, Devil's Bit 153
  Field 168, *168*, 169
  Lesser Field 168–9
  Sheep's Bit 153
Scammony 169, *169*
Scented Mayweed 75
Scilla maritima 183, *183*
Scotch Thistle 64
Scots Pine 76, 144
Scrophularia auriculata 26
  nodosa 76, *76*
Scullcap 160, 174, 195
Scurvy-grass 170, *170*
Sea Beet 158
  Holly 69
  Onion 183
  Wormwood 204
Sedum acre 102, *102*, 184
  album 184, *184*
  rupestre 102
  telephium 137, *137*
Self-heal 170, *170*
Sempervivum tectorum 101, *101*
Senecio jacobaea 153, *153*
  vulgaris 90, *90*
Senna, Common Bladder 171
  Red-flowered Bladder 171, *171*
Shallots 45, 83

Sheep's Bit Scabious 153
   Rampion 153
   Sorrel 178
Shepherd's Purse 171, *171*
   Rod 172, *172*
Sickle-wort 33
Silver Birch 28
Silverweed 172, *172*
Simson, Blue 173, *173*
Sinapis alba 132, *132*
Sisymbrium officinale 80, 131, *131*
   sophia 80, *80*
Sium angustifolium 139, *139*
   latifolium 139
   nodiflorum 139
   sisarum 173, *173*
Skirret 173, *173*
Slippery Elm 68, 113, 121, 169
Sloe Bush 174, *174*
Smallage 12, 174, *174*
Smilax 165, *165*
   officinalis 165
Smooth Sow-thistle 180
   Sumach 187
Smyrnium olusatrum 14, *14*
Snakeweed 29
Snapdragon 80
Sneezewort 175, *175*
Solanum 30
   dulcamara 30, *30*
   nigrum 133, *133*
Solbegrella 34
Soldier, Common Water 176, *176*
Solidago virgaurea 87, *87*
Solomon's Seal 176, *176*
Sonchus arvensis 181, *181*
   oleraceus 180, *180*
   palustris 181, *181*
Sorrel 18, 60
   Common 177, *177*
   Field 178
   Mountain 177, *177*
   Sheep's 178, *178*
   Wood 178, *178*
Southernwood 179, *179*
   Field 179, *179*, 204
Sowbread 180, *180*
Sow's Fennel 71, 139
Sow-thistle, Common 180, *180*
   Marsh 181
   Perennial 181
   Smooth 180
   Tree 181, *181*
Sow-thistle Tree
   Marsh 181, *181*
Spanish Bugloss 14
Spear Mint 125, 126
Speedwell 80, *80*
   Heath 80
Spignel 182
   Broad-leaved 182, *182*
Spikenard 79, 162, 182, *182*
   Ploughman's 146
Spinach 156, 183, *183*
   Mountain 17
Spinacia oleracea 183, *183*
Spiny Rest-harrow 155

Spoonwort 170
Spiraea ulmaria 123, *123*
Spruce Fir 76
Spurge, Laurel 109
   Mezereon 124–5
   Sun 188
Squill 183, *183*
Squinancy Woodruffe 201
Squinancywort 201
Stachys officinalis 27, 27
   palustris 48, *48*
Stratiotes aloides 176, *176*
Staves-acre 184, *184*
Stellaria media 44–5, *44*
Sticta pulmonaria 116–17
Stinging Nettle 17
Stinking Iris 85
   Mayweed 122
   Chamomile 122
Stonecrop 184, *184*
   White 184
Storax Tree 185, *185*
Strawberries 46, 185, *185*
Styrax officinalis 185, *185*
Succisa pratensis 57, *57*
Succory 12, 68
   Wild 91, 186, *186*
Sulphur-wort 71
Sumach 186–7, *186*
   Smooth 187
   Sweet 187
Summer Savory 166, 167
Sun Spurge 188, *188*
Sundew 187, *187*
   Common 187
   Great 187
   Round-leaved 187
Sunflower
   Wild 67
Swallow-wort 188–9, *188*
Sycamore Tree 189, *189*
Symphytum officinale 50, *50*
Syrian Bindweed 169

Tanacetum parthenium 74, *74*
   vulgare 189, *189*
Tansy 16, 50, 51, 70, 189, *189*
Taraxacum officinale 56, *56*
Tarragon 190, *190*
Taxus baccata 205, *205*
Tea 190, *190*
Teasel 172, 191, *191*
   Common 172
   Small 172
Teucrium
   chamaedrys 84–5, *84*
   scorodonia 162–3, *162*
Thistle, Blessed 31, 38
   Down 64
   Cotton 64
   Holy 38
   Scotch 64
Thorn-apple 191, *191*
Throatwort 76
Thyme 60, 192, *192*
   Garden 192
   Wild 192, *192*

Thymus serpyllum 192, *192*
   vulgaris 192, *192*
Tilia europaea 114, *114*
   x *vulgaris* 114, *114*
Toadflax 78, 204
Tobacco 192–3, *193*
Tormentil 193, *193*, 197
Tragacanth 87
Tragopogon pratensis 86, *86*
Treacle Mustard 202
   Wormseed 202
Tree Sow-thistle 181
Trefoil 194, *194*
Trientalis europaea 89, *89*
Trifolium pratense 194
   repens 194, *194*
Trigonella foenum-graecum 72, *72*
Trillium pendulum 63
Triticum 199, *199*
   repens 194, *194*
Tropaeolum majus 58
True Maidenhair 118
   Wild Valerian 195
Tubular Water Dropwort 64
Turn-hoof 13
Turnip 118, 158
Tussilago farfara 49, *49*
   hybrida 36, *36*
Twitch 62

Ulmus fulva 68
   minor 68, *68*
Umbilicus rupestris 105, *105*
Umbrella Plant 82
Upright Water Parsnip 139
Urginea maritima 183, *183*
Urtica dioica 132–3, *133*

Vaccinium myrtillus 28, *28*, 187
Valerian 127, 128, 160, 195
   Greek 194, *194*
   True Wild 195, *195*
Valeriana officinalis 195, *195*
   sylvestris 195, *195*
Velvet-flower 15
Veratrum album 93
   viride 93, *93*
Verbascum nigrum 129, *129*
   thapsus 130, *130*
Verbena officinalis 195, *195*, 196
Veronica beccabunga 32, *32*
   officinalis 80, *80*
Vervain 59, 127, 196
   Common 195, *195*
Vicia faba 25, *25*
Vinca major 144, *144*
   minor 144
Vine Tree 196, *196*
   Grape 196
Viola odorata 196, *196*
   tricolor 92, *92*
Violet 196, *196*
   Water 197, *197*
   White 196
Viper's Bugloss 197, *197*
Viscum album 127, *127*
Vitis vinifera 196, *196*

Wake Robin 52
Wall Germander 84
   Pennyroyal 105
Wallflower, Common 198, *198*
Wall-wort 55
Walnut 22, *198*
Wary 56
Water Agrimony 11, *11*
   Betony 26–7
   Dropwort 64
   Figwort 26
   Gladiole 85
   Hemlock 64
   Hemp 11
   Lily 113
   Mint 126
   Pimpernel 32
   Soldier, Common 176
   Violet 197
Watercress 32, 108
Water-pepper 18
Wayside Dock, Common 60
Wheat 22, 167, 199, *199*
White-rot 142
Wholesome Aconite 9
   Wolf's-bane 9
Whortleberries 28
   Black 28
   Red 28
Willow 118, 127, 200, *200*
   White 200
Willowherb, Hairy 199, *199*
   Rosebay 200, *200*
   Yellow 115
Wind-flower 15
Winter Cherries 42–3
   Green 89, *89*
   Savory 167
Wintergreen 89, 201, *201*
   Chickweed 89
   Common 201
   Large 201
Witch Hazel 197
Wolf's-bane 83
   Wholesome 9
Wood Anemone 15
   Betony 27
   Sage 162–3
   Sorrel 178
Woodbine 98
Woodruffe, Squinancy 201, *201*
   Sweet 201, 202, *202*
Woody Nightshade 30
Wooly Faverel 70
Wormseed, Treacle 202, *202*
Wormwood 12, 124, 203, *203*
   Field 179
   Roman 203, *203*
   Sea 204, *204*
Woundwort, Clown's 48
   Marsh 48

Yarrow 109, 126, 175, 195, 197, 204, *204*
Yew 205, *205*
Yucca 205, *205*
Yucca gloriosa 205, *205*